FIRST-TIME MOTHERHOOD
Experiences from Teens to Forties

Ramona T. Mercer, R.N., Ph.D., F.A.A.N., is a Professor in the Department of Family Health Care Nursing of the University of California, San Francisco. She first became interested in the transition to motherhood during her staff nurse experiences in Alabama and New Mexico and began her research career in this area when she was Assistant Professor at Emory University in Atlanta, Georgia from 1965 to 1969.

She is the author of over fifty articles, book chapters, and books. Her books *Nursing Care for Parents at Risk* and *Perspectives on Adolescent Health Care* each received the *American Journal of Nursing's* Book of the Year Awards. She has shared her research findings in the areas of adaptation to breastfeeding, mothers of infants with anomalies, adolescent mothers, perceptions of the birth experience, and maternal age differences in the transition to motherhood with national and international audiences.

Dr. Mercer received the Maternal Child Health Nurse of the Year Award from the American Nurses' Association Division on Maternal Child Health Practice and the National Foundation March of Dimes in 1982. In 1984 she was the Fourth Annual Helen Nahm Lecturer at the University of California, San Francisco.

She received a diploma in nursing from St. Margaret's Hospital School of Nursing in Montgomery, Alabama, a B.S. from the University of New Mexico in Albuquerque, an M.N. from Emory University in Atlanta, Georgia, and a Ph.D. in maternity nursing from the University of Pittsburgh in Pittsburgh, Pennsylvania. Her mentor was Reva Rubin, author of *Maternal Identity and the Maternal Experience.*

First-Time Motherhood
Experiences from Teens to Forties

Ramona T. Mercer
R.N., Ph.D., F.A.A.N.

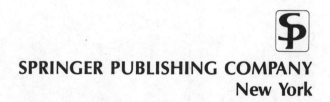

SPRINGER PUBLISHING COMPANY
New York

Springer Publishing Company, Inc.
536 Broadway
New York, NY 10012

86 87 88 89 90 / 5 4 3 2 1

Library of Congress Cataloging-in-Publication Data

Mercer, Ramona Thieme.
  First-time motherhood.

  Bibliography: p. 357
  Includes index.
  1. Pregnancy—Psychological aspects. 2. Motherhood
—Psychological aspects. 3. Children, First-born.
4. Maternal age. I. Title. [DNLM: 1. Age Factors.
2. Child Development. 3. Mother-Child Relations.
4. Mothers—psychology. WS 105.5.F2 M554f]
RG560.M47 1986   155.6'463   86-4437
ISBN 0-8261-5160-4

Printed in the United States of America

Contents

v

Preface

Mothering is one of the most difficult yet most satisfying roles in a woman's life. Part of the difficulty in mothering results from the many additional roles that must be managed along with mothering. Because mothering styles differ from culture to culture and from generation to generation, role models and support persons are often scarce. Two mothers summarized these dilemmas: "If the person giving you advice doesn't have an infant two years or younger, what she has to say is not relevant"; "It was cold turkey; I did not know anyone who had a career and also mothered."

In addition to cultural and generational differences regarding mothering practices, many have suggested differences by maternal age. Teenagers have often been described as incompetent mothers without comparisons with older women. However, the gratifications and losses described by a sample of teenage mothers over their first year of motherhood sounded very similar to those of older women. This led to the study reported in this book, in which direct comparisons could be made to determine how the teenagers' mothering contrasted with that of older women. Funding was obtained through Maternal and Child Health Research Grants (Social Security Act, Title V), Grant MC–R–060435, to compare the experiences of the younger first-time mother with the 20- to 29-year-old mother and with the 30- to 42-year-old mother.

This comparative study affirmed earlier informal observations: all mothers responded similarly in describing the joys and challenges during the first year of motherhood. The two older groups of women were consistently somewhat more adaptive or competent in mothering behaviors, but the oldest group of women did not derive as much satisfaction from the mothering role as did the younger women.

Although the older women scored higher on a continuum of more adaptive or competent maternal behavior, the younger group was not incompetent. There seemed to be trade-offs as to which age group may have been at an advantage. The younger-age group's birth process required less medical intervention, and teenagers recuperated more quickly following birth and described less fatigue than the older age groups. The older women had greater financial assets that allowed them more freedom of choice, and their worries about managing in day-to-day situations were not so acute as those of the younger groups.

Obviously, the three age groups of women differed in many ways, such as in their educational background, financial resources, and marital status. However, developmental and attitudinal differences were also evident; these differences accounted for the variation in gratification from mothering, as well as in differences in competency behaviors.

This book describes all of these differences that were observed over the first year of motherhood. Two unmarried and two married women from each of the age groups are presented at each of the test periods as paradigm cases to illustrate how motherhood affected the women's lives and how they managed and coped, along with their difficulties and their joys. These illustrative paradigm cases indicate how motherhood was perceived at each particular period and illustrate some of the quantitative findings.

Additional theories and research are presented along with the study findings to provide an overall context, as well as to highlight agreement or disagreement with other research. Discussions of the findings are followed by implications for nurse clinicians or other health care providers who are working with the diverse group of first-time mothers. The literature more often suggests strategies for promoting the psychosocial development of the teenage mother, with the assumption that "adult women" need little help in these areas. This was not the case among the 294 women who were studied; all of the women dealt with conflicting internal drives to achieve or excel in other roles in their lives apart from mothering.

The first chapter presents an overview of the study, the theoretical framework, and general methodology. The reader who is interested in the research methodology has access to detail about measures and statistical analyses in the Appendix. When findings are reported as significantly different, this means that statistical differences were $\leq.05$. The second chapter describes the women's background, personality traits, and attitudes. The third chapter details the women's pregnancy, birth, and early events following birth. Their infants' health status, temperament, growth, and development are described in the fourth chapter, along with how their mothers compared them to an average infant. Chapters 5 through 8 present the major findings of each test period following the initial interview after birth at 1, 4, 8, and 12 months. Chapter 9 addresses the change in maternal role behaviors over the year and patterns that emerged. Chapter 10 highlights maternal age differences and discusses their implications.

The book offers suggestions to the clinician, raises questions for clinician and researcher alike, and adds to knowledge about the harsh reality of what the experience of mothering is like in this society. Our children are our most important resource for the future, yet we continue to provide the least economic, educational, and social support for the adults who take on this most important task without previous experience, any prior knowledge of what is entailed, or much insight about the process. Yet, against these odds, because of intense motivation to do what is right, deepest love, and commitment to their child, most parents succeed admirably.

Acknowledgments

The project Factors Having an Impact on Maternal Role Attainment the First Year of Motherhood provided the data base for this book. The project was supported by Maternal and Child Health (Social Security Act, Title V) Grant MC-R-060435. Appreciation is expressed to this Research Grants Program for their support and to Dr. Gontran Lamberty, director of the Maternal and Child Health Research Grants program.

Several persons contributed valuable time and consultation during the planning phase of the project. Important contributors were Dr. Kathryn Barnard, University of Washington; Dr. Mildred Disbrow, University of Washington; Dr. Susan Gortner, University of California, San Francisco; Dr. Susan Virden, University of Washington; and Dr. Eugenia H. Waechter (deceased), University of California, San Francisco.

Individuals who generously shared instruments that they had developed in their own research greatly enhanced the project's aims. Appreciation is expressed to Drs. Kathryn Barnard, University of Washington; Marion Blank, Yeshiva University, Bronx, New York; Elsie R. Broussard, University of Pittsburgh; William Carey, University of Pennsylvania; Stella Chess, New York University; Bertram J. Cohler, University of Chicago; Mildred Disbrow, University of Washington; Daniel F. Hobbs, University of Georgia; Virginia Larsen, Truman Restorative Center, St. Louis; Myra Leifer, Illinois Institute of Technology, Chicago; Katherine Nuckolls, University of North Carolina; Candyce Russell, Kansas State University; Irwin G. Sarason, University of Washington; Alexander Thomas, New York University Medical Center; and Susan Virden, University of Washington.

Special thanks goes to Dr. Bertram J. Cohler, University of Chicago, for his contribution of time in the analyses of the Maternal Attitude Scale data. Dr. Mary Mittleman, Columbia University, shared the computer program for creating the temperament categories from the Young Adult Temperament Questionnaire. Dr. Jack Gandour and Ms. Mary Jane Gandour shared their computer program for scoring the Infant Temperament Questionnaire.

Special appreciation is expressed to the 294 mothers who contributed their time and completed the battery of instruments during their very busy first year. Their openness and willingness to share their thoughts and feelings about their experiences made it possible to achieve the study aims.

Special recognition goes to Kathryn C. Hackley, research associate, who directed the project and assured continuity in the research team. Her optimistic outlook was always appreciated, and her hard work in meeting heavy schedules was outstanding. Dr. Alan Bostrom, biostatistician, translated all of the written requests into computer programs and conducted all of the analyses. His constant availability for consultation was critical in all phases of the project.

Research assistants who were in the field conducting interviews, in addition to the research associate, were Dr. Janice Majewski, Ronda Miller, Anne Patton, Linda Robrecht, and Barbara Wylie. Without their superb help the rich data for the vignettes and qualitative analyses would not have been possible. Other research assistants who worked during coding and analysis were Dr. Vivian Gedaly-Duff, Dr. Colleen Stainton, and Cynthia Williams.

Dr. Gilbert A. Webb, who was chairman of the Department of Obstetrics and Gynecology, sponsored the project at Children's Hospital in San Francisco. His most valuable help and participation contributed greatly to the recruitment of teenage mothers.

Nursing staff and hospital administrators at Children's Hospital, Moffitt Hospital (University of California), and San Francisco General Hospital were all helpful in facilitating the recruitment of mothers for the study.

Departmental administrative assistance from Patricia Rodden and Maria Elena Sotela was most faithful and persevering. Project secretaries who made sure that the 294 women were interviewed at the appropriate time over the five test periods played an extremely important role in setting up appointments and assuring smooth operations. They included Diana Hemstreet, Nan Milner, and Anne Ossulton; each participated for a part of the 3-year period.

I am particularly grateful to the experts who critiqued the manuscript and provided constructive suggestions. These very important editors included Ruth Chasek, Nursing Editor, Springer Publishing Company; Mary Margaret Gottesman, neonatal clinical nurse specialist, Moffitt Hospital, University of California, San Francisco, and doctoral candidate, University of Rochester; Rebecca Johnson, doctoral student, University of California, San Francisco; Camille Ronay, free-lance writer, Decatur, Georgia; Deanna Sollid, private practice as clinical specialist and consultant for antepartum and postpartum care, co-producer and co-owner of an audiovisual production company, childbirth educator, and project director, Antepartum Stress: Effect on Family Health and Family Functioning, University of California, San Francisco; and Catherine Wittenberg, head nurse, Moffitt Hospital Intrapartum and Antepartum/Postpartum Unit, University of California, San Francisco.

My deepest appreciation is expressed to all of the persons who made the book possible.

R.T.M.

CHAPTER 1

Transition to the Maternal Role

Although women assume many roles over a lifetime, one of the most significant and time-consuming is the maternal role. Because of advances in contraceptive technology women now have the choice to delay motherhood until the timing seems right in relation to other life goals. Although the timing of fatherhood has usually been after the establishment of a career, the sequencing of motherhood has been more varied. The majority of women become first-time mothers while in their twenties, just under one fifth during their teenage years; and increasing numbers of women are postponing motherhood until a career is well established. Career opportunities and the economic necessity of continuing employment following the child's birth add to the difficulty in deciding on the optimal time to have a child.

Making the decision to become a mother usually involves weighing the advantages and disadvantages of motherhood at each particular period of life. Sometimes the decision may be a less conscious one, such as a contraceptive failure due to carelessness, and abortion is not viewed as an acceptable option. Others may wish to become a mother "someday" and not use any contraceptive.

Women who do make a deliberate decision in timing their motherhood role have little information about how the personal experience may vary at different stages in life, such as during the teenage years, in the twenties, or after 30. The problems of teenage parenting have long been of interest, but few comparative studies are available to describe whether the problems of early-age parenting are really different, and if so, how they are different. Do the problems of teenage parenting relate to psychosocial deficits rather than age per se?

1

The increased rate of births for women 30 years and older since 1975 raises questions about the advantages and disadvantages for motherhood after 30. Women are aware of increased medical risks for childbearing after the age of 35, but little is known about how the experience affects other facets of a woman's life. This book reports a study of the first year of motherhood, in which three age groups of women shared their experiences in achieving the mothering role and tell how their lives were affected.

This first chapter presents the theoretical framework on which the study was based and the context in which it was interpreted. The study aims and a description of the methods used conclude the chapter.

THEORETICAL FRAMEWORK

The study was approached from the belief that the way in which women perceive their day-to-day experiences represents their current living situations, which may either facilitate or otherwise affect their work toward achieving the maternal role. Women adapt their mothering behaviors according to their infants', families', friends', and other important persons' responses to their actions. Thus, new mothers proceed by trial and error or success as the mothering role evolves; appraisal from the persons in their social world helps to shape the final outcome. Both role and developmental theories provided the overall framework for examining the variables that were theoretically linked with mothering behaviors (Mercer, 1981).

Maternal Role Attainment

Roles are culturally defined; this is particularly true for the maternal role. Within the context of the United States society, the rich diversity of cultures have blended, remained fixed, or followed the most current local trends. As a result, in contrast to career roles, which have specific guidelines and expected behaviors set by an employer (sometimes in writing as "job descriptions"), such specificity is lacking for the mothering role. The mother's cultural group has general expectations and lets her know if she errs but less often informs her when she is excelling. Thus, the mothering role lacks clarity, specificity, and consensus, all of which make transition to any role more difficult (Burr, Leigh, Day, & Constantine, 1979). A father of Hispanic heritage may have very different ideas about child rearing than his mate of Irish heritage.

Additionally, finances are a major concern in families with an infant; many mothers are working outside the home as early as 4 months following the birth of their first child (Barnard & Eyres, 1979). Unless parenting responsibilities are shared with a trusted, reliable person, outside employment adds to the mother's tasks, and the potential for role strain is increased. If the husband agrees with the wife regarding the saliency of roles other than motherhood, and if there is adequate child care and adequate emotional support, career mothers are less likely to experience role strain (Van Meter & Agronow, 1982).

In addition to commitment to other roles and the mate's view of their importance, the ease of moving into the mothering role is also affected by her level of commitment to the role, felt competency in the role, conflict of the maternal role with her other roles or personal values, power within the role (Nye & Gecas, 1976), value of the role in society and to the individual, earlier socialization for the role, and resources available (Burr et al., 1979). Career mothers were observed to handle role conflict either through redefining the maternal role or by expanding it (Van Meter & Agronow, 1982). Role expansion in which the mother attempts to be all things to all people can lead to burnout and dissatisfaction with other roles, whereas redefining a role to expect less from herself is less likely to lead to burnout.

The earliest socialization for mothering behaviors begins during early childhood of being mothered and observing mothering within the family context (Uddenberg, 1974). Formal anticipatory socialization for the mothering role begins during pregnancy (Leifer, 1977, 1980; Rubin, 1967a, 1967b, 1977). Becoming a mother means taking on a new identity. Taking on a new identity involves a complete rethinking and redefining of self.

Redefining self is a very active process that involves the total self system: the *ideal image,* i.e., who the woman would like to be like or what she would like to do; the *self-image,* i.e., how the woman sees herself at this particular time in this specific situation; and the *body image,* i.e., her bodily accommodations to the fetus and body functioning and capacities (Rubin, 1967a). The process of redefining self in assuming the maternal role has been described as occurring through four operations: *taking-on* behaviors, which involve mimicry and role-play; *taking-in* behaviors, which involve fantasy about what it will be like as a mother and introjection–projection–rejection

(or acceptance) in which the woman mentally tries for herself behaviors that she sees others exhibit, tests the behaviors against her
values and style, and either rejects the observed behaviors as unacceptable or accepts the behaviors as how she would like to be;
letting-go behaviors, which involve grief work in the roles that must
be relinquished for the maternal role; and *maternal identity,* the final
stage when the maternal role has been internalized, and she comfortably says, "I do," or "I think," with much confidence and a
sense of competency (Rubin, 1967a). Her own mother is usually her
prototype role model; however, the mother may be too threatening
as a peer. Peers and others, such as those viewed on television or
read about in books, or nurses, physicians, and work colleagues
are more frequently used for the pregnant woman's reflections of
who-she-once-was, who-she-is, and who-she-will-be (Rubin, 1967b).

During pregnancy the woman accepts the fetus into her self system (Bibring, Dwyer, & Valenstein, 1961; Rubin, 1972). For several
years, researchers have reported the emotional attachment to the
fetus beginning and following an orderly sequence during pregnancy (Caplan, 1959; Carter-Jessop, 1981; Cranley, 1981a, 1981b;
Josten, 1981; Leifer, 1977; Lumley, 1982). The mother communicates with her fetus both verbally and tactilely and indicates knowledge of her fetus's sleep/wake cycle and temperament (Stainton,
1985a). Importantly, these early maternal interactions with and attachment to the fetus, along with the mother's adjustment to the
pregnancy, appear to contribute to maternal adaptation during the
postpartum (Leifer, 1977; Shereshefsky & Yarrow, 1973).

Toward the end of pregnancy the woman begins to experience
her fetus as a separate individual who will soon exist apart from her
(Bibring et al., 1961). Following birth, maternal role identity continues to evolve as the mother deepens her emotional involvement
with an infant who now offers visual input. A final conceptual
separation of mother–infant pair occurs following birth and was
called *polarization* by Rubin (1977) because the process is analogous to the stage in cell reproduction before final separation of the
mother–daughter cells. *Identification* of the infant, the first phase
of polarization, occurs during the first 4 postpartal weeks. As the
mother identifies the infant, she identifies *herself* and *her behavior*
in relation to that particular infant. Gottlieb (1978) observed the
same identification process but called the behavior a discovery process. *Claiming,* a process in which the mother links characteristics
of her infant to family members, also occurs during this period.
Claiming behaviors by other family members are reaffirmation to

the mother that her intimate social unit accepts her infant. She is especially sensitive to whether important persons in her family and social sphere claim her child in the same way they have claimed her.

Following her exclusive possession of her infant during pregnancy, the mother must share her infant with others after birth. During the first month, multiparous mothers tend to perform most of the caretaking tasks for their new infants themselves, allowing fathers or others to participate very little; they also enjoy placing the infants on their abdomens (Stainton, 1985b). The mother's placement of the infant on her abdomen may be a step in the process of polarization; resting the infant over the area in which she lived internally the previous 9 months may be comforting to both mother and infant and ease the separation somewhat.

In the final phase of polarization, the mother is able to perceive her infant as distinct, no longer a part of her body boundaries, either physically or conceptually. A restoration of the woman's own intactness, completeness, and wholeness as an individual are seen as prerequisite to her ability to view her infant as intact, complete, and whole (Rubin, 1977, 1984). Gottlieb's (1978) observations also suggested that positive input such as the mother's personalized contact with her infant, physical well-being, and positive feedback from others are facilitators of the discovery process; whereas negative input, such as physical problems, inhibit the process. Others observed that intense, unanticipated fatigue, disorganization, and feelings of inadequacy hampered early mothering; approximately one third of the 62 women in Shereshefsky and Yarrow's (1973) study had difficulty in assuming care of their infants.

Robson and Moss (1970) described a sequential, temporal process in maternal attachment behaviors of 54 primiparous women, aged 18 to 34 years, from birth to 3 months. Attachment was defined "as the extent to which a mother feels that her infant occupies an essential position in her life" (p. 977). Components of attachment included feelings of love, possession, devotion, and protectiveness toward the infant, along with a need for, and pleasure in, prolonged interactions with the infant. The women responded vaguely and impersonally in describing their infants the first 4 days following birth. Like Rubin and Gottlieb, Robson and Moss were impressed with the "mother's need to deal with their infants' anonymity. Soon after birth, in a variety of ways, mothers attempted to create some sense that their babies were unique individuals who belonged to them" (p. 978). Robson and Moss also described the claiming process in which almost half the sample identified a physical similarity of their infants to a close family member during the hospitalization. The majority of the mothers in the study did not experience intense attachment until 4 to 6 weeks later, when the infants became more responsive. By 9 weeks most of the mothers felt that their infants became persons and recognized them. By the end of the third month most of the women felt strongly attached to their babies. Both early and late attachers were observed in this sample, with 2% remaining detached.

In addition to the psychodynamic aspects of the attachment process, Cogan and Edmunds (1980) suggested a linguistic component of the developing maternal role. They observed a change in the type of pronouns used to describe the infant, with movement from the neutral *it* to the gender pronouns *he* or *she,* as attachment developed.

In addition to being the time when strong attachment to the infant had developed (Robson & Moss, 1970), 3 months was also the time when 20- to 25-year-old mothers were observed to internalize the maternal role as a part of their identity (Highley, 1967). A longer period of time seemed to be needed by teenagers for internalizing the maternal role; they reported that they did not feel like mothers until the infant was 6 to 10 months of age (Mercer, 1980).

In summary, *maternal role attainment* is defined as a process that has been observed to occur over a 3- to 10-month period. Major components of the mothering role include attachment to the infant through identifying, claiming, and interacting with the infant, gaining competence in mothering behaviors, and expressing gratification in the mother–infant interactions. Empirical evidence suggests that maternal adaptation may be delayed or hampered if the woman's health status is less than optimal, such as complications from childbirth or chronic illness.

VARIABLES IDENTIFIED AS HAVING A RELATIONSHIP WITH MATERNAL ROLE ATTAINMENT

A review of reported research was done to identify relevant variables for study. Variables that were identified repeatedly as influencing the mothering role provided further theoretical basis for the study.

Maternal Age at First Birth

A wide range of handicaps for teenage parenthood have been described, including long-range financial, educational, and family structural impediments (Hofferth & Moore, 1979; Kellam, Adams, Brown, & Ensminger, 1982; Moore & Waite, 1977). A critical review of early research in the 1950s and 1960s by Grant and Heald (1972) concluded that young maternal age was not the sole determinant of higher perinatal morbidity and mortality; rather, the situations of malnutrition, poverty, and lack of prenatal care that were often prevalent among teenage pregnant populations appeared to contribute to higher morbidity and mortality. When variables associated with prematurity, low birth weight, lower Apgar scores, and higher morbidity and mortality have been controlled, age differences have not been found (Scholl, Decker, Karp, Greene, & DeSales, 1984; Zuckerman et al., 1983). Infants of younger mothers had higher Apgar scores than infants of older mothers among a sample of blacks and Hispanics (Rothenberg & Varga, 1981). Merritt, Lawrence, and Naeye (1980) reported the lowest perinatal mortality rates among the 16- to 19-year-old group when compared with both younger and older age groups and suggested that from a medical viewpoint the optimal time to give birth is from 16 to 19 years.

Analysis of data from 44,386 pregnancies found that perinatal mortality rates increased progressively with maternal age, from 25/1,000 at 17 to 19 years to 69/1,000 after 39 years (Naeye, 1983). Accounting for the increase were stillbirths (92%), congenital malformations (14%), disorders associated with uteroplacental hypoperfusion (i.e., abruptio placentae, large placental infarcts, and placental growth retardation) (50%). Naeye concluded that sclerotic lesions in the myometrial arteries were possibly the cause of hypoperfusion because the proportion of arteries with these lesions increased from 11% at 17 to 19 years to 83% after 39 years.

Although previous research regarding developmental differences of teenagers' children has not been in agreement (Broman, 1981; Hardy, Welcher, Stanley, & Dallas, 1978; Mercer, 1984; Oppel & Royston, 1971), more recent research has agreed with Hardy and associates (1978) in finding no developmental differences between children of teenagers and children of older parents (Finkelstein, Finkelstein, Christie, Roden, & Shelton, 1982; Roosa, Fitzgerald, & Carlson, 1982a, 1982b). Many factors could account for failure to find developmental differences among children. Family support for the mother-infant couple and psychosocial assets are both important factors. Women who are unaware of infant developmental capabilities during the first year of life do not encourage or promote these skills or behaviors (Snyder, Eyres, & Barnard, 1979).

Readiness for mothering also would influence commitment to mothering and mothering activities such as stimulating the infant.

Although Jones, Green, and Krauss (1980) based their findings on a lower socioeconomic status (SES) sample, they suggested that there may be a "critical" age when an individual develops a readiness for mothering. They reported that mothers 19 years or older demonstrated greater maternal responsiveness than mothers 18 years and younger.

Other studies without control groups of older mothers suggested that teenage mothers were impatient with the growing child's behaviors (DeLissovoy, 1973; Jarrett, 1982; Mercer, 1980). Wise and Grossman (1980) observed that the adolescents' ego strength and the infants' behavior were the variables most strongly related to early mother–child interactions and attachment.

Much less is known about the first-time mother over 30 years old who may have achieved a greater sense of readiness for the maternal role. Grossman et al. (1980) did not find that age was predictive of psychological adaptation to mothering among women who were 21 to 34 years of age. Others also failed to see differences in maternal behavior as a function of age among women aged 17 to 30 years (Svejda, Campos, & Emde, 1980). Ragozin, Basham, Crnic, Greenberg, and Robinson (1982) observed that when demographic and psychosocial variables were controlled, the older the mother, the greater the satisfaction with parenting, the greater time commitment to the role, and the more optimal the observed behavior. Their subjects included mothers ranging in age from 16 to 38 years. In contrast others have observed that the older the woman, the less gratification she derived from the parenting role (Russell, 1974; Steffensmeier, 1982).

A higher level of education may account for differences in older women's mothering behaviors. Mothers over 29 years who had graduated from college, and who had attended graduate school had more adaptive behaviors than younger mothers described in Ralph's (1977) study.

Uddenberg (1974) found that a greater number of women over the age of 27 years had postpartum depression than women who were 18 to 26 years. They related depression to negative attitudes toward pregnancy, conflicts with their mothers, and denial of sensations connected with pregnancy (Uddenberg & Nilsson, 1975). Negative attitudes about pregnancy and conflicts with the mother could be influential in a woman's postponing motherhood.

Pickens (1982) studied 30- to 33-year-old first-time mothers the first 4 months following birth to describe the process through which career women formulated a new identity. She observed that the women experienced an identity crisis characterized by ambiguity when they felt they were neither career women nor mothers. They experienced discontinuity with many of their former attributes; the former competent self was perceived as incompetent postpartally, and the former independent self was perceived as dependent. In attempting to maintain continuity with former selves as planners and organizers, the mothers planned and organized for integrating the maternal role into their identities. They had been knowledgeable in career roles, so they took prenatal classes and read extensively to experience continuity in being knowledgeable. Pickens observed less identity confusion at 4 months postpartum, along with increased rewards of motherhood and increased self-confidence.

In summary, when demographic and psychosocial variables are controlled, the teenager's child does not experience either greater health problems or developmental deficits than children of older women. By contrast, with increasing maternal age there seem to be greater health risks for the fetus and neonate. The more mature woman, although handicapped by an aging cardiovascular system, has greater assets in her educational preparation and perhaps readiness for and commitment to the maternal role. However, there is an indication that the older first-time mother may be more vulnerable to depression and may experience greater identity conflicts in synchronizing her career and maternal roles.

Perception of the Birth Experience

Childbirth is viewed as the first act of motherhood, and a woman's perceptions of her performance during labor and birth may be viewed by her as an indication of her later capabilities in the mothering role (Deutscher, 1970). Perception of the birth experience may be affected by many variables. Accurate knowledge and realistic expectations for childbirth seem to contribute to positive feelings (Charles, Norr, Block, Meyering, & Meyers, 1978; Clark, 1975; Doering and Entwisle, 1975). Maintaining control during labor and delivery also is linked with satisfaction with the experience (Chertok, 1969; Humenick & Bugen, 1981; Oakley, 1980).

Support persons, particularly help from the mate during labor and delivery, are very important (Lederman, Lederman, Work, & McCann, 1979; Norr, Block, Charles, Meyering, & Meyers, 1977; Sosa, Kennell, Klaus, Robertson, & Urrutia, 1980; Westbrook, 1978). The mate's emotional support during childbirth was the major predictor of positive perceptions of the experience, accounting for 20% of the variance (Mercer, Hackley, & Bostrom, 1983). The husband's satisfaction with the marriage and maternal anxiety level during pregnancy were the strongest predictors of maternal adaptation during labor and delivery and also were correlated with post-partum well-being and mother–child interaction at 2 months (Grossman et al., 1980).

The woman's level of awareness during childbirth was related to her satisfaction with the experience (Entwisle & Doering, 1981); however, others did not find this relationship (Slavazza, Mercer, Marut, & Shnider, 1985; Tilden & Lipson, 1981). Women desire a range of anesthesia and pain relief for the birth of their child; and when desires are not met, negative feelings may result.

Women delivering by cesarean birth were observed to have lower self-esteem than women having a vaginal birth (Cox & Smith, 1982). Delivery by cesarean birth appears to contribute to body image distortions and feelings of inadequacy (Birdsong, 1981; Mercer & Marut, 1981). However, one of the critical determinants of the mother's perception of her cesarean experience relates to whether the cesarean was anticipated.

Women delivering by unanticipated cesarean birth had a less positive perception of the birth experience than those delivering vaginally (Cranley, Hedahl, & Pegg, 1983; Marut & Mercer, 1979; Mercer, Hackley, & Bostrum, 1983). They also described their infants less positively (Mercer & Marut, 1981). However, when the cesarean was anticipated, women perceived the birth experience similarly to those delivering vaginally (Cranley et al., 1983).

The birth experience was an important predictor of attachment in Peterson and Mehl's (1978) study, but early maternal-infant separation was the greatest predictor. Maternal-infant separation was the second predictor of positive perception of the birth experience (after mate emotional support) in another study, with type of delivery entering the regression model last and accounting for only 1% of the variance at a nonsignificant ($p = .09$) level (Mercer et al., 1983). With cesarean birth, early maternal-infant contact is more difficult, less extensive, and more likely to be delayed than with vaginal births. One study compared mothers delivering by cesarean who had early extended contact with their infants with mothers delivering by cesarean who had only brief contact the first 12 hours after birth and found that early differences in maternal perceptions were short-lived (McClellan & Cabianca, 1980). The early extended contact group had more positive maternal perceptions of their infants the first 1 to 2 postpartum days, but there were no differences at 1 month. Canadian mothers who had a cesarean birth did not show differences in their feelings toward their infants (Bradley, Ross, & Warnyca, 1983), nor was the type of birth predictive of either maternal adjustment or psychological functioning during the postpartum period (Bradley, 1983).

Mothers' slow recuperation postpartum following a cesarean birth could delay the polarization process of identifying and conceptually separating out from the infant because their physical intactness and competence would be less robust than women having a vaginal delivery. More abused children were delivered by cesarean birth than were delivered by cesarean in the general population (Helfer, 1974; Lynch & Roberts, 1977). Retrospective data must be viewed with caution, however, since factors contributing to a cesarean birth may relate to factors within the environment, and child abuse has been related to the interaction of stressors within the environment, the child, and the parent (Green, Gaines, & Sandgrund, 1974; Millor, 1981).

Higher fatigue levels from longer labors that sometimes end by cesarean birth also deplete a woman's energy for early interactions with her infant. Fatigue tends to lower the pain threshold, and pain relief may afford some rest; women delivering vaginally who had epidural anesthesia made more positive remarks about their infants immediately following birth than those who had local anesthesia or no anesthesia (Slavazza et al., 1985).

In summary, the perception of the birth experience as the formal entry to motherhood has much meaning for a woman. A woman's view of the process is related to her knowledge of childbirth, expectations, the amount of control maintained during labor and birth, and the presence of her mate and other support persons. An unanticipated cesarean birth results in less positive feelings about the birth experience. The type of birth experience also influences the extent of early mother–infant separation, another variable identified as influencing early mothering.

Early Maternal-Infant Separation

Retrospective studies of abused infants show that a disproportionate percentage were premature and/or ill at birth and were separated from their mothers for an extended period of time as a result of the required special care (Fanaroff, Kennell, & Klaus, 1972; Lynch & Roberts, 1977; Stern, 1973). The maternal differences of those who tend to deliver prematurely in all probability contribute more to dysfunctional mothering behavior than the early maternal–infant separation, however. The maternal characteristics of those delivering prematurely include a more stressful life, neglect and/or desertion by their mothers, poorer physical and mental health, greater emotional immaturity, and negative attitudes about pregnancy (Gunther, 1963; Newton, Webster, Binu, Maskrey, & Phillips, 1979).

Early maternal–infant separation such as occurs in premature birth does not necessarily lead to different outcomes for the infant. Bakeman and Brown (1980) found no relationship between early mother–infant interaction and the premature infant's social and mental development at 3 years, indicating that an infant within broad normal limits may be buffered against any long-term consequences of interaction during the first few months of life.

Differences in attachment behaviors between small samples of mothers of full-term infants who had early and extended contact the first hours following birth (N = 12 to 22) and those who did not have this early contact have been reported (DeChateau, 1976; Klaus et al., 1972; Kontos, 1978). Campbell and Taylor's (1979) study with a larger sample (N = 50) noted that an extra hour of early contact had no effect on maternal perceptions of their infants at 3 days or at 1 month.

Others have failed to find later maternal behavioral differences when extra early contact with the infant was provided (Lamb, 1982). Antecedent variables of race, marital status, parity, education, and age influenced the mother's acceptance of her infant, more so than the amount of early contact (Siegle, Bauman, Schaefer, Saunders, & Ingram, 1980). Extended contact in the hospital along with home intervention measures to promote maternal attachment failed to make a difference between groups (Siegle et al., 1980).

Rooming-in was introduced (O'Connor, Vietze, Sherrod, Sandler, and Altmeier, 1980) to study its effect on parenting adequacy. Rooming-in mothers had the baby placed in their rooms for as long as 8 hours daily after the baby was 7 hours or older. Mothers not rooming-in saw their babies at delivery and after 12 hours for feedings only. Although rooming-in was correlated with fewer subsequent cases of parenting inadequacies 12 to 21 months following birth, 90% of the women *not* rooming-in had *no* demonstrable parenting deficiency. Svejda and associates (1980) also failed to confirm differences in attachment with early and enhanced contact.

In summary, while early maternal–infant contact has been associated with greater attachment behaviors, early contact is confounded by the type of delivery, the condition of the infant, and the infant's ability to respond. Further, the lack of consistent, valid, and reliable attachment measures makes it difficult to compare research reports or to make any generalizations. Research reported in the 1980s with full-term infants has failed to confirm any differences with early maternal-infant contact and routine care. Lamb's (1983) critical review of the literature on the bonding phenomenon concluded that claims regarding the effects of early mother–infant contact on attachment have not been well supported, and although short-term effects have been observed for some mother–infant pairs in some situations, data are too inconsistent to identify the characteristics of those affected.

Social Stress

Social stress has been linked with difficulties with pregnancy and parenting. Lynch (1975) identified diffuse, difficult-to-define, long-term social problems among parents of abused children. Others have observed family characteristics of social isolation, serious marital problems, inadequate child care arrangements, dependent personality styles, and lack of child spacing to be associated with child abuse (Green, 1976; Hunter, Kilstrom, Kraybill, & Loda, 1978). A family history of child abuse and neglect is common for abusive parents (Hunter et al., 1978; Stern, 1973). Conger, Burgess, and Barrett (1979) found an interaction between life change stresses and childhood punishment; abusive parents were far more likely than nonabusive parents to have experienced many life changes in a short period of time. Life change stress had the greatest impact on those abusive parents whose parents had been severely punitive.

Egeland, Breitenbucher, and Rosenberg (1980) observed that the relationship between life events and child abuse and neglect was dependent on the mother's anxiety level, personality characteristics, and competence in interacting with her infant. They noted that the mother's ability to see herself as completely separate from her infant affected her ability to deal with stressful situations; unless a mother has a clear concept of her ego boundaries, she is unable to isolate stress from the stress-causing event or stressor.

Maternal exposure to stress factors during pregnancy or the neonatal period seems to deplete the mother's capacity to view her infant as an intact and rewarding person to care for; the mother's depletion may be markedly disproportionate to the extent of the stress per se (Cohen, 1966). The stress of meeting the needs of a new baby, along with loss of sleep and fatigue, plays an important role in postpartum adjustment (Larsen, 1966).

Both mothers and fathers have reported increased personal stress after the birth of a child (Miller & Sollie, 1980). Personal and marital stress was observed to be higher at 8 months than at 1 month post-birth for mothers, and personal stress was higher at 8 months for fathers. Personal well-being was lower for both parents at 8 months, indicating the need for information and support during the first year of parenthood.

Social stress has often been linked to the onset of illness (Holmes, 1978). However, Nuckolls, Cassel, and Kaplan (1972) established that women who experienced higher life-change scores but also had high psychosocial assets experienced only one third of the medical complications that women who had high life-change scores and low psychosocial assets experienced. Others also found that social support had a mediating effect on stress and pregnancy outcome (Norbeck & Tilden, 1983). Thus, the impact of social stress may be tempered by the social support system.

Social Support

Social support is a term that has been used widely and indiscriminately without adequate definition of what is meant. Thus, there has been little consistency in how support has been measured in research (Bruhn & Philips, 1984; Rock, Green, Wise, & Rock, 1984). There tends to be general agreement about four types of support—emotional, informational, instrumental or physical, and appraisal (House, 1981). *Emotional support* is defined as feeling loved, cared for, trusted, and understood. *Informational support* helps the individual to help herself by providing information that is useful in dealing with the problem and/or situation. *Physical support* is a direct kind of help, such as baby-sitting, lending money, etc. *Appraisal support* is information that tells the role-taker how she is performing in the role; it enables the individual to evaluate herself in relationship to others' performance in the role. Each type of support meets different needs, and little is known about the type of support needed during the first year of motherhood. Cronenwett and Kunst-Wilson (1981) presented hypotheses about the transition to fatherhood related to these four types of support, noting that fathers have traditionally had little access to support. The access to support is often limited for women also because of the mobile structure of society.

Wandersman, Wandersman, and Kahn (1980) reported that emotional and network support were positively related to maternal well-being and marital interactions at 3 and 9 months postpartum. However, support had little predictive potential (7%) of postpartum adjustment in their sample. Women with close family relationships, strong emotional support from husbands, and good care from professionals did not become overly distressed by social stressors and deprivations (Cohen, 1979). Kahn and Antocucci (1980) maintained that strong supportive relationships facilitate coping with environmental stressors. Importantly, a person who is capable of eliciting a support system has been socialized to accept supportive help from others and to trust that others will be helpful (Henderson, 1977).

Others have noted the high correlation between spousal support and maternal functioning (Grossman et al., 1980; Shereshefsky & Yarrow, 1973; Westbrook, 1978). The absence of social support has been linked with postpartum depression (Paykel, Emms, Fletcher, & Rassaby, 1980). Perceived stress and social support were significant predictors of maternal attitudes and the quality of mother–infant interactions over the child's first 18 months (Crnic, Greenberg, Robinson, & Ragozin, 1984). Younger mothers reported less intimate support (mate support), less community support, and greater stress; however, maternal education and number of children in the family did not influence reports of stress or support (Crnic et al., 1984).

Mothers who interacted more with their infants in the premature nursery had greater support from spouse and friends (Minde et al., 1978). Others observed that the mother's social support system had a positive effect on affectionate mother–infant behaviors (Ainsfeld & Lipper, 1983). Women with greater social support showed similar affectionate behavior regardless of extent of early contact; however, women with less social support who had early contact with their infants exhibited more affectionate behavior than those with a low social support and less contact.

Having a large support network does not assure that social support is forthcoming in a positive manner, however. The network, or those persons available for support, seems to be more helpful to women assuming the maternal role if the support persons are acquainted and see each other regularly (a tight network) because information and help are less likely to be conflictual (Abernethy,

1973). Women in a loose network (network members do not know or interact with each other) do not have clear feedback regarding their mothering and have to deal with a larger scope of conflicting opinions about child rearing.

Support offered may also be in conflict with the individual's beliefs and values, or it may be undesired. Barrera (1981), who studied 86 pregnant adolescents, argued that the teenager's major source of support was also her major source of strain. Since he found a high positive correlation of social support with the total symptom score and stressful life events, he suggested that his support measure also served as a barometer of the amount of stress the adolescents experienced. Data from other research also suggest that the size of the support system is an indicator of the extent of the stress experienced. Mothers (aged 16 to 36) who had extra help were five times more likely to be categorized as experiencing extensive to severe crisis in the transition to parenthood than those in the slight-to-moderate crisis category (Hobbs, 1965). Distressed women in single-parent families had unusually large networks, but this was interpreted as an unsuccessful attempt to establish security through seeking more persons to help (McLanahan, Wedemeyer, & Adelberg, 1981).

Barrera (1981) observed a positive relationship of total somatic and psychic symptoms with the size of the conflicted network (number of persons who were sources of intrapersonal conflict) and a negative relationship between the unconflicted network and symptomatology. Thus, the unconflicted network appears to have a buffering effect or to lead to fewer illnesses, whereas the conflicted network does not. Colletta and Gregg (1981) observed that adolescent mothers who had high levels of support reported lower levels of stress than did those with less support.

Older, better educated mothers were more likely to continue in a postpartum support group (Cronenwett, 1980). Cronenwett suggested that more highly educated women may require more emotional work in adjusting to the parenting role because other avenues may offer more self-fulfillment than parenting. Or the older, better educated mothers' continuation in a support group may relate to their efforts to maintain continuity with their former selves as well-informed, knowledgeable persons, as was observed by Pickens (1982).

To summarize, the number of persons identified as being in a person's social network does not necessarily indicate the amount of support that may be forthcoming. Conflict within the network and a loose network in which members do not know or interact with each other may not be the most conducive to fostering maternal role attainment. It is the quality and appropriateness of the network rather than its size that influences maternal adaptation most significantly. Some types of support, either emotional, physical, informational, or appraisal, may be more helpful at some times than others. From the empirical evidence to date, emotional support from a mate appears most important in the transition to the mothering role.

Personality Traits

A lack of fit between maternal and infant personality traits may add to the difficulty in the transition to the mothering role. As noted earlier, the maltreatment syndrome of children may be viewed as the end result of current environmental stress, the abuse-prone personality of the parent, and the child's characteristics (Green et al., 1974; Millor, 1981). Research has related maternal traits of temperament, empathy, and rigidity to mothering behaviors.

Burks and Rubenstein (1979) describe the temperamental style of an individual as an automatic and habitual response to the environment. Their work is based on that of Thomas and Chess (1977) who identified nine categories of temperament that reflect an individual's behavioral style: (a) *activity level,* the motor component of functioning and the proportion of activity and inactivity; (b) *rhythmicity,* the regularity and predictability or unpredictability in time of a function; (c) *approach or withdrawal,* the nature of a response to a new stimulus; (d) *adaptability,* the ease in which responses are modified to new or altered situations; (e) *threshold of responsiveness,* the intensity level of stimulation that is necessary to evoke a response; (f) *intensity of reaction,* the energy level of a response; (g) *quality of mood,* the amount of pleasant or unpleasant behavior; (h) *distractibility,* the ease with which environmental stimuli affect ongoing behavior; and (i) *persistence,* the continuation of activity in the face of obstacles. Parent–infant and parent–parent interactional misfits of temperamental styles may lead to problems in socialization and in harmonious relationships (Burks & Rubenstein, 1979).

Buss and Plomin (1975) defined emotionality, activity, sociability, and impulsivity as four temperament categories that reflect the style and nature of behavior. Ralph (1977), using an adaptation of Buss and Plomin's Temperament Survey, found that infants who were rated as fussy and as having a negative mood were associated with mothers who rated themselves as highly impulsive.

Empathy, being able to place oneself in the other's situation, is an important behavior in role-taking. Caulfield, Disbrow, and Smith (1977) found that abusive and neglectful parents were low in empathy. One of the most important maternal tasks of the first 4 to 6 weeks is meshing her behavioral responses to her infant's cues (Sander, 1962); empathy appears to be a salient trait in this task.

Rigidity is a developmental construct; with increasing development, an individual moves from rigid behavioral responses in particular situations to increasingly greater flexibility in responses. The ability to respond with flexibility greatly facilitates adaptation in unusual circumstances (Baldwin, 1967). The person who is better organized and more stable is also more flexible (Werner, 1948). Larsen and associates (1966) observed that mothers with more child-care experiences responded to their infants less rigidly.

To summarize, innate traits, such as temperament, and traits that may be socially learned, such as empathy and flexibility, may influence maternal role-taking. Particularly important is the ability to put oneself in the place of the other.

Self-Concept

Self-regard, or self-concept may be defined as the overall perception of self that includes self-satisfaction, self-acceptance, self-esteem, and congruence or discrepancy between self and ideal self (Wylie, 1974). A woman's feelings about herself are reflected in her relationships with others; if a woman does not trust her own abilities or feels unworthy or incapable of performing mothering tasks, it is difficult for her to trust others, including her infant's response to her (Kennedy, 1973). Some of the women who expressed negative feelings about themselves were demonstrably aggressive toward their 2-week-old infants (shaking or yelling at them).

A woman's self-concept may become more positive and integrated at a higher level as a result of motherhood (Leifer, 1977). Others reported an overall decrease in self-concept 8 months following birth (Miller & Sollie, 1980). Deutsch (1967) suggested that pregnancy in early adolescence may be crippling to an immature personality, whereas motherhood in late adolescence has the potential either to consolidate maturity or to inhibit maturation.

Performance of maternal role behaviors and self-regard appear to be closely related. Shereshefsky and Yarrow (1973) observed that the woman's ego strength, self-confidence, and nurturant qualities were the basic determinants of her capacity as a mother. Curry (1983) reported that women who adapted easily to motherhood had an increase in self-concept; difficult adapters did not experience an increase. As mentioned earlier, Wise and Grossman (1980) found ego strength to be an important variable in the teenager's early adaptation to the maternal role.

Maternal self-acceptance has been linked with child acceptance (Medinnus & Curtis, 1963). A positive relationship between maternal self-esteem and perception of the neonate was observed by Roberts (1983), supporting the earlier finding.

A mother's self-concept may influence how her child perceives herself. The mother's self-concept was positively related to her kindergarten and first-grade child's self-concept (Tocco & Bridges, 1973).

To summarize, a positive self-concept that is acceptable to the individual appears central to her ability to relate positively to another person and to the environment in general. Motherhood has been suggested as contributing to a more positive self-concept for some; however, only those who adapted to the maternal role more easily had an increase in self-concept in Curry's (1983) study. Questions are raised about other factors that may be operative in facilitating adaptation to the maternal role and that also enhance an individual's self-concept.

Child-Rearing Attitudes

A pattern of consistency appears to exist in whether the mother interacts a little or a lot with her infant (Minde et al., 1978). Child-rearing attitudes, how parents reported they handled irritating child behaviors, parent–child interaction, empathy, and parent–child communication all sharply differentiated 55 abusive families and 54 nonabusive families (Caulfield et al., 1977). Maternal attitudes or beliefs about child rearing are believed to have a direct effect on the child's socialization (Cohler & Grunebaum, 1981).

The work of Cohler and associates (1970, 1976, 1980) has supported the effect of child-care attitudes on adaptation to the maternal role and on the child's cognitive development among both well and mentally ill mothers. The mentally ill mother believes less in the infant's ability to respond in a reciprocal mother–child relationship, is less differentiating between her own and her child's needs, and is more likely to deny negative or ambivalent feelings about child care.

Health Status

Maternal illness associated with the pregnancy may decrease the woman's feelings of self-esteem or drain energy that would be available otherwise for mothering (Mercer, 1977). Problems with bodily functioning or ill health also delay the early identification and claiming process (Gottlieb, 1978; Rubin, 1977). A higher incidence of gestational illnesses and medical complications during labor and delivery was found among births of abused siblings than among nonabused siblings (Lynch, 1975). Mothers who were later abusive experienced a higher rate of gestational illness and made later postpartum visits to the nursery than did nonabusive mothers (ten Bensel & Paxson, 1977). Of 10 abusive mothers, 7 had been isolated from the nursery because of their illnesses. Since illness led to early separation from the infant, conclusions may not be drawn as to which variable may have had greater impact. Maternal and infant health complications were higher among the group of abusive parents compared with nonabusive parents in another study (Caulfield et al., 1977).

Maternal child-care attitudes were adversely affected by pregnancy and birth complications in the Cohler et al. (1980) study. This supports the conclusion that attitudes, which are reflected in mothering behaviors, are reactive to health complications.

Infant Variables Affecting Maternal Role Attainment

Two infant variables have been consistently identified as impacting on the mothering role: infant temperament and the infant's health status.

Temperament Feiring (1976) observed that mothers who rated high in adaptive maternal behavior had infants they rated as having an easy temperament. The infant with a difficult temperament is hard to read for cues and therefore leads the mother to feel incompetent and frustrated. The converse is also true. Parents who perceived their infant as having more smiling and laughing behaviors were more content and thankful, whereas depressed and anxious parents described their infants as less soothable and more distressed in Ventura's (1982) study.

Roberts (1983) reported that infant obligatory behavior that was operationalized by variables indicative of temperament (predictability of behavior, frequency of obligatory behaviors, frequency of satisfaction responses, sleep patterns, and time required for feedings) related negatively to both ease of transition to motherhood and parental perception of the infant. A positive relationship between infant obligatory behavior and normative life-style change suggested that a difficult infant disrupts the parents' life-style more so than an easy infant. The greater the normative life-style change, the more difficult the transition to motherhood and the more negative their perceptions of the infant.

Reporting infants as difficult was associated with having major concerns and large family adjustments (Kronstadt, Oberklaid, Ferb, & Swartz, 1979). However, early negative perceptions of infant behavior continued to affect the maternal-child relationship even though perceptions of infant behavior changed in a more positive direction (Campbell, 1979).

Mothers interacted with preschool children differently depending on their assessments of the children's temperaments (Simonds & Simonds, 1981). Mothers with difficult children or children who were slow to warm up were more likely than mothers of easy children to use negative parental behaviors, such as controlling the child through use of guilt, temper, or detachment.

Findings regarding effects of infant temperament must be viewed with caution. For example, the Carey Infant Temperament Questionnaire may be an assessment of maternal characteristics and attitudes as well as of maternal perception of infant temperament (Vaughn, Taraldson, Crichton, & Egeland, 1981). The mother's social status, anxiety level, and mental health status all related to temperament ratings on the Carey Infant Temperament Questionnaire at 4 months (Sameroff, Seifer, & Elias, 1982). Although child behavior measured both at home and in the laboratory related to temperament, the mother effects were much more powerful. In another study social class, gender, and birth order were not related to the temperament of 160 children at 6, 12, and 24 months of age (Persson-Blennow & McNeil, 1981). Others reported that multiparous, extroverted mothers tended to rate their infants as easy (Bates, Freeland, & Lounsbury, 1979). Women who had prior experience with infants and greater empathy less often rated their easy and average infants' cries as spoiled, but more often rated their difficult infants' cries as spoiled (Lounsbury & Bates, 1982).

In summary, the infant who is easy to care for and who is predictable appears to create less of a life-style change for parents and enhances the parents' feelings of competency in infant care. Thus, the easy infant is associated with an easier transition to parenthood and is described more positively by the parents. Questions are raised, however, as to whether the mother's greater experience and psychosocial assets lead to both her more positive rating of infant temperament and her greater ease in the transition to motherhood.

Health Status As is the case in maternal illness, the effect of infant illness on later maternal behavior is confounded by the maternal-infant separation that accompanies both. Infant illness may interfere with the attachment process in two ways. The mother may delay identification and claiming behaviors because of less opportunity to interact with her infant, and she may avoid attaching to her infant if she is afraid the infant will die. A higher rate of infant illnesses has been reported as a factor in child abuse in several studies (Lynch, 1975; Stern, 1973).

At 2 months postpartum the infant's health, along with the mother's emotional well-being, lack of anxiety and depression, and good marital adjustment, correlated with maternal adaptation(Grossman et al.,1980). The ill infant requires additional caretaking and also may threaten the parents' sense of competence.

Confounding Variables

Variables influencing maternal role attainment and those that impact on maternal role attainment are viewed as confounding variables. These include the women's ethnic background, marital status, and socioeconomic status (SES), which is determined in part by educational level.

Mothering behaviors differ from culture to culture; behavior judged as "good mothering" in one culture may be frowned on in another culture (Brink, 1982). Patterns of mothering evolve to socialize a child for a specific culture. There are no data to support the supposition that any one pattern of mothering or of expressing affection is superior to any other. Dysfunctional parenting patterns are not unique to any ethnic or socioeconomic group.

Empirical evidence to date has not been in agreement about the relationships of SES and mother–child interaction. Grossman et al. (1980) did not find SES predictive of the quality of mothering. They observed that lower SES was correlated with greater comfort with parenting at 2 months postpartum. Attitudes, which in turn affect behavior, reportedly differ by SES. Lower-SES mothers tended to believe that infants acquired cognitive skills later than did higher SES mothers; consequently, they began cognitive stimulation activities later (Ninio, 1979).

Harmon and Kogan's (1980) findings indicated that social class could not be used as a predictor of any differences in maternal-child interactions. Others observed that middle-SES mothers did not do more for their infants than lower-SES mothers but that they responded differently to different infant cues (Lewis & Wilson, 1972). Middle-SES mothers vocalized when their infants vocalized, touched or held their infants when they were fretful, and watched their infants play. In contrast, lower-SES mothers tended to touch their infants when their infants vocalized and to vocalize when their infants were fretful or playing.

Russell (1974) noted that more highly educated parents experienced more of a crisis in the transition to parenthood and enjoyed the parenting role less than parents who had less education. Steffensmeier (1982) also observed that more highly educated parents derived less gratification in the parenting role.

Well-educated and poorly educated mothers differed from the time of their infants' birth in their knowledge of infant capabilities, style of interaction, and control techniques (Barnard & Eyres, 1979). Married white women with a higher level of education rated higher on measures of teaching, feeding, and providing a stimulating home environment (Barnard & Eyres, 1979).

Maternal education was concretely related to the quality of mothering in Nigeria (Caldwell, 1981). Maternal education was the single greatest determinant of child mortality; educated mothers defied tradition and were less fatalistic about illness, consequently seeking earlier health care, which resulted in lower mortality rates. More highly educated persons may feel more comfortable relying on their own judgment and observations of their infants.

Marital status appears to affect both the children and the mother. The presence of both parents in the family has had a stress-reducing effect on children when compared with one-parent families (Sandler, 1980). Single teenage mothers had lower self-concepts than married school-age mothers (Zongker, 1980). Much of the research related the marital relationship positively to later mothering behaviors, as well as feelings about self in the mothering role (Grossman et al., 1980; Shereshefsy & Yarrow, 1973; Westbrook, 1978).

Except for gratification in the mothering role, maternal education has been consistently related to more positive mothering behaviors irrespective of SES. Maternal education also may have a relationship with ethnic background, maternal attitudes about child rearing, age, and self-concept.

Summary of Theoretical Framework for the Research

The comparative study of maternal role attainment for the three age groups of women was planned within the broad framework of role and developmental theories. Maternal role attainment is an interactional and developmental process occurring over a period of time, during which the mother becomes attached to her infant, acquires competence in the caretaking tasks involved in the role, and expresses pleasure and gratification in the role. Role-taking involves the active interaction of the role-taker and the role partner; each responds to cues from the other and alters behavior according to the other's response.

Empirical findings related age, perception of the birth experience, early maternal-infant separation, social stress, social support, maternal and infant temperament, empathy, rigidity, self-concept, and maternal and infant health status to maternal role attainment. All of these variables appear to interact with one or more of the other variables in affecting maternal role behaviors. There was no evidence, however, to support the conclusion that any one variable would be more influential on maternal role attainment. Therefore, it was important to study all of these variables as they occurred in the process of mothering without assigning priority to one variable over another.

ASSUMPTIONS

Assumptions for this study included the following: (a) there is a relatively stable "core self," acquired through lifelong socialization that influences how a mother defines and perceives events (Turner, 1978); and her perceptions of her infant's and others' responses to her mothering, along with her life situation, are the real world that

she responds to (Mead, 1934); (b) in addition to the mother's socialization, her developmental level and innate personality characteristics
also influence her behavioral responses; and (c) the mother's role
partner, her infant, will reflect her competence in the mothering
role via growth and development.

RESEARCH AIMS

The major aim of the research project was to determine whether
there were age differences in mothering behaviors and responses to
the maternal role. Variables identified by previous researchers as
influencing the maternal role were studied in addition to maternal
age to determine their relationship to maternal role behaviors. These
variables included perception of the birth experience, early maternal-
infant separation, stress, social support, personality traits, self-concept, health status, child-rearing attitudes, and infant variables of
temperament and health status. A second aim of the study was to
determine the significance of these variables in predicting maternal
role behaviors over the year. A third aim was to identify other factors that appeared to influence maternal role behaviors as they
emerged from interviews and observations over the five test periods.

METHODOLOGY

Design

To study maternal role attainment as a developmental process, a
longitudinal design was planned with cross-sectional analyses of test
periods to detect any change over time. Since the range for attaining
the maternal role was reported to be from 3 to 9 months, a period of
1 year was selected as inclusive. However, despite the additional margin of 3 months, 6% of the women in this study indicated that they
had just begun to feel comfortable in the mothering role at 1 year,
and 4% stated that they were still working toward that end.

Five sets of measurements were taken: initially during the early
postpartum period prior to discharge from the hospital and at 1, 4,
8, and 12 months following birth. The measures for each of the variables are described in the Appendix. The three-group design allowed
comparison of the three age groups of mothers on each of the variables, and stepwise multiple regressions were done at each test period

to determine the best predictors of maternal role attainment behaviors for the total sample. The longitudinal analyses involved
modeling the maternal role attainment variables across the time
periods.

Sample

Comparisons were made between mothers aged 15 to 19 years,
mothers aged 20 to 29 years, and mothers aged 30 to 42 years.
Consequently, any differences observed in either the younger or the
older age groups may be contrasted to the age group (20 to 29 years)
in which the majority of first births in the United States occur.
Characteristics of the women are described in Chapter 2.

A sample of 294 women were interviewed and completed the
initial set of instruments during their postpartum hospitalization;
276 continued at the 1-month test period, 264 at 4 months, 250 at
8 months, and 242 at 12 months. Women who dropped out of the
study did not differ from those who continued by marital status,
racial group, self-concept, or personality integration *within* each of
the three age groups. Women from the 20- to 29-year-old group who
dropped out had less education. When differences were studied for
the *total* sample, those who dropped out had less education, were
less likely to be married, and had a less integrated personality than
those who continued through the year.

Attrition rates differed dramatically by age group; 39% of the
teenage women dropped out, 17% of those aged 20 to 29, and only
2% of those aged 30 to 42. Thus, the initial sample of 66 aged 15
to 19 (Group 1), 138 aged 20 to 29 (Group 2), and 90 aged 30 to 42
(Group 3) was reduced to 40 in Group 1, 114 in Group 2, and 88 in
Group 3 by the fifth test period at 1 year, an overall attrition rate of
18%.

Selection Criteria

Originally, selection criteria were that the woman was in the age
range of 13 to 39 years, had given birth to her first live-born infant
without a diagnosed anomaly at birth (all classifications of abortion
and previous stillbirths were included), was fluent in English, and
lived in the San Francisco Bay area. The special problems that

mothers encounter with either infants who are born prematurely or who have an anomaly introduces additional problems and challenges beyond the scope of this project. The intent was to study the development of the maternal role in more normal circumstances.

As primiparous mothers over 39 years were encountered, the decision was made to delete an upper age limit for the older group because the project was concerned with how the women who had postponed motherhood would deal with motherhood in comparison with the two younger groups of women. Only one person under 15 (14 years) met the criteria for participation, and she refused to participate.

In order to follow up for the four subsequent test periods in the mother's home or a place specified by her, residence within the Bay Area was limited to an hour's travel from the setting in which they delivered. The university hospital where all except 41% of Group 1 were recruited is a high-risk referral center for the region, and many patients did not meet the study criteria. Nine percent of Group 1 were recruited from a private hospital, and 32% were recruited from a county hospital; both hospitals are affiliated with the university.

All mothers who met the study criteria were invited to participate in the study on Mondays through Fridays. Since some families opt for early discharge, a few women who delivered Friday afternoon or later and who went home before Monday were missed. However, most women delivering at the university hospital during the 16-month recruitment period had an opportunity to participate in the study. The refusal rate was 48%; fewer in Group 3 refused to participate (31%, compared with 53% in both groups 1 and 2). Refusal rates differed by racial group also: Asians, 70%; Hispanics, 69%; blacks, 58%; Caucasians (Anglo-whites), 40%; and others, 36%. One-fourth of the women gave as their reason for refusal that they were moving, either out of the area or out of the state, during the coming year; 35% gave no reason; 16% weren't interested; 15% said they would be too busy; 4% said their mates or a family member objected; 3% stated they were uncomfortable being interviewed; and 2% were already in a research project.

Procedure

Interviewers were all registered nurse graduate students majoring in an area of maternal-child health, except for the full-time research associate and the principal investigator, who had graduate degrees in maternity nursing. Except for the principal investigator, all were under 30 years of age. All interviewers were Anglo-white.

The interviews had both structured and open-ended questions. Answers were written verbatim on the interview schedule; at times key words were written and the data filled in immediately following the interview. At each interview the infant was weighed, and the length and head circumference were measured. A set of instruments was mailed to each woman about 2 weeks prior to the scheduled interview so that they could be completed at a time more convenient for her and were picked up at the time of the interview.

Most of the women were interviewed initially on their first or second postpartum day after informed consent was obtained. The first postpartum day begins the first midnight following the infant's birth. Some who had a cesarean birth, or were otherwise busy or fatigued, were interviewed as late as the third or fourth postpartum day. A few women who opted for early discharge were interviewed on the day of delivery. These initial interviews were held on the postpartum unit at the woman's bedside.

The women were visited in their homes or another setting convenient for them at 1, 4, 8, and 12 months following birth. The setting for the interview varied more with the teenagers, Group 1. Single mothers in Group 1 sometimes selected their mother's home, an aunt's or cousin's home, or a boyfriend's apartment. Some women had other persons living with them and chose settings away from home for more privacy for the interviews. Pizza and ice cream parlors were a favorite for the younger group who elected outside settings. A physician's office or a clinic was selected by some if they had appointments near the date for the interview. The public settings did not seem to interfere with the mothers' sharing their feelings about the mothering role. They usually had their infants with them.

The women in groups 2 and 3 as a whole were very attentive to the interview and tended to keep distractions to a minimum. However, this was not true for some of the teenagers: the interviewer vied with the television for attention or at times had to ask questions in competition with a very loud stereo. The teenagers also were the greatest offenders in failing to keep interview appointments. Even though calls were made to verify the visits prior to leaving, occasionally by the time the interviewer arrived the young mother had left to "get a haircut" or to "go to the store." As many as five or six attempts were made for some interviews. Single women in Group

1 had several other interests to distract them, and participation in a research project was not a high priority. The married, employed teenagers were an exception; they kept appointments and demonstrated more interest in the interviews, although they were pushed for time like all of the mothers.

As a guest in the women's homes, the interviewer accomplished the goals with whatever restrictions were placed. Phone calls and drop-in visits by friends or neighbors were interruptions that occurred most often, second only to interruptions that were necessary for the infant's care.

Initial interviews averaged 55 min; interviews with groups 2 and 3 were lengthier, as the older women either were more comfortable elaborating on their feelings or felt freer to discuss their feelings. By the fifth test period at 1 year, the interviews averaged 78 min; interviews were most often 60 min, but the older women's interviews continued to be longer. The average length for the interviews was 69 min for Group 1, 79 min for Group 2, and 81 min for Group 3. With increased contact with the interviewers the women either felt more comfortable sharing their feelings and thus talked more, or with increasing experience in the mothering role they had more information to share.

Beginning at 4 months, 41% of the women had returned to work, so it was necessary to schedule interviews in the evenings or on weekends. Some women dropped out of the study then because of lack of available time. Stress, a variable under study, was also a factor that contributed to withdrawal from the study. For example, one woman left her husband and could not be located. Another had a family member die and withdrew from the study.

Hawthorne Effect

An unavoidable result of any longitudinal project is a Hawthorne effect to some extent; that is, the observed behavior was somewhat different as a result of participation in the study. Women were asked at the final test period if they had done anything differently as a result of participating in the study. About half (51%) said no (Group 1, 65%; Group 2, 47%; and Group 3, 51%). Over one third (37%) said yes. The examples of how they were influenced included "becoming more aware," "thought of different/more ways to do things," and "became more in touch with my feelings." Just over one tenth (12%) said no but qualified their response with additions such as "partici-

pation had provided an opportunity to vent feelings" and "participation had increased awareness." Thus, it appears that some women,
particularly those in groups 2 and 3, may have altered their maternal
role behaviors because of their participation in the project. A more
obvious example of how interview items influenced the mother was
the item "What things are you helping your baby to learn at this
time?" At 1 month, some of the mothers said, "Oh, the baby is able
to learn now," and by the next interview they had gone to the
library and read about infant development or had bought a book so
that they had a repertoire of activities to report.

All of the women in the study generously shared their perspectives
on the joys and trials of the first-time mother and supplied colorful
illustrations from day-to-day activities to illustrate both. There was
a feeling of generosity in their sharing because of the possibility of
their experiences being of help to future mothers in similar situations.

CHAPTER **2**

The Mothers

Because this was a study of maternal age differences spanning an age range of 15 to 42 years, developmental differences were expected in addition to different life situations and demographic differences. This chapter focuses on the characteristics of the three age groups of mothers, 15 to 19 years (Group 1), 20 to 29 years (Group 2), and 30 to 42 years (Group 3). First an overview of adolescent and adult developmental theory is presented. The characteristics of the mothers, including demographic characteristics; personal and social histories; life events stress experienced during both the year prior to birth and the first year of motherhood; self-concept; personality traits of empathy, rigidity, and temperament; and child-rearing attitudes, are compared by age group. Implications for nursing interventions conclude the chapter.

ADOLESCENT AND ADULT DEVELOPMENTAL CONCEPTS

Interactionist role theory views self-development as an ever-changing and dynamic process of evolving self-awareness and self-definition that occurs through actions and interactions with others; culture and environmental situations also influence this process (Burr et al., 1979). Competence in role-taking increases as a person's knowledge of cultural symbols, ability to take the role of others, and self-complexity increases. Developmental theories are in agreement with these major role concepts of increasing self-complexity and greater competency in adapting to the environment as the individual develops over time. A teenager with less experience in role-taking could be expected to be less competent in mothering skills, yet with a supportive environment she may do well. An older woman who is very skilled in role-taking but who has an unsupportive environmental situation may experience difficulty with the mothering role.

Developmental Concepts

Werner (1957) defined development as progression from a state of relative diffuseness and lack of differentiation to a state of increasingly greater differentiation, articulation, and hierarchic integration. For example, a child experiences objects (including persons) as discrete as opposed to having several qualities. With increasing articulation, an individual begins to see separateness to object parts as well as the coordination of parts. A child's functioning is both rigid and labile. The important rituals that a child enjoys repeating over and over are an example of rigidity. In some cultures where inventions or new ways of responding to the environment are not valued, rigidity is adaptive. A child also displays erratic and unpredictable responses as well as rigidity. By adulthood a person is able to view complex situations in a flexible manner apart from personal experiences and to respond with more consistent behavior. According to Werner's developmental theory, the teenage group of mothers would be expected to be more rigid in their maternal beliefs than Group 2, who would be more rigid than Group 3. Likewise, more consistent behavioral responses could be expected from the older mother.

Erikson's (1959) developmental theory stressed the importance of both the timing and the sequencing of development. According to Erikson's theory, a ground plan is inherent from which parts and/or ability to function arise at a specific time until all parts and/or abilities are complete to form a functioning whole. Despite cultural variations, a child is said to develop within "the proper rate and the proper sequence which govern the growth of a personality as well as that of an organism" (p. 52). Eight stages of development with major tasks for each stage were described by Erikson. Characteristically, the successful completion of tasks of each earlier stage makes it easier to achieve tasks at a later stage. During infancy, the major task is to learn trust; if trust is not learned, mistrust may be the outcome. During toddlerhood, the major task is autonomy versus shame and doubt; during play or preschool age, initiative versus guilt is the major task. During school age, industry versus inferiority is the major task. The major task of adolescence is identity achievement versus identity diffusion; the young adult masters intimacy versus isolation. During adulthood, generativity versus self-absorption is the major task, and during the mature age of later adulthood, integrity versus disgust and despair are central. Three of Erikson's developmental stages are relevant to this study—adolescence, young adulthood, and adulthood. The teenage mother has moved from the task of internalizing an identity to generativity in rearing the next generation, often without having achieved a true sense of intimacy. The question could be raised whether the woman 30 years and older who has had a period of self-absorption in a career might find it more difficult to adapt to the unexpected and uncontrollable events of motherhood.

Based on a study of 40 men, Levinson, Darrow, Klein, Levinson, and McKee (1978) proposed four eras in the life cycle. An era was defined as much broader and more conclusive than Erikson's developmental stages but provided an overview of the life cycle similar to acts in a play. The eras included childhood and adolescence, ages 0 to 20 years; early adulthood, 17 to 45 years; middle adulthood, 40 to 65 years; late adulthood, 60 years and older. Eras were observed to overlap so that as a new era began, the earlier era was ending. This overlap of eras is called a *transition* and occurs as follows: early childhood transition, 0 to 3 years: early adult transition, 17 to 22 years; an age-30 transition; midlife transition, 40 to 45 years; and late adult transitions, 60 to 65 years. The early adult era is the most relevant to this study, as are the early adult and midlife transitions.

Tasks defined for a novice phase of the early adult era included forming a life's dream, forming mentor relationships with experienced, established adults to help young adults achieve their dream, forming an occupation, and establishing love relationships and a family. The age-30 transition provides a second chance to establish a life structure more congruent with the life's dream. The age-30 transition may help to explain the career woman's decision to become pregnant if her life's dream included the role of mother. A comment by one of the older mothers supports this idea: "Before I had him, I was in the mid-thirties crisis. The problems I was having stopped when I decided to have a baby. Now I am more satisfied. I was bored with my work, and I asked myself, 'What do I want to do; is this all there is?' " The *transition* to motherhood facilitated the age-30 *transition* for this woman; by making an appraisal of her life and asking herself what her goals were, she made a decision that motherhood would make up for the void that she was experiencing. Many persons make career changes at the age-30 transition.

When Levinson's framework was tested in a study of women, a greater variability in the sequencing and accomplishment of early adult developmental tasks was found than was observed in men (Stewart, 1977). The variability Stewart observed is represented in this study of three age groups of women, those who formed a stable marriage and family life in their twenties, and those who remained single and/or pusued a career during this decade. The formation of a satisfactory early adult life structure was far more complex and difficult for women than for men because of the devaluation of traditional female roles in this culture, along with severe sanctions when women did not succeed in them (Stewart, 1977). All transitions are more difficult when they occur out of sequence for cultural norms or expectations (Neugarten, Moore, & Lowe, 1965).

Women's difficulty in the transition to the maternal role might also vary depending on the cultural norms and stereotypes that either value or devalue motherhood; some cultures value early motherhood, whereas others value career achievement. Some women in this study faced this kind of cultural conflict:

- I feel guilty that I am not a traditional Chinese wife; I can't be that.
- In the Philippines we have maids, nannies; here everything is on my shoulders.
- I have no part of my husband's life. Children don't fit into this life style . . . I think he is blaming me for not being with him.
- I lost a little self-esteem being home and not working or not seeing people. I've had to pull myself out of that at times.

Motherhood and Development

Motherhood has been described as a developmental stage (Schectman, 1980), a developmental task (Cohler, 1984), and a developmental phase (Benedek, 1959). Schectman describes developmental processes accompanying motherhood as occurring simultaneously and equally on social, biological, emotional, and cognitive levels. As such, the growth that accompanies the transition to parenthood is synonymous with adult development.

Benedek's (1959) notion of parenthood as developmental also focuses on change within the individual. Benedek argued that parenthood is a developmental phase that enables parents to achieve a higher level of intrapsychic integration. At each stage of the child's development, any of the parent's unresolved conflicts of that stage may re-emerge and present an opportunity to resolve the conflict at a higher level.

The reproduction of society is dependent on families having children. Cohler (1984) stated, "Parenthood represents the cardinal social role and major developmental task of adulthood, beginning with the birth of the first child and continuing through old age" (p. 119). The conception of motherhood as an adult developmental task and a major social role presents different facets of development. Establishing love relationships and a family is one of several tasks Levinson et al. (1978) identified for the novice phase of the early adult era for men that was discussed above.

Women, regardless of their age, have described the transition to motherhood as entry to adulthood (Leifer, 1977; Shereshefsky & Yarrow, 1973). Women in all three age groups in this study supported the notion that the first year of motherhood was a maturing process for them:

Group 1 (15 to 19 years)
- Being a mother makes me feel good mentally more than physically; I have someone to grow up with me. Watching him grow makes me feel important.

Group 2 (20 to 29 years)
- I feel power in being able to reproduce. It put me in touch with basic values, and I take a stand a lot more and don't back down.
- I feel older, an adult role of mother, a responsible adult member of society.

Group 3 (30 to 42 years)
- I feel a lot different; there is a lot of redefining of yourself. Other people see me as a mother.
- I feel complete; I had done what else I wanted to. A sense of sharing my life, a sense of posterity.

These comments verify the different developmental perspectives discussed above: An inner development occurred within the woman that included mental and physical accomplishments and a redefinition of self; an adult task was achieved in considering basic values, gaining a sense of power, and feeling complete; and a major social role was fulfilled in becoming a responsible member of society in which a continuity of self to future generations was experienced.

DEMOGRAPHIC CHARACTERISTICS

As would be expected, the characteristics and life situations of the three groups of women were quite diverse. However, within each age group characteristics and situations were more similar. The older the age group, the more likely they were Caucasian (Anglo-white), were married, and had a college degree.

The teenage group was 30% Caucasian; 28% reported some college, 31% had high school diplomas, and 42% had not completed high school; only 32% were married. Group 2 was 67% Caucasian; 35% had baccalaureate or graduate degrees, 44% had some college, 17% had high school diplomas, and 4% had not completed high school; 76% were married. Group 3 was 80% Caucasian; 63% had baccalaureate or graduate degrees, 30% had some college, 6% had high school diplomas, and only one had not completed high school; 79% were married.

The non-Caucasians included Asians (0%, 6%, and 9%, respectively, from the youngest to the oldest group), blacks (41%, 12%, and 2%), Filipinos (8%, 4%, and 0%), Hispanics (9%, 3%, and 2%), and others (12%, 10%, and 8%). Fewer non-Caucasians postponed motherhood until age 30.

Income levels during the first year of motherhood also reflected both the educational differences and the hardships of minority groups from the younger to the older group of women. Two-thirds of the teenagers were in families that had annual incomes of $12,000 or less, two-thirds of Group 2 had an income of $18,000 or higher, and two-thirds of Group 3 had incomes of $22,000 or higher, with 10% having an income of $70,000 or higher.

The religious preferences of the teenagers were 42% Catholic, 26% no preference, 16% Protestant, 3% Jewish, and 13% other. Group 2 were 30% Catholic, 29% no preference, 22% Protestant, 5% Jewish, and 14% other. Group 3 were 20% Catholic, 25% no preference, 30% Protestant, 13% Jewish, and 12% other. Because the largest religious group was Catholic (28%) and the second largest group (Protestant, 20%) was much more diverse in beliefs and socialization, groups were divided into Catholic and non-Catholic when relationships were examined between religion and mothering variables.

PERSONAL AND SOCIAL HISTORY

Type of Household

The three groups of women lived in different types of households. Older women were more often living with the father of the baby (Group 1, 61%; Group 2, 91%; and Group 3, 92%). More teenagers than older women lived in households with relatives and their mothers; some teenagers and their mates lived with their parents.

Parenting Background

Because the first role model for mothering comes from the woman's earliest experiences of being mothered, it was important to learn whether she had parental role models. Women who were separated from their parents through the age of 11 years were observed to have greater child-rearing and family problems than those who were not separated from their parents (Frommer & O'Shea, 1973a, 1973b). Child abuse as a way of coping with stress is also learned in the process of being parented (Conger et al., 1979).

Significantly more of the teenagers (47%) were separated from either one or both of their parents before the age of 12 years than those in groups 2 (26%) and 3 (18%). Eleven percent of the teenagers, 8% of Group 2, and no one from Group 3 were separated from *both* parents before they were 12 years old. Women more often reported being separated from their father; 31% of the teenagers, 16% of Group 2, and 13% of Group 3 had been separated from their fathers before the age of 12. Divorce was the most frequent reason for the separation from a parent.

There were no significant age group differences in whether either the woman or a sibling had been severely punished as a child. Nineteen percent of the total sample reported that either they or a sibling had been severely punished as a child ($\underline{N}$ = 52); another 13% ($\underline{N}$ = 36) would not say one way or another. Two women who were abused as children continued to be abused by their mates. A teenager who had been living with her husband since she was 13 years old reported that he hit her in the chest and threw her against the closet door while her infant watched and cried hysterically; she had to be hospitalized. A woman from Group 2 reported that her boyfriend had fractured her hand twice.

Disciplining methods that women described their parents as using were in the order of the frequency reported: talked to, 61%; spanked, 52%; privileges withheld, 25%; restricted mobility (grounded, stood in corner), 24%; beating with belt, hangar, sticks, 10%; yelled at, harsh words, 8%; too strict, too much, 5%; never punished, 6%; and rewarded for good behavior, 2%. Teenagers reported being talked to less often and being grounded more often than the two older groups of women; otherwise, there were no group differences in type of punishment that women reported receiving as children.

Employment Status

Women's plans to work following the birth of their infants was related to whether they had jobs to which they wished to return and their financial need. Fifty-eight percent of the teenagers reported that they were either not employed or held unskilled positions prior to their pregnancy, compared with 20% of Group 2 and 9% of Group 3. At early postpartum, 40% of the teenagers stated that they did not intend to work, compared with 18% of Group 2 and 22% of Group 3. Forty-five percent of the two older groups indicated they planned to return to their previous jobs, compared with 13% of the teenagers. Financial need was the reason most frequently given for plans to seek employment following birth; 21% of Group 1, 36% of Group 2, and 17% of Group 3 gave that reason.

Twice as many of the women in Group 3 as in groups 1 and 2 indicated they wanted to return to work, which probably reflects their greater progress in career development. Fewer in groups 1 (10%) and 2 (11%) than in Group 3 (20%) indicated they planned to return to work because they wanted to. About one third in each group listed both the financial need and the desire to work as their reasons for plans to go to work.

The women's projections of their plans to return to work because of financial need and their desire to return to work were reflected in the percentage who were employed in each age group. By 4 months postpartum, 41% of the women were employed (from youngest to oldest group, 21%, 42%, 50%, respectively). At 8 months postpartum, 55% of the total sample were employed, 40% of the teenagers, 59% of Group 2, and 55% of Group 3. At 1 year, 62% of all of the mothers were employed (32%, 72%, 61%, respectively).

Overall, groups 2 and 3 tended to be employed 1 month earlier than Group 1. The average age of infants when all of the mothers became employed was 15 weeks. By age group, the average infant in Group 1 was 20 weeks old; Group 2, 15 weeks; and Group 3, 14 weeks.

Friends as Support Network

Although peers are extremely important to teenagers, they tended to have a less close network of friends. The two older groups of women more often had a close friend who lived in the Bay Area than did those in the teenage group. The teenagers went to parties or on picnics with friends less often than the two older groups of women. More of the teenagers never had a friend visit them in their homes (29% compared with 3% and 5%).

Whereas 97% of Group 3 and 95% of Group 2 had someone living in the Bay Area whom they could call on for any kind of help, only 82% of the teenagers had such a person. Of those who had such a person, the two older groups of women more often noted that this person could be counted on to do everything possible to help. Thus, not only were the younger group handicapped by fewer educational and financial resources, they had fewer social resources in the way of friends.

The teenagers' lack of social support from friends was not offset by increased support from parents. There were no significant differences by age group reporting that their mothers or fathers would be living with them the first month after discharge from the hospital or listing their mothers as one of the persons who would be helping them after discharge.

Stressful Life Events the Year Prior to Birth

Life events that had occurred the year prior to the birth were scored by the woman as either positive (good) events or negative (bad) events and were rated according to the felt impact of the event. The life event that all of the women had experienced was pregnancy; 267 (93%) reported it as a good event, and 9 (3%) reported it as a bad event. Twelve (4%) of the women failed to check pregnancy. Marriage was the life event reported second most frequently by the women; 120 (41%) checked marriage as a good event, and 4 (1%)

as a bad event. A major change in eating habits was noted as a good event by 125 (43%) and as a bad event by 47 (16%); 122 (41%) did not rate this as a change.

Group 2 reported more life change the year prior to birth than either of the other groups. Group 2 reported a greater average positive (good) life events score (13.11) than groups 1 (10.21) and 3 (10.95), who did not differ significantly from each other. Group 2 also had a greater average negative life events score (5.14) than Group 3 (3.33), but Group 1's score (4.84) did not differ significantly from either.

Stressful Life Events Occurring the First Year of Motherhood

Group 2 also reported a greater average positive life events score (13.00) the first year of motherhood than did Group 3 (10.05), with Group 1 (12.53) scoring between the two and not differing significantly from either.

The teenagers who were handicapped educationally and financially were also handicapped by greater negative stress during the first year of motherhood. Their negative life events score (11.03) was significantly higher than groups 2 (7.78) and 3 (6.30), who did not differ significantly from each other. Negatively perceived life events are more stressful to persons and produce greater negative effects (Sarason, Johnson, & Siegel, 1978). Others observed that younger mothers reported both greater stress and less social support during the first 18 months of motherhood (Crnic et al., 1984).

SELF-CONCEPT

A total positive self-concept score, which reflects an individual's overall level of self-esteem, and a personality integration score that indicates the level of adjustment were measured during the first few days postpartum and again at 8 months postpartum.

At early postpartum, Group 2 (356.62) and Group 3 (361.41) had significantly higher self-concepts than did the teenage group (334.73); however, the scores of groups 2 and 3 did not differ significantly from each other. Teenage mothers' self-concept scores were similar to married teenage mothers' scores (332.60) in Zongker's (1980) study and higher than he reported for single mothers (314.71). Mothers in the single group tended to be younger (youngest, 12 years) than mothers in the married group (youngest, 15 years). Arnold (1980) reported that adolescents aged 16 to 17 years had higher self-concept scores than adolescents aged 13 to 15. Group 2's self-concept scores were similar to those reported by Curry (1983) for women aged 20 to 31 years during the last trimester of pregnancy (354); scores for both groups 2 and 3 are well above the established norm (345.57) (Fitts, 1965).

The personality integration mean score was significantly higher for each older age group, which supports the conclusion that personality integration represents a developmental construct. The mean scores for the teenagers (8.48) was somewhat lower than Zongker's (1980) group of married teenage mothers (9.20) but was higher than the single group of teenage mothers (6.55). The Group 2 mean (10.13) was similar to the norm (10.42) (Fitts, 1965), and Group 3's was higher (11.49) than the norm.

An unexpected overall decrease in self-concept occurred at 8 months postpartum for all three age groups, although the personality integration score did not change significantly (Mercer, 1986a). If motherhood contributes to overall adult development, resulting in a feeling of greater maturity, an increase in self-concept could be expected. An increase in self-concept was observed in 33% of the teenagers, 37% of Group 2, and 30% of Group 3. Entwisle and Doering (1981) also observed that that 120 primiparous women had deteriorating views of themselves during the 6 months postpartum. They reported that following birth women viewed themselves in the wife role more favorably, but they rated themselves less favorably in the mother role. These less favorable views of self were thought to contribute to postpartum depression.

At 8 months postpartum, the teenage group mean score for self-concept was 327.38. Group 2's mean score was 349.99, and Group 3's was 350.97, which are lower than Curry (1983) reported for mothers at 3 months who adapted to motherhood easily (364.1) but higher than was reported for those who had difficulty adapting (336.8).

Personality integration, which appears to be a developmental construct, was also more stable. The slight decreases were not significant. The mean scores were Group 1, 8.21; Group 2, 9.75; and Group 3, 11.22.

The cultural milieu and general support systems apparently did not provide the kind of feedback to the majority of the women during the first 8 months that enabled them to feel as good about themselves as they did shortly following birth. The challenges of the more assertive and mobile infant, and additional roles such as employment, also affected how the women viewed themselves at 8 months. Comments made by the women indicate some of the problems with self-concept at 8 months:

Group 1
- I ain't doing nothing but take care of him; I don't like it that much.
- Everyone in my family is "the mom"; I'm just a little mom.

Group 2
- My mother-in-law made me feel terribly inadequate as a mother; I wonder if I was really meant to be a mother.
- I didn't do anything I should do; I feel bad about that [had sent baby to Taiwan for family of origin to rear].
- Am I a woman or am I a mother? I can't decide whether it's worth fixing myself up. Will anybody notice?
- Having a baby takes a lot out of you; I feel so vulnerable—so fragile.

Group 3
- I still don't see myself as a mother. I'm performing the role. My mother is a mother. The whole dependence of infancy is hard.
- I don't have a picture of myself at this stage. I am living a sheltered life.
- As a mother–housewife you feel like you are less than you were before. You're isolated and its hard to feel good about what you are doing.

Motherhood for the majority of the women in this study had contributed to feelings of isolation, inadequacy, vulnerability, and devaluation of self-regard. This is in opposition to a higher level of development as an adult in which a person experiences a higher level of integration and organization.

EMPATHY

Teenagers had significantly less ability to imagine the feelings of other persons in different situations than the women in their twenties had (mean score, 36.29; higher score indicated less empathy).

An unexpected finding was that Group 3's empathy score (34.03) reflected less empathy than Group 2's (33.17) and did not differ significantly from either Group 1's or Group 2's.

Both role and developmental theories support the idea that empathy could be expected to increase with increasing age, so this finding is difficult to interpret. Different cognitive styles may influence empathetic responses, and data on cognitive style were not collected. Persons high in empathy view others more discriminatingly and less stereotypically, and are more often firstborns (Hansson, Mathews, & Disbrow, 1978). The empathy instrument's reliability was low with this sample and may not have adequately tapped the construct of empathy.

RIGIDITY

As was expected, the older the age group, the more flexible they were in child-rearing attitudes. Group 1's mean rigidity score was 53.99, Group 2's was 44.78, and Group 3's was 40.37. This finding supports the developmental theory that flexibility increases with increased development and it indicates that older mothers have the potential to respond less rigidly to their infants and to view each situation in respect to the unique nuances that may be present.

MATERNAL TEMPERAMENT

Findings from this sample indicate that maternal temperament is not a developmental construct and offers support that it is an innate characteristic. There was no significant age group differences in the activity, rhythmicity, approach–withdrawal, and threshold to stimulus categories of temperament. The two groups of older women scored higher on adaptability (4.78, 5.26, 5.27, respectively, from youngest to oldest), lower on intensity (3.64, 3.23, 3.28), and more positively on mood quality (4.40, 4.72, 4.63) than the teenagers.

The two older groups' higher scores on the temperament trait of adaptability indicate that their responses to new or different situations are more easily modified; this is an asset in any role transition but particularly so for the transition to motherhood. The lower intensity scores of groups 2 and 3 indicate that they have a lower energy level of response to situations than Group 1. The higher scores on mood quality of groups 2 and 3 indicate that they exhibit a greater amount of pleasant behavior than Group 1.

Group 2 scored higher (4.71) on persistence than the teenagers (4.34), but Group 3 (4.47) did not differ significantly from either. This indicates that Group 2 will continue an activity in the face of obstacles more so than Group 1, suggesting that Group 2 will keep going when the going gets tough more so than the teenagers. Group 3 scored higher in distractibility (4.42) than Group 2 (4.09), but Group 1 (4.29) did not differ significantly from either. This indicates that Group 3 will be more likely to allow environmental stimuli to affect their behavior than will Group 2, and thus, Group 3 is vulnerable to greater disturbance from changes in their environment as a result of the infant.

CHILD-REARING ATTITUDES

Early Perinatal Attitudes

Attitudes about preparation for pregnancy, birth, and mothering differed significantly by maternal age, which probably indicates a different level of readiness for pregnancy as well as developmental differences in planning for the future. Over half of the teenage group (52%) *did not* attend any prenatal classes, compared with 23% of the 20- to 29-year-olds and 8% of the older group. The older career woman may be more oriented to preparing for roles trhough classes and study. The teenagers less often had someone to attend classes with them, and that also may have affected their attendance; 48% reported that no one attended the classes with them, contrasted with 22% of Group 2 and 8% of Group 3. Only 29% of the teenagers reported that baby's father attended classes with them, compared with 67% of Group 2 and 81% of Group 3.

Prenatal classes that offer content to help prepare a woman for labor and delivery and early child care may be too threatening for the younger woman. The teenager also may fail to see a need to attend prenatal classes if she feels comfortable caring for children. Teenagers reported more previous experience than the older women in caring for infants. Only 8% of Group 1 reported no previous experience, whereas 20% of Group 2 and 26% of Group 3 reported no previous experience.

The older the woman, the more likely she chose to breast-feed her infant; 62% of the teenagers, 72% of Group 2, and 93% of the older group elected to breast-feed. From younger to older groups, the respective percentages of breast-feeding at 1 month were 34%, 76%, and 91%; at 4 months 21%, 56%, and 74%; at 8 months 16%, 36%, and 58%; and at 1 year 5%, 23%, and 28%.

Attitudes About the Parenting Role

Attitudes pertinent to the parenting role were measured in four areas—role reversal, low boiling point, strict disciplinarian, and sadistic (Disbrow, Doerr, & Caulfield, March 1977, 1977). Role reversal attitudes focus on whether parents use their infants to meet their own needs and perceive their infant's negative behavior as a deliberate attempt to hurt them. Boiling point or emotional lability attitudes focus on parents' levels of stress and their ability to cope with their stresses. Strict disciplinarian attitudes focus on parents' beliefs in and use of physical punishment with greater concern for supervising the child than on caring for her. Sadistic attitudes focus on whether parents use cruel and unusual forms of punishment or carefully plan retaliative actions to fit the child's crime.

One Month Postpartum At 1 month postpartum, Group 2 scored significantly more adaptive on role reversal than the teenage group; the Group 3 score fell between those two groups without differing significantly from either. However, the reliability of this subscale was extremely low at 1 month, and this finding must be viewed cautiously. There were no significant group differences on low boiling point or sadistic attitudes, but the older the age group, the more favorable the disciplinarian attitudes. This suggests that with increased maternal maturity the ability to utilize methods of punishment other than physical may occur. This is also congruent with the finding that flexibility increased with maternal age.

Eight Months Postpartum At 8 months postpartum, both of the older groups of women were more adaptive in role reversal than the teenage group and did not differ significantly from each other; again the reliability of this subscale measure was so low that this finding must be viewed with caution. There were no group differences in low boiling point attitudes. However, at this time both of the older groups scored significantly more favorably on sadistic attitudes than the teenage group. Consistent with attitudes at 1 month, the older the age group, the more favorable the strict disciplinarian attitudes, supporting the theory that the older woman was consistently less likely to believe in physical punishment for her child.

Maternal Attitudes in Relation to the Growing Child at 1 Year

Several subscales of maternal attitudes and five major factors focusing on tasks confronting the mother during the first three years of the child's life were measured (Cohler et al., 1970; Johnson, 1976). Maternal attitudes subscales included adaptation, reciprocal exchange, directed activity, focalization on the mother, self-assertion, instructive activity, challenge to the mother, exploration, body image, early sex role differentiation, female sexuality, attitudes about childbirth, lie scale, anxiety, infant feeding, suffering, threatening impulses, acceptance of the child's impulses, naivete, infant sexuality, and maternal satisfaction. The five major factors included appropriate versus inappropriate control of child's aggressive impulses (believes that child's impulses may be directed into socially appropriate channels rather than inhibited); encouragement versus discouragement of reciprocity (acknowledges infant's ability to communicate and seek social interaction with the mother and to respond to the infant in doing so); appropriate versus inappropriate closeness with the child (attains gratification missing in her life through the infant or views the infant as a narcissistic extension of self); acceptance versus denial of emotional complexity in child care (acknowledges that motherhood is sometimes more work than pleasure and that mothers do not always know best); and feeling of competence versus lack of competence in perceiving and meeting the baby's needs (understands what the infant wants and provides these needs).

There were no age group differences on the initial adaptation to baby's needs, female sexuality, and childbirth attitudes' subscales or for the factors of appropriate versus inappropriate closeness and competence or comfort versus incompetence in perceiving and meeting the infant's physical needs.

The older the age group, the more favorable or adaptable were their maternal attitudes on the subscales of early directed infant activity, sex-role differentiation, and conventional naivete toward child rearing. The teenage group scored significantly less adaptable than the two older groups, who did not differ significantly from each other, on reciprocal exchange and interaction with infant, infant's focalization on mother, self-assertion/negativism, destructiveness and initiative, challenge to the mother, encouragement of widening reciprocal interchange, consolidation of body image, maternal anxiety, comfort in the feeding situation, maternal control of threatening impulses, and sensitivity to infant sexuality.

Group 2 had significantly more positive attitudes on the maternal satisfaction subscale than Group 3. This finding is in agreement with those of other researchers who reported less gratification among more highly educated mothers (Russell, 1974; Steffensmeier, 1982), and with the findings in this study at 1 year when Group 2 reported significantly greater gratification in the mothering role than did Group 3 (see Chapter 8). The teenage group scored in between the other two groups for both the maternal satisfaction subscale and gratification at 1 year, without differing significantly from either.

Group 3 women were significantly more adaptable in their attitudes of acceptance of the child's impulses than the two younger groups of women. Their greater personality integration and flexibility were probably contributing factors here. This is also congruent with their attitudes toward using less physical punishment.

The older the age group, the more adaptive the women were for the factors of appropriate control of the child's impulses, encouragement of reciprocity, and acceptance of the emotional complexity of child rearing. The teenager may feel too vulnerable to admit that motherhood is sometimes more work than pleasure and that their decisions may not always be the best.

SUMMARY OF MOTHERS' BACKGROUNDS AND CHARACTERISTICS

The older the woman, the higher the level of her development, as indicated by a higher level of personality integration and greater flexibility. With increased age, temperament traits of adaptability and positive mood quality were higher, and many child-rearing and parenting attitudes were more positive. Older women also had social advantages of a higher education, higher income, and greater likelihood of being married. In addition to developmental, maturational, and social disadvantages, teenage mothers in this study experienced greater stress from negative life events during the first year of motherhood.

Although motherhood seemed to enhance self-concepts in one-third of the women, the majority experienced a decrease in self-concept by 8 months following birth. This decrease in self-concept is in opposition to the notion that motherhood is developmental; however, 8 months may be too early for many potential developmental changes to have occurred, especially since the possibility exists for these changes to occur through her child's adolescence. Comments made by the women suggest that cultural values place greater priority on roles outside the home, but the mothering role isolates them from outside resources. There may be societal messages to have a child, but once the child is born, there is a lack of social support to help with the mothering role.

IMPLICATIONS FOR NURSING CARE

Any transition is a period of change and disequilibrium for the individual; transition to the maternal role presents dramatic change from the nonmother state. Interventions for individuals experiencing any transition need to take into consideration prior experience of the individual, the way the transition is viewed by the individual's social network, and what learning opportunities are available (Silverman, 1982). Role models, legitimation of feelings, help in the form of resources and information, and the availability of a peer who has had a similar experience facilitates the transition process (Silverman, 1982).

Many different levels of resources are helpful in the transition to the maternal role. Help from family, friends, and neighbors, voluntary and community support groups, and health professionals are all important for new mothers, and each provides a different kind of resource. However, the assumption cannot be made, when a large number of persons are available to help, that the kind of help that is needed is available or that the help does not also represent conflict. For example, Smith (1983) reported that families incorporating a teenage mother and her infant into the household exhibit a range of patterns of responses—role sharing, role blocking, and role binding. In role blocking the teenage mother does not assume the role either because she relinquishes it or another family member takes it over; family dynamics then prevent the daughter from growing into the maternal role or gaining competence in child rearing. In role binding, the family delegates total responsibility to the teenage mother, severely restricting the teenager's options. Role-binding families were characterized by poor parental health, emotional unavailability of the grandmother, unclear generational boundaries due to alcoholism or other problems, and one-parent households. In role-sharing families the family functions as a unit to meet the infant's needs as well as the needs of other family members. Although the teenage mother gains adult status by bearing a child, she does not gain independence in all areas of her life but must abide by parental requests. Depending on the type of family pattern, the support that the adolescent is receiving and the nursing interventions are very different.

Barrera (1981) also noted that the teenagers' greatest source of help was often their greatest source of conflict. Teenagers had not reached the developmental level of the two older groups of women; thus, they are handicapped by fewer internal and fewer external resources. Crawford (1985) argued that persons who do not have many relationships in which they give as well as receive support may lack the opportunity to let others know the kind of help that is needed, thereby resulting in incongruent support and conflict.

Postpartum depression has been linked with less emotional and instrumental support from mates, less emotional support from confidants and mothers, and less ability to *give* instrumental support to mates, confidants, and mothers (O'Hara, Rehm, & Campbell, 1983). Depressed women also reported greater conflict with their mates. Conflict in the support system contributes to anxiety, depression, and increased somatic symptoms (Barrera, 1981; Crawford, 1985).

The majority of all groups of women experienced a decrease in positive feelings of self-regard at 8 months postpartum, indicating that their needs were not met in making the transition to the maternal role. The social support network may not have provided the kind of appraisal and reassurance of their efforts in their new role that was badly needed. There may not have been sufficient role models or adequate opportunity for legitimation of their feelings.

Support groups have been particularly helpful in providing role models, legitimation of feelings, and valuable information for new mothers (Cronenwett, 1980; Wandersman, 1978). Support groups for new mothers offer practical help from other women with hints that have worked for them, as well as an opportunity for them to see that the problems they are facing are not unique to them. Many types of support groups may be available within the community; therefore, it is important for the nurse to be aware of these resources and have printed lists available for parents to use for later reference. Explanation of the different kinds of support is also important. For example, some groups may meet with mates and infants; others may meet with mothers only. The time and frequency of meetings are also important for busy new mothers.

The teenage mother needs additional support that will enable her to continue her own growth and development as well as that of her infant. When parent training was provided for 80 low-income black teenage mothers the first 6 months following birth, the growth and development of their infants was superior to infants whose mothers had not received training (Field, Widmayer, Greenberg, & Stoller, 1982). Two programs of training were tested; half were visited bi-weekly in their homes and taught care giving and sensorimotor and interaction exercises, and half were trained as paid teacher's aides in a nursery that provided care for their infants and infants of medical faculty. Infants of teenagers in the paid teacher aide program were somewhat ahead of those trained in the home; repeat pregnancy rates were lower and return to either work or school was higher for mothers in the paid programs.

Teenagers may need help in identifying their goals and resources and in assessing their living situation. Referral to the social worker is very important if one is available in the setting. If none is available, it is important to be aware of possible residences, foster homes, or other resources to provide the kind of home environment conducive to growth and devlopment. A teenager in a characteristic family structure for role binding will need help in getting into an environment in which she can develop and learn to become independent. One group of researchers found that teenage mothers of high-risk infants were not using available resources because they did not know about available resources or how to identify them, did not know how to use existing resources, lacked trust in social service providers, or had no access to the services (Levinson, Hale, Tirado, & Hollier, 1979). Porter (1984) reported a parenting enhancement program (PEP) model for teenage parents, based on a philosophic framework of belief in human potential, respect for human dignity, recognizing potential of individual decision making, and enhanced opportunity for self-direction. The PEP has three phases—prenatal, natal, and postnatal.

Fewer teenagers elected to breast-feed. This may have been because they had inaccurate knowledge about possible deleterious effects of breast-feeding (Berger & Winter, 1980). Information about breast-feeding may be incorporated in school health programs or presented to pregnant adolescent groups.

Long-term follow-up is warranted because the health care system may be a major provider of social support in some very impoverished situations. The present-oriented teenager learns relevant information for the practical application at the time. Older women also need the long-term follow-up as indicated by the decrease in self-concept at 8 months.

CHAPTER 3

The Pregnancy, Birth, and Early Events Following Birth

Following a theoretical overview of pregnancy and childbirth, this chapter focuses on the mothers' descriptions of the pregnancy, their birth experiences, how they felt their birth experiences compared to their mothers', their feelings since birth, and their thoughts on what motherhood would be like. Alice, Alison, Amy, and Alma from Group 1; Betty, Barbara, Bea, and Bonnie from Group 2; and Carrie, Cynthia, Cathryn, and Carmen from Group 3 are introduced in this chapter. Vignettes of their experiences will be used to illustrate the mothers' feelings and responses and the areas for nursing intervention for this initial and subsequent interviews.

PSYCHODYNAMICS OF PREGNANCY

Pregnancy is the beginning of an important transition period during which the woman experiences many physiological and emotional changes. This 9-month period allows for the woman's restructuring of her life and adaptation on several levels: Her body adapts to physiological demands of the fetus; she adapts to the idea of being a mother, or a mother of two, three, or more children; and she begins the necessary adaptation to incorporate another person into her family and social sphere. Physical changes occur slowly as the increasing weight of the fetus and its support system necessitate gradual adaptation in posture and movement. Many cognitive and emotional changes also occur, slowly during pregnancy and continuing after the infant's birth, as the woman makes the transition from non-mother to mother or from mother of one or more to mother of two or more children.

Although a woman may be ambivalent initially about whether this is the "right time" for the pregnancy, she gradually resolves this cognitive dissonance and becomes excited about the coming child. The experience of fetal movement usually dispels doubts about readiness or desire for a child at this particular period of her life. Fetal movement (quickening) is the first positive sign or glimpse of reality to reaffirm any doubt that she is indeed carrying a child, unless she has had a sonogram in which she saw the fetus. Prior to the experience of fetal movement, the absence of an event (menstruation) is the major symptom indicating that she is pregnant.

Change in Cognitive Functioning

As pregnancy progresses, the woman who is pregnant for the first time becomes increasingly preoccupied with herself and the growing fetus. Multigravidas do not focus so much on self and continue to focus on environmental events more so than primigravidas (Grossman et al., 1980). Although there may be a decrease in a pregnant woman's social activity and in the range of persons she usually interacts with, her mental state is increasingly active. Particularly critical are changes in the woman's cognitive functioning that seem to facilitate her adaptation to the pregnancy and changes in her life to incorporate a child. A disequilibrium between the ego and id occurs so that the usually repressed instinctual wishes, fantasies, and urges of the unconscious (id) are allowed to surface by the ego (conscious self that mediates with the real world) into consciousness (Caplan, 1959). Unconscious material emerges during pregnancy with less anxiety than is experienced when the same material surfaces during nonpregnant periods.

The pregnant woman is well aware that her fantasies are fantasies. She may experience fantasies in either daydreams or night dreams (Sherwen, 1981). The unconscious work of dreams may have some beneficial effects for labor. Winget and Kapp (1972) found that the presence of anxiety and threat in dreams was associated with a shorter labor; they suggested that dreams may be an adaptive mechanism for coping with an impending normal crisis. Dreams during pregnancy do not appear to be linked to adaptive responses following birth, however. Gillman (1968) failed to find a significant correlation between dream content during pregnancy and maternal adaptation.

Many emerging fantasies during pregnancy are thought to represent earlier childhood conflicts (Caplan, 1959; Deutsch, 1945); therefore, there is potential for growth because superior solutions for dealing with these conflicts may be found. The Colmans (1973/74) referred to pregnancy as "the epitome of positive growth experience" (p. 7).

The phenomenon of change in the woman's intrapsychic (mental) work during pregnancy is referred to by different terms. The Colmans (1973/74) described the pregnant woman's alternate style of experiencing her conscious world as an "altered state of consciousness." They viewed pregnancy as removing the pregnant woman's illusion of separateness and as reminding her of her interconnectedness with others. Rubin (1970) referred to this changing intrapsychic state as the "cognitive style of pregnancy." Winnicott (1958) saw the introspective "primary maternal preoccupation" as prerequisite to later contingent maternal-child behavior, just as Caplan (1959) suggested that the disequilibrium permitted a reorganization to include a new individual in the woman's life. Winnicott noted that in the woman's state of heightened sensitivity she becomes preoccupied with her infant to the exclusion of all other interests and thus becomes sensitized to her infant's uniqueness. This special sensitization enables her to respond to subtle infant cues and to meet her infant's needs. Leifer (1977) observed this total preoccupation with the infant to continue throughout the first 2 months following birth.

Maternal Tasks of Pregnancy

Accomplishment of identified maternal tasks of pregnancy appears to facilitate both the postpartum mother-child relationship and the woman's maturation. Bibring and associates (1961) first described and the Colmans (1973) later verified three major intrapsychic tasks, all centering around the woman's relationships with her child, her husband, and her mother. The first task of pregnancy is to accept the fetus as part of her self-image as she matures both personally and in her relationship with her mate. This initial acceptance by a woman may provide the initial attachment to a particular child. A second task occurs after fetal movement in which the woman differentiates the fetus as an individual and prepares for the physical separation at delivery and for establishing a relationship with the infant after birth. Sonography now allows the woman to visualize the fetus, and amniocentesis reveals the infant's gender, possibly enhancing this process (Kohn, Nelson, & Weiner, 1980; Milne & Rich, 1981).

The third task is for the woman to move from a child-mother relationship to a peer relationship with her mother. When childhood conflicts of remorse, guilt, ambivalence, and resentment toward the mother are resolved, an adult-adult relationship is then possible. Ballou (1978) observed that women who resolved dependency conflicts in relationship to their mothers could allow themselves to be dependent on their mothers during pregnancy and childbirth. Acceptance of the infant's dependency was also possible. The husband appears to play a large role in the woman's reconciliative process with her mother through providing the psychological context (Ballou, 1978). The husband functions both as a maternal figure (the oedipal father) who appreciates his wife's sexuality while protecting her from her mother.

The interplay between daughter and mother during the daughter's pregnancy is thought to foster both reconciliation with and separation from her mother. Girls fail to differentiate from their mothers as boys do during the oedipal stage, and according to Chodorow (1978), this boundary diffuseness continues throughout a woman's life. Lebe (1982) argued that the period between the ages of 30 and 40 years may be the normal time developmentally for women to complete the individuation from their mothers. If this is true, in a study of women aged 15 to 42 years, those women who are 30 years and older would have greater developmental advantage in separating from and moving to peer relationships with their mothers.

The grandmother's availability, acceptance of her daughter's pregnancy, respect for her daughter's autonomy, and willingness to reminisce with the daughter about her own childbearing experiences play an important role in the daughter's transition to motherhood (Lederman, 1984). These findings substantiate Ballou's belief that in some cases, the milieu provided by the husband plays an important role in the resolution of mother-daughter conflicts. Some grandmothers, particularly if the daughter is very young, may refuse to recognize her autonomy or to accept and be pleased about her pregnancy.

Deutsch (1945) stressed the importance of the pregnant woman finding synchrony with her future-directed identification with her child and her past-directed identification with her own mother. Deutsch argued that the woman's failure to identify with her fetus may result in rejection, and her refusal to identify with her mother may weaken her capacity for mothering.

In addition to the woman's relationship with her mother influencing the identification with the motherhood role, Lederman (1984) reported that a poor marital relationship was associated with earlier admission to the labor unit, receiving sedatives and tranquilizers during early labor, and prolonged labor. Other dimensions of maternal development in psychosocial adaptation during pregnancy identified by Lederman included acceptance of the pregnancy, identification with a motherhood role, preparation for labor, dealing with prenatal fear of loss of control in labor, and dealing with prenatal fear of loss of self-esteem in labor.

Rubin (1975, 1984) described four maternal tasks during pregnancy: seeking safe passage for self and for child during pregnancy, labor, and delivery; ensuring that the child is accepted by significant persons in her social world; binding-in (attaching) to the child; and learning to give of herself. These tasks reflect a sense of commitment to self and child through assuring a healthy child as well as assuring a nurturing environment for the child. Josten (1981) operationalized these tasks with public health nurses who then scored women's work toward the accomplishment of tasks during pregnancy. The nurses were able to predict from the pregnancy behaviors, with 87% accuracy, whether the woman would be an excellent or an inadequate mother. Rees (1980) also developed measures of feelings of motherliness, conception of the fetus as a person, and appropriateness of fantasies about the baby-to-be during pregnancy for predicting postpartum adaptation. Her measures reflect congruence with the notion of the interdependence of maternal identity and attainment of the maternal role.

Father's Responses to Pregnancy and His Role

Ballou's (1978) observations also offer some explanation for the positive impact of the woman's relationship to her mate on later mothering that has been observed repeatedly. The husband's roles of confidence building and sustaining the woman were strongly related to maternal functioning, and the husband–wife relationship was significantly related to maternal adaptation during pregnancy and through 6 months postpartum (Shereshefsky et al., 1973).

The husband's anxiety level during pregnancy and his satisfaction with the marriage were significantly related to the woman's psychological health and the quality of her interactions with her infant at 2 months postpartum (Grossman et al., 1980). These husband traits were also the strongest predictors of the woman's adaptation during labor and delivery. At 1 year, the infant's mental development was higher when the father was more sexually active and satisfied, enjoyed his marriage more, was better adapted in his own life, and had less anxiety during early and late pregnancy. Thus, the infant's cognitive and social functioning was strongly predicted by the psychological health and marital satisfaction of the parents during pregnancy.

The woman's prenatal perception of the father's involvement during pregnancy was positively related to her involvement and responsiveness to the child during the first 4 years of life (Barnard, 1981). Unfortunately, men either may not have been socialized to be actively involved with pregnancy or may be unready for pregnancy and such involvement.

The ability of the man to support the woman during pregnancy is highly variable. Some fathers experience conflicts with their parents similar to those women experience with their mothers (Ballou, 1978). Over half of the fathers that Ballou observed during pregnancy experienced disequilibrium to some extent. Three styles of detachment/involvement were exhibited by husbands during pregnancy—observer, expressive, and instrumental (May, 1980). The observer-style husband maintained an emotional distance from the pregnancy and viewed himself as a bystander. The expressive-style father saw himself as a full partner and was very emotionally involved in the pregnancy. The instrumental-style husband focused on the physical tasks and served as caretaker or manager. The instrumentalist downplayed any emotional impact but enjoyed fulfilling the traditional roles of fatherhood. The range of husband involvement in a pregnancy may also relate to the man's ability to fulfill the maternal or parental functions in his wife's reconciliation process with her mother.

LABOR AND DELIVERY

Unlike the 9-month pregnancy period, which offers gradual adjustment to events, labor occurs unannounced at unexpected and undesirable times. Within a few hours birth may occur so that many events have to be assimilated within a very short period of time. A long-held belief that the shorter the labor, the easier it would be viewed by the woman was disproved in this study; the rapid, precipitous labors (3 hr or shorter) failed to allow the women time to adjust to what was happening and to get in control of the very hard and frequent uterine contractions.

Social support is strongly linked to satisfaction with labor and delivery by many researchers. Labors were shorter, women were more alert, and they smiled and talked to their infants more when a lay female support person was with them during their labors (Sosa et al., 1980). Westbrook (1978) observed that women with positive marital relationships had fewer negative attitudes, had fewer problems in labor, and expressed little rejection of the infant. Women who had negative marital relationships were hostile and defensive and expressed rejection of their child. A positive relationship with the husband and preparation for delivery were linked to a shorter labor (Lederman et al., 1979). Grossman and associates (1980) found that the husband's satisfaction with the marriage and maternal anxiety during pregnancy were the strongest predictors of adaptation during labor and delivery. Entwisle and Doering (1981) determined that husband participation, the woman's preparation level, worst pain during the first stage of labor, and the level of awareness predicted 52% of the woman's satisfaction with the birth experience.

A sense of mastery and control in the situation are also related to satisfaction with the childbirth experience (Humenick & Bugen, 1981; Marut & Mercer, 1979). If a woman is able to maintain a sense of herself as the person having the infant and has high social suppports, she has more of a sense of being a victor as opposed to being a victim (Oakley, 1980).

With increased numbers of women limiting childbearing experiences to one or two children, effort toward increasing the quality and meaning of the experience has increased. Closely related to the meaning of the childbirth experience, or to how much a woman can enjoy the experience, is the extent of the pain that she experiences; a high negative correlation ($\underline{r}$ = -.57) was observed between pain and enjoyment of childbirth in a sample of 249 women (Norr, Block, Charles, Meyering, & Meyers, 1977). Variables that were associated with the women's enjoyment in childbirth were less pain, Lamaze preparation, husband's help, feeling better during pregnancy, marital closeness, use of pain control techniques, higher socioeconomic status (SES), and absence of more than local anesthesia in delivery. Variables associated with greater pain included low self-concept, less marital closeness, feeling less well during pregnancy, higher pregnancy complaints, increased worry about childbirth, lack of Lamaze preparation, longer labor, less help from husband and staff, failure to use techniques to control pain, analgesia in labor, and anesthesia in delivery. Women with higher SES, less traditional attitudes toward sex roles, and greater marital closeness were more likely to prepare for childbirth and have less pain, more enjoyment, and help from their husbands during labor and delivery. However, others reported no differences in self-esteem or feelings about the childbirth experience between women who attended childbirth classes and those who did not (Slavazza et al., 1985).

Pain is a subjective experience, and an individual's threshold to pain may be lowered by fatigue, isolation, disorientation, or loss of control. The cultural context defines socially acceptable ways of expressing pain, so that laboring women may express pain in quite different ways. Racial and age differences in pain tolerance were reported: Pain tolerance decreased with age; whites tolerated more pain than Asians; and blacks' pain tolerance scores were between those of whites and Asians (Woodrow, Friedman, Siegelaub, & Collen, 1972). Melzack, Kinch, Dobkin, Lebrun, and Taenzer (1984) observed that older women reported less pain in labor; prepared childbirth training, absence of menstrual difficulties, and lower prepregnancy weight per unit of height were associated with lower pain scores. Pain increased over the course of labor.

Many physiological factors contribute to pain during labor. During strong uterine contractions, some hypoxia to the myometrium contributes to the pain; contractions usually are stronger, may come more frequently, and may last longer as labor progresses. A major source of pain during the first stage of labor results from the stretching of the cervix and lower uterine segment (Bonica, 1960). Pain during the second stage of labor is produced by the distention of the birth canal, vulva, and perineum and is transmitted by sensory output that are part of the pudendal nerves (Bonica, 1960).

The experience of increased pain as labor progresses contributes to increased anxiety. Increased anxiety contributes to increased secretion of catecholamines, which may have harmful effects on mother and fetus (Levinson & Shnider, 1979). Anxiety and plasma epinephrine during labor were significantly correlated with fetal heart rate pattern, and the fetal heart rate pattern was significantly correlated with Apgar scores at 1 and 5 min (Lederman, Lederman, Work, & McCann, 1981). Coping mechanisms and adaptation during labor include a withdrawal from social interactions with others as labor progresses and a constriction of the ego such that only immediate survival is dealt with (Rich, 1973).

Following birth the woman gradually expands her social sphere and may begin by a review of her birth experience with someone who can fill in the missing pieces of information (Affonso, 1977). She tends to view her childbirth experience more positively with the passage of time (Slavazza et al., 1985).

THE WOMEN'S EXPERIENCES DURING PREGNANCY

Although a criterion for the study was that this was their first live birth, 45% of the women had experienced pregnancy before (30% of Group 1, 45% of Group 2, and 53% of Group 3). The older women in Group 3 with more earlier pregnancies tended to have had more therapeutic and spontaneous abortions; two reported having had a stillbirth. Over one-fourth (27%) of the women had experienced one therapeutic abortion (18%, 29%, and 30%);[1] 14 (6%) from groups 2 and 3 had experienced two or more. Spontaneous abortions were reported by 15% of the women (9%, 12%, and 17%); group differences were significant. The abortion rate was higher for these women than in a comparison group from Calgary, Alberta (Mercer & Stainton, 1984).

Teenagers' pregnancies were 3 to 4 days shorter than those of the older women; differences were significant between Group 1 and Group 2 (39.7 weeks compared to 40.3 weeks). Group 3 women did not differ significantly from either of the two younger groups in length of pregnancy (40.1 weeks). Others have reported shorter pregnancies among teenagers with infant birth weights similar to that of older women (Horon, Strobino, & MacDonald, 1983).

The women rated their overall feelings about their current pregnancy from 1 (very bad) to 5 (very good). Group differences were significant; 75% of Group 1 rated their feelings about the pregnancy as good or very good, compared with 87% of Group 2 and 90% of Group 3. Group differences were not significant in feeling surprised at discovering that they were pregnant. However, the older the woman, the more often she had hoped that she was pregnant, felt proud versus ashamed, was less worried, and felt that the pregnancy was just as welcome as planned and at a good time.

---

[1] Series of three figures in parentheses indicates percentages for the three groups from the youngest to the oldest, respectively.

The most frequently reported time for first feeling fetal movement was 4 months, with a range of from 2 to 8 months. The great majority (84%) of the women reported that they were excited with fetal movement; 13% stated that fetal movements made them realize that a baby was really there. Only 2% of the women reported no change in their feelings at the time of fetal movement. There were no group differences in these feelings.

Teenagers reported that they thought about having a boy significantly more often than did the older women (58% compared with 29% and 28%). Interestingly, they were more likely to have a boy (62% compared with 39% and 54%). Thirty-nine percent of the total reported thinking about having either a boy or a girl equally (20% of Group 1, 43% of Group 2, and 46% of Group 3). The majority (82%) reported that they had picked out a name for their child during pregnancy.

When the women were asked what their pregnancy had been like, the overall response ranged from terrible (13%); worried and stressful (11%); OK (27%); easy (24%); good, happy, excited, or ideal (19%); other (6%). The older the woman, the more positively she had viewed pregnancy. The teenager had had less time to assimilate body image changes from pubertal growth before having to incorporate the changes occurring with pregnancy and may have been overwhelmed in dealing with pregnancy body image changes. Also, the older the woman, the more deliberate had been her planning for the pregnancy, which probably influenced her feelings about the experience.

However, there were no age group differences in the types of anxieties or concerns during pregnancy; 59% expressed body image concerns, and 41% described feelings of vulnerability. The most frequently mentioned body image concern had to do with feelings during the last 2 to 6 weeks of pregnancy, which were described as feeling miserable and a slowed pace in activities (23%). Seventeen percent voiced multiple kinds of body image and body function concerns; 10% were concerned about their hugeness or awkwardness, 5% noted that they had stayed small, and 2% felt they were ugly or fat. Feelings of vulnerability came from fear of illness or of harm to self (12%), fear of fetal abnormality (10%), previous stillbirth or miscarriage (4%), death of a loved one (1%), and a variety of other responses (14%). These were all spontaneous comments in response to "What was your pregnancy like?" and some women may have experienced these concerns but failed to comment on them.

There were no significant group differences in the number of physical symptoms reported during pregnancy. Three-fourths of the teenagers did not report a physical symptom, compared with 58% of the 20- to 29-year-olds and 71% of the 30-and-older group. Physical symptoms spontaneously reported (no checklist was given nor were symptoms solicited) were heartburn, 2%; morning sickness, 25%; edema, 6%; fatigue, 11%; backache, 5%; difficulty sleeping, 3%; and hemorrhoids, 2%.

Teenagers (Group 1) were significantly less likely to describe emotional symptoms during pregnancy (50%, compared with 55% of Group 2 and 75% of Group 3). Over one fourth (29%) of all women said they were depressed during pregnancy; the older the woman, the more often she reported that she was depressed (17% of Group 1, 29% of Group 2, and 40% of Group 3). Nineteen percent described mood swings, and 17% said they were happier or more serene during pregnancy. Group 3 women more often described their emotional state as serene (3%, 2%, and 18%). Ten percent enjoyed the attention they received during their pregnancy.

There were no significant group differences in the complications spontaneously mentioned: overall 31% spoke of a complication. However, their medical records indicated that 40% had experienced a problem during pregnancy (47% of Group 1, 41% of Group 2, and 35% of Group 3). Younger women less often talked about pregnancy complications when describing their overall pregnancy. Nine percent of all of the women reported premature labor with this pregnancy (5% of Group 1, 9% of Group 2, and 10% of Group 3), and 4% reported a threatened abortion. Seven percent reported pre-eclampsia (6%, 10%, and 3%). Nineteen of the women (6%) reported they had been hospitalized for a complication of pregnancy (6% of Group 1, 7% of Group 2, and 6% of Group 3). Four percent of the women reported a chronic illness (4% of Group 2 and 6% of Group 3).

THE BIRTH EXPERIENCE

The younger the woman, the more likely that she had a spontaneous vaginal delivery. Teenagers also tended to have their infants earlier in the day than the older women. The average time for the teenage births was 10:00 a.m., compared with 12:25 p.m. for Group 3 and 12:40 p.m. for Group 2. Three-fourths of the teenagers' labors began spontaneously, compared with 59% and 60% of the two older groups. The majority (80%) of the teenagers delivered spontaneously, compared with 58% of Group 2 and 41% of Group 3 (Mercer et al., 1983). Similarly, the older the woman, the more likely she had a cesarean birth (6%, 18%, and 31%). There were no significant group differences in complications experienced during labor and delivery. Although differences were not significant, 44% of the teenagers experienced a laceration with the episiotomy, compared with 30% and 32% of groups 2 and 3.

There were no significant differences in the total length of the labor as recorded on the medical records among the groups (13.1, 13.5, and 13.3 hr). By stage, there were no significant differences in the length of the first stage (11.0, 12.0, and 11.8 hr). The teenagers who had the greater number of spontaneous births also had a shorter second stage of labor (49 min, compared with 75 and 79 min). However, the teenagers' third stage of labor was significantly longer (an average of 8.7 min compared with 6.3 and 5.4 min).

The Women's Descriptions of Their Birth Experiences

When asked what their labor and delivery experience had been like, 7% described it in highly negative terms such as horrible, hell, shattering, horrendous, anguish, terrible, and close to death. The older woman more often described the labor as long or not normal (26%, 46%, and 45%). Fifteen percent noted that they had been scared, freaked out, worried, or anxious (24%, 10%, 16%). Twelve percent described the overall experience in terms of fatigue—tired, exhausted, exasperated, and weak. Two-thirds mentioned the pain as intense, hard, rough, or particularly bothersome (71%, 66%, and 61%). Forty-one percent used some positive terms in describing the experience such as a good experience, incredible, easy, hard to believe, quick, exciting, super, beautiful, or great. Women often used more than one category in describing their overall experience, such as horrible and long or long and fatiguing.

The women were then asked whether they would do everything the same way or whether they would make a change for their next delivery if given a choice. Nine of the 20 (45%) who described their labors as horrible said that they would not change a thing. Forty-five of the 120 (38%) who noted that their labors were too long said they would not change a thing. Eighteen of 44 (41%) who said they were scared stated that they would not change a thing. Eleven of 35 (31%) who spoke of extreme fatigue stated they would not change a thing. Ninety-one of the 191 (48%) who described their labor in posi-

tive terms would not change anything in a future labor. There seemed to be a reluctance to tempt fate if a live, normal child was the
outcome and the mother survived. However, those who viewed the
experience more positively were even less likely to state a desire to
change anything in a future labor.

Comer and Laird (1975) reported that people who chose to "suffer" after expecting to suffer and were then given an option not to
either changed their view of themselves or of the situation during
the waiting period. Some people seemed to make the choice to suffer
because they came to see themselves as heroic figures who would
endure discomfort willingly for the good of science. Others believed
they deserved the suffering. The third group decided if they were
going to endure it that it could not really be that bad after all. The
expression made by so many women on studying their babies during
early days following birth—"When I see her/him, it was worth all of
the pain and suffering"—suggest a willingness to endure pain for the
good received. Taylor (1983) proposed a theory of cognitive adaptation to threatening events that also may explain a woman's commitment to not change anything about a negative birth experience
if given the choice next time. The theory states that when individuals experience a threatening event they respond with adaptive efforts
that allow them to return to or exceed their earlier level of psychological functioning. They search for meaning, which includes finding
a casual explanation. Mastery of the event is maintained by attempts
at gaining control over the event. Finally, a degree of self-enhancement occurs through finding personal gain from the event and making comparisons of behavior with those who did not do so well in a
comparable event. Taylor maintains that these cognitive restructur-
ings are based largely on illusions that protect the individual and lead
to constructive thought and action. A woman who has mastered a
painful, horrible childbirth experience sees herself as even stronger
in such future events, especially if her behavior surpassed others in
her family or her circle of friends. A 20-year-old stated at 1 year following birth, "I feel power in being able to reproduce. It put me in
touch with some sort of basic values. I faced an extreme situation in
labor and I survived it. Labor was very hard; it was like facing death—
the pain was that bad." This woman's comments reflect self-enhancement as a result of giving birth.

For women who said they would want a future childbirth experience to be different, 6% desired less pain, 6% would take childbirth
classes, 5% desired a shorter labor, 3% would opt for natural child-

birth or the alternative birth center, 3% would take anesthesia or medication, 3% would prefer a vaginal delivery to a cesarean birth, and 1% preferred a cesarean birth rather than a vaginal birth.

The Women's Overall Self-Ratings of the Childbirth Experience

The 20- to 29-year-old group had significantly more positive perceptions of the birth experience than the teenage group. The 30- to 42-year-old women's scores fell between the two groups and did not differ significantly from either group (Mercer et al., 1983). This is in contrast to the findings of Norr et al. (1977), who reported that the older the woman, the greater her enjoyment of the childbirth experience. In a Calgary sample of women aged 17 to 32 years, the younger the woman the more positively she tended to perceive her birth experience (Mercer & Stainton, 1984). Almost one third of the women in the 30- to 42-year-old group had cesarean births, and that may have diminished the group's enthusiasm for or positive perceptions about the experience.

At 1 year post-birth, some comments reflected strong unresolved feelings about the birth experience. Comments by the group 30 years and older include the following:

- I never went through such unbearable pain. Was told in Lamaze that it would be like menstrual cramps. They lay a trip on you that it's not that bad. I was totally unprepared for what happened before, during, and after birth.
- I was disappointed I didn't have a vaginal delivery, but was glad it was over. Delivery was not satisfying, but something to get over. My mother had a vaginal birth.

Kutzner (1984) reported that 3 to 4 years following birth, some women described their experiences so vividly that it was hard to believe that they had not just occurred.

Comparisons of Birth Experience with Their Mothers'

At 1 year following birth, the women were asked to rate whether their labor and delivery was easier, harder, the same as, or not discussed with their mothers, and whether it was more satisfying, less satisfying, the same, or not discussed. There were no group differences in how the women compared the ease of their birth experience with their mothers' experience: 34% judged their experience as easier; 38% as harder, 14% as the same; and 14% had not discussed it.

There were significant group differences in whether the childbirth experience was judged as more satisfying. Teenagers more often reported that their experience was the same as their mothers' (38%, 23%, and 19%), less often reported the experience was more satisfying than their mother's (35%, 61%, and 51%), and more often reported their own experience was less satisfying than their mothers' (15%, 9%, 10%).

The teenager who had an easier birth in regard to medical intervention rated her childbirth experience the least positively compared with other groups. Developmental differences must be considered here because a stressful experience such as labor poses threats to body image and body function for all women. The more youthful woman may also have more difficulty in resolving the maternal task of moving to an adult relationship with her mother; consequently, the mother continues to be an awesome role model for her.

EARLY THOUGHTS ON WHAT MOTHERHOOD WOULD BE LIKE

Although one-fourth of the women stated they did not know whether they wanted another child, only one woman stated she did not. Twenty percent indicated they wanted one additional child; 34% wanted two additional children; 14% wanted three additional children; and 7% wanted four or more children.

The women were asked during their postpartum hospitalization what they thought it would be like as a mother. Overall, 22% of the women stated that they were looking forward to motherhood, saw it as satisfying, and had good feelings about it. However, only 9% of the teenagers made this response, compared with 25% of Group 2 and 28% of Group 3. Almost one fourth (23%) were unsure. Over one-fifth expected motherhood to be fun, exciting, or easy. Fewer (14%) presented realistic viewpoints incorporating both the positive and negative aspects of parenting as "difficult and rewarding," or "a lot of work but worth it." Almost one-fourth (23%)

were very cautious in their replies: "I think positively," "OK," "I hope it'll be nice." Seven percent admitted they were scared by the prospect of motherhood, felt insecure, and were concerned that they would do something wrong. Four percent held frankly negative views and made comments such as "I don't think I'll be a good mother."

In describing what they expected motherhood to be like, half of the women described goals that they had in mind for their mothering. The most frequently mentioned goal centered around how they planned to mother (30%); they mentioned their personal traits and specific behaviors such as patience and teaching ability. Nine percent mentioned goals for the infant; these often focused on the infant's development or later education. A few (3%) of the women had as a goal maintaining a balanced family with time for husband, self, and infant (0%, 2%, and 8%). Twelve percent spoke of their career goals at this time (2%, 11%, and 22%). Three percent mentioned goals for returning to school (8%, 2%, and 0%).

Thus, multiple roles—mother, career, student, and wife or mate roles—were being contemplated during the postpartum hospitalization. It was unrealistic to view motherhood in isolation or apart from the numerous other roles.

WORK TOWARD MATERNAL ROLE ATTAINMENT DURING POSTPARTUM HOSPITALIZATION

Early attachment to the infant begins during pregnancy; however, with the birth of the infant, the process becomes transactional—each individual's behavior affecting the other—through the visual modalities that were unavailable prior to birth. Physical touch becomes skin to skin rather than through an abdominal wall, and voice sounds are more direct.

The woman's emotional response to the cue "Tell me about your baby"; whether she referred to the baby as it, the baby, he/she, or by name; and her acquaintance behaviors of identifying her infant's uniqueness were recorded. Although the women did not differ by age group on the factor weighted by these three measures, there were group differences for acquaintance behaviors. The older the woman, the more she was likely to describe unique features of her infant— 31, 45, and 52%. Women in this study identified their infants similarly to the process described earlier by Rubin (1972) and Gottlieb (1978). The women focused largely on describing their infants' appearance (44%), unique responses (45%), how good or quiet the baby was (25%), the infant's gender (7%), and the infant's health or feeding problems (10%).

Eighty-five percent of the women were pleased or excited in their emotional responses when telling about their infants. Only two women, both in the oldest group, called their baby by name; 95% referred to their babies by either he or she. Gender identity was common during this early period; calling by name apparently comes later. Very few (4%) referred to the baby as "it" or "the baby."

Only 15.9% of the variance in the women's attachment behavior was predictable at early postpartum. Her educational level predicted 6.1%; the positive life events experienced the year prior to birth predicted 5.2%; negative life events predicted 2.6%, and racial status predicted 2%. Higher attachment was associated with a higher level of education, greater positive and negative life events, and being Caucasian. Positive life events the year prior to pregnancy included such events as marriage (41%), outstanding personal achievement (35%), pregnancy (93%), and new job (24%). These types of events provided social support and probably enhanced positive feelings about themselves. The fact that pregnancy was perceived as a positive life event indicates early positive feelings toward the infant. Negative life events such as an illness may have increased feelings of appreciation for a live, healthy infant.

The identified attachment behaviors apparently do not indicate attachment in non-Caucasian groups. Some cultures believe that excitement over identifying their infants' features invites the "evil eye." Change in use of type of pronouns from *it* to *he* or *she* (Cogan & Edmunds, 1980), to use of the infant's name may not indicate attachment. Because two-thirds of the teenage group were non-Caucasian, cultural differences may account for fewer acquaintance or identifying behaviors.

SELECTED WOMEN'S EXPERIENCES

Two married and two single women from each of the age groups were randomly selected to illustrate life-style changes in the transition to motherhood. Women whose names begin with an *A* are from

Group 1; those whose names begin with a *B* are from Group 2, and those from Group 3 have names beginning with a *C*. The first two from each group, Alma, Alison, Betty, Barbara, Carrie, and Cathryn indicated that they were unmarried at the first interview.

Alma

Alma, a 16-year-old Filipino still in high school, was all smiles and happy at the time of her postpartum interview. She noted that it was hard for her to believe that her son was "out of her," but that it was nice to have him around. When asked whether she wanted other children, she said she'd like to have one more—a girl. In her own words:

> Labor was hard, but delivery was easy [spontaneous]. It was all worth it. I had a hard time not pushing. My boyfriend was more tired than I was. I felt so relaxed after the birth. I was glad it was a baby boy. My boyfriend was so happy too. It's hard to believe that he came out of me. He weighed eight pounds.
>
> Both my mother and my mother's mother will help me when I go home; that's too much, but it's nice to know it's there. I think I can manage on my own, really.
>
> When I was pregnant, I felt like I needed someone closer to me all the time. I didn't like my boyfriend going out with his friends.
>
> I think it will be fun having kids around. It will be hard I know, but it will be worth it. I won't be able to do as much as I have been—going out. I'll be going back to school in January. People say you won't be able to go to parties or dances. I can do that when he's older. People feel you can't care for your baby if you're too young. If you love them, you can do it.

Alison

Alison, an 18-year-old single Caucasian high school graduate, was also feeling great during her postpartum interview. She described the time since her baby's birth as exciting. She described her labor and spontaneous delivery:

> The beginning was OK, but the last two hours were the worst. The head

wouldn't come out; it kept going back up. I couldn't believe when he was born what had happened. I couldn't believe it was mine.

My mother and father will help me when I go home. I feel like that will be enough.

My pregnancy was very emotional—the effect it had on me. I got upset at everything. It is going to be an experience being a mother.

Alice

Alice, a married, 19-year-old black woman with some college educa-tion who delivered her son with only three pushes was quite proud. After prodromal labor for a day and a night in the hospital, she went home and lounged around half a day. Her labor progressed rapidly when rehospitalized.

I dilated three centimeters in one hour; I had the willpower. At a later check I was five centimeters; then I asked the doctor to check me again. I said, 'I'm eight centimeters.' He said, 'How did you know?' I was so ex-cited. My husband was in the room with me all of the time; Mom came in and out. The next check was an anterior lip. I turned on my side, and it was gone. I pushed twice in the labor room and once in the delivery room, and had him.

He's cute, still has a pushed in face. The swelling doesn't bother me. His complexion is changing.

My mom and stepfather live with us. I'm not scared to say I don't know. My mom will do a lot at first; I have a lot of confidence in my mom.

I lost twenty to twenty-five pounds the first three months of pregnan-cy; I was in school. Some days I was pregnant, some days not; couldn't enjoy it. Got married at five months, then started to be pregnant. Had a lot of school problems that put a strain on pregnancy. I was at UC Davis and he worked at USF. The last month I was home, bored stiff. I wrote five letters a day.

I think I'll be a good mom. My baby will be spoiled. He's been wanted since I was twelve. I wanted a little girl, and my husband wanted a boy. It makes me feel good to give up something to accommodate him. I plan to go back to school in September.

Amy

Amy, an 18-year-old Filipino who is married and has a high school diploma, reported that it had been painful for her since the baby's birth. She said she had been in bed for two whole days. She noted that if she had it to do over, she'd not change a thing about her labor, but it was quite difficult.

Labor hurt. I was screaming. That's why my voice sounds like it does. Labor was hard. I kept pushing, but it wouldn't come out. When we was in the delivery room, they kept saying to push. They vacuumed it out [vacuum extraction]. They gave me a shot to numb the bottom.

I just now held him. When I first seen him, they let me hold him. I didn't want to hold him. He's so skinny—he looks so hopeless.

Nobody is going to help me when I go home. I hope I'll have enough help.

My pregnancy didn't feel good, especially around the eighth or ninth month. You can't do what you want to do. I wanted to have a lot of kids—six. But I won't—just this one [laughs].

As a mother you have a lot of worries. That's all—worries about your baby. Responsibility.

Betty

Betty, a 22-year-old single Caucasian with a high school education, had a spontaneous delivery. She was all smiles during the interview and described the time since the baby's birth as a tremendous experience. "Yesterday I had him circumcised, and I cried 'cause I love him so much and he is such a part of me." She felt that Lamaze classes were a lot of help during her labor:

You need a really strong coach; I had my girlfriend and my father. My water broke at four thirty p.m., and at eleven p.m. labor started. I had to walk for three hours. At three a.m., contractions were one minute apart and I was three centimeters dilated. I was going nuts—losing control. I had a shot of Nisentil, and I could rest between contractions. At five a.m. I was complete. I was in the delivery room only five minutes and pushed twice, and there he was. I compared it with having my wisdom teeth pulled. I felt the pressure and I didn't know they had been pulled. I missed the moment. I saw him when his head and shoulders were out. I wouldn't change a thing. Perfect! It could have been a lot worse. I just couldn't believe it.

He's precious. He's a good breast-feeder. He's quiet, hardly ever cries. He doesn't have any special characteristics yet. He stares at me when I hold him.

I'm staying with my mom for six weeks. I'll be fine. My mom is great.

I was disappointed with my pregnancy. At first I was really sick. I experienced it to the fullest. I didn't enjoy it because everyone was so worried because he was so small . . . They never could say that the baby was just a little baby. Dad was really upset too. He kept saying it would be all right and tried to help. No one else would reassure me.

I want at least three children. I want a little girl too. I have a feeling I'm going to like being a mother very much. I've always wanted to be a mother.

Barbara

Barbara, a single 26-year-old who has done some graduate study and works as a theater lighting designer, had a spontaneous delivery. She is continuing the relationship with the father of her infant who is black; she is Caucasian. She described the time since her baby's birth as wonderful. She described her experiences:

Labor was long—very long. It was smooth, but it was rough—transition and delivery. I had three support people—father of the baby, girl friend, and a labor coach. Someone was always with me. I had to push much harder than I expected. It was almost completely what I expected, except the first stage was much longer than I expected. It was incredible when she was born. I was surprised—felt "There's a baby inside of me!" I knew it all along, but suddenly she was there. I felt during pregnancy that she was a separate person. I see it already. If I had it to do over, I'd practice breathing techniques better and more often. I feel good about it though.

She is an incredibly responsive, healthy baby. I thought she was a boy in my pregnancy. I had only one dream that she was a girl. The rest were about boys.

My old man and two friends will help me out when I go home. I know I'll need help the first two weeks.

My pregnancy was wonderful. No problems, never sick, worked up till one month prior to delivery. I was large, couldn't sleep. Overall, it was an excellent pregnancy. I had a good diet, enough sleep. This is the only child I want.

I love children. I feel like a mother. It's exciting to raise a child; I'm a career woman. It's easier to integrate one child with a career rather than two.

Bea

Bea, a married 21-year-old Caucasian, delivered her son by low forceps. She had some college education. She rated her relationship with her husband as excellent. Her major concern since birth was anxiety about her son, who was undergoing tests to rule out infection (her membranes had been ruptured for 27 hr prior to birth). She described her childbirth experience:

It was hard and long. I got so much support from my family. My mother and husband were in the labor and delivery room. My mom wasn't sure she'd be able to stand the pain and blood. It was a really touching experience when he was born. We were all touching and hugging each other. It made James special. I had a hard time. I really was exhausted. They gave me Pitocin; I didn't want it. I was having contractions every three minutes, but they weren't strong enough. The Pitocin didn't work. I had to take something for an hour's rest. I was reassured that it would only make James sleepy for about half an hour. I felt OK that I wasn't taking any big pain killers. He was very alert when he was born—screaming and crying.

He really is a good baby—picked up on breast-feeding. I was amazed. One of my friends had a difficult time with breast-feeding. He's not fussy at all except when wet. He loves to be cuddled—lovable and cuddly.

My mother is going to help me when I go home. I'll have plenty of help.

My pregnancy was fine. The first three months were kind of hard. I had morning sickness. He is a ten-month baby. The last month was hard because he was overdue. The due date came and I was getting frustrated; I wanted him out.

I'd like two children—maybe. After the labor, I'm not sure that I want another one [laughs].

Motherhood will be enjoyable. I love my son already. I loved him in my belly, and I love him now. It'll be hard and sad and happy. I know that I gave my mother some trouble. I feel like I'm starting down a new path of life.

Bonnie

Bonnie, a 28-year-old married black woman with a baccalaureate degree, delivered her daughter by low forceps. She rated her relationship with her husband as excellent. She described the couple of days since her daughter's birth as painful and delightful. She described her childbirth and later experiences:

> Everyone kept saying I was so brave. Even one of the teachers told her students I was so brave. I was in labor six days. Once I ran into a sensitive doctor who gave me morphine. At first, I didn't know—if this wasn't labor, how would I know what labor is? This was painful. I had an epidural with pain. They gave me pitocin and the baby still wouldn't come down. Finally they used forceps and tore me in five different parts. The baby came and I didn't see it. My husband did and was so elated. I wouldn't ever do it again. I'm just destroyed— almost. I don't think I took care of myself. During this pregnancy I was so careful. I stopped work in June and went to school in September. I stopped school in December. In January I waited and gained a lot of weight. Three of my girlfriends' babies died. I was ten days late.
>
> Every day she gets prettier. She seems to have her father's disposition— strong. She's loving. She seems to recognize my scent and her father's. She focused the first day. She's brave too. She's jaundiced.
>
> My mother, grandmother, aunt, and sisters will all be helping us when we go home. There'll probably be times when I want to be alone.
>
> My pregnancy was so normal. I was sick the first three months. But it was normal. I could dance. But last month I could hardly walk.
>
> I don't want any more children. My husband wants another one; he'd like a son. We might adopt one. I wish I could be brave and have another one.
>
> Motherhood is so natural for me. I love kids—it's a natural part for me. I know it won't be a bed of roses.

Carrie

Carrie, a 33-year-old Caucasian with a graduate degree, had separated from her husband for a year at the time of the birth of her daughter. They both thought she was sterile because of long-term use of an intrauterine device. They dated during their separation, and it was at this time she became pregnant; her husband wanted her to have an abortion, but she refused. She rated relationship with her husband as poor (the lowest possible rating). She described her first day after birth as "out of it." She had a difficult delivery (vacuum extraction) and had needed the time to recover. She had been to visit her daughter in the intensive care nursery the last evening; "She recognized my voice. She might need an exchange transfusion. She is Rh positive and I am negative." Carrie described her childbirth and pregnancy experiences:

It was very painful. I had a small pelvis and she was a facial presentation. I pushed for hours, and it didn't really do any good. I had taken the Bradley class, but most items weren't applicable. I wish an anesthesiologist had been at class to explain the different medications available. I was in the delivery room for one and a half hours, and they couldn't get her out; several doctors tried to get her out. They all had too big of hands—couldn't believe this was happening. Finally, a Japanese doctor with small hands could turn her head and then she came out. The anesthesiologist was most helpful—helped me with timing and when to push. I was pushing so hard I would get faint.

I felt like I was on TV also. Ten people were waiting; they knew the baby had Rh antibodies. I felt the whole hospital was in my room. They all helped me past a cesarean section which would have scared me a lot.

She looks strong—weighed seven pounds, eight ounces—has black hair, dark brown eyes, and looks like her father. She is very pretty, seems peaceful. She coos. I tried to do my bonding this morning since it was unavailable to me yesterday.

I share a house with another woman who also has a daughter. She and friends that I have, along with her father, will help me for a week or so when I go home.

My pregnancy was real healthy. I'd like to have two children eventually.

I think motherhood is going to be really nice. I have wanted a baby for a long time. Your life doesn't have many peaks; this is like a peak for me, a very high experience. I know not everyone's on this wavelength to understand, but I'm glad I'm open to it, and I'm astounded to see my baby.

Cathryn

Cathryn, a 36-year-old single woman of Russian background, rated her relationship with the father of her baby as very good. Cathryn has a baccalaureate degree and still lives with her parents. At the time of the postpartum interview Cathryn was, in her words, "ecstatic—just living in another world. I don't have the words to say it. It's the complete opposite of when you're giving birth—all the anger and the complete sense of hopelessness is gone. I feel like I had it coming. I had a stillbirth six years ago. Even though I thought I got over things, I'll see if it'll take another child to get over it. It sure influenced my life then. I broke up with a man I had been with for seven years; I don't know if the relationship ended because the child didn't live." She described her experiences:

I was late, high-risk percentage, so the doctor felt I should be induced. I was induced all day Friday, Monday, and Tuesday again. I was pretty discouraged because I thought I'd have to go home again. Then at two p.m. the water bag broke. The next two hours the contractions were on top of each other—getting stronger and stronger. The doctor came in to measure me and said I was ready to push. I was at ten centimeters. That was great. It was a big thrill. Once I could push, I forgot about medication.

I went to the delivery room, and for the next hour and fourteen minutes I pushed. I was angry and helpless. I was cursing the baby inside. But I had my coach, and I was squeezing her hand to bits . . . In between pushing I was like passing out. Certain words, certain voice tones are really important. I wouldn't have even minded if someone scolded me then. The really important things—mind over body. Pain is inevitable. The minute it's over the physical thing doesn't really matter—just gets better and better. I think that I was very lucky—didn't have any stitches or medication to deal with afterwards.

I'm just getting to know my son. I haven't given him a name yet. I want to get to know him first. Already I thought he'd be a quiet one, but he isn't. I've never met anyone like him before. It's like the most open person I've met. It's like total commitment and also total discovery. You can't have any preconceptions. It's all in the making. All the time you think you're controlling, but incredibly they are their very own being. I'm sure I'll feel guilty and down a lot of the time. He's very interested, quite observant and focused. He spent his first moments after birth looking at me; it seemed like a long time that they let me have him.

My mother will help me when I go home; it will be more than I want. My mother is very practical—earthy. She should have been a nurse.

The pregnancy was very good. The only thing, I was a bit sick in the beginning. The first pregnancy I told everyone right away, but this time I was more superstitious. I didn't have a pregnancy test until three months. I knew I wanted to keep the baby. The father of the baby was away at the time. I didn't tell my friends either—that's the way I wanted it. Very healthy pregnancy—I worked. I wore a big sweat shirt and jeans and nobody ever knew. It was kind of interesting. . . . I found some interesting things. If I socialized I didn't feel that sick, but if I was on my own I felt more sick.

I think I'll be a pretty good mother. It'll be exciting. At thirty-six I'm not sure if I could have another one. Maybe I'll have one more.

Cynthia

Cynthia, a 40-year-old married Caucasian, is a registered nurse with credit toward a baccalaureate degree. She rated her relationship with her husband as very good. She noted that she was just recovering from her cesarean birth and was doing OK. She described her experiences:

I labored twelve hours. The cervix was fully dilated, but the baby didn't descend, so they decided to go on and do a cesarean. I had taken Lamaze classes. It was discouraging to go that far and not be able to deliver vaginally. They had me pushing for about an hour and a half. I just wanted to get it over with.

My son looks alert. They say he's doing really well. I've been starting to breast-feed him and he does really well. My husband and my mother will be helping me when I go home.

I guess my pregnancy was OK. I probably will want one more. I think motherhood will be a good experience.

Carmen

Carmen, a 31-year-old Mexican-American with a graduate degree, rated her relationship with her husband as very good. She had a cesarean birth and described the time since birth: "I feel great just to see him. Up until delivery I was tired and kind of discouraged. I had a long labor. After the baby was born, everything was great." She went on to describe her experiences:

I started labor at one a.m. but went to the hospital at five a.m. My water was broken, and the doctor told me to stay and see how things developed. I stayed like that for hours; then the pains were coming more frequently until I wanted to yell. It was so painful. I wanted an epidural. I didn't want to take one, but it was really hard, especially because it took so long. After that I rested for about half an hour when I felt the pressure. At twelve thirty p.m. the doctor checked me again—I was five centimeters. By one p.m. I was really dilated. From there it took an hour and a half. The baby's heartbeat was going down so they helped me.

We had made up our minds that we'd have everything natural. I was really suffering; my husband was worried about me. I felt discouraged about having the epidural and felt that the doctors and nurses were also discouraged.

My son is beautiful. He weighed seven and a half pounds. I just wanted to see him. After I had the baby, I was holding him awhile, and then my husband held him. I just couldn't believe that I had the baby. My sister-in-law will help me when I go home.

My pregnancy was pretty normal—no problems. I was worried because I had a miscarriage five years ago. I was really sick [nauseated] at first. I took antinausea pills. I felt guilty, but then I felt awful. You hear so much about the pills—both good and bad. I may want two or three more children, but I'm not sure.

Motherhood will be different—all changes. I already feel different. I've seen change in my husband. He's so worried about the baby. He's afraid he'll drop the baby.

IMPLICATIONS FOR NURSING CARE

The interview data from the 12 women present a variety of situations that dramatize the individuality of nursing care needs during childbirth and early postpartum. Implications for nursing care are presented first based on the overall findings, followed by specific examples from the 12 women's situations.

Care of the Teenager

Several implications are evident in providing care for the teenager during pregnancy and childbirth. The teenagers tended to talk less about her pregnancy, particularly in regard to discussing emotional changes or identifying complications. Either she was less sensitive to emotional changes and health problems during pregnancy, or the changes and health problems held little significance for her. This finding emphasizes the importance of going beyond the routine oral health history with the adolescent. When planning care, it is important to refer to ongoing medical records or to verify health data with a parent. The teenager has moved from concrete thinking to abstract conceptualization for only a short time. Implications of bodily or emotional change may be beyond her usual reasoning abilities or practices.

A question is raised about whether teenagers tend to experience less nausea and vomiting during the first trimester than older women, or do they not remember it? Or is it that this younger group that is less ready for pregnancy tends to deny all possible signs during early pregnancy? The age group differences only approached significance (p = .08); 17% of the teenagers, 30% of Group 2, and 22% of Group 3 mentioned nausea and vomiting when asked what their pregnancy had been like. Cathryn reported that if she socialized she felt much better; perhaps the teenagers were busy socializing with school or other activities so that they felt better.

Amy described the eight and ninth months of her pregnancy as hard because she could not do what she wanted to do then. The restrictiveness of the increased body bulk may be much more problematic for the younger, more active group than earlier pregnancy symptoms.

The need for closeness to supportive persons during pregnancy was stressed by Alma, who didn't want her boyfriend going off with friends and leaving her. Alison described how pregnancy was a very emotional time for her. These data stress the importance of securing support systems for the teenager during pregnancy. Persons who can be understanding, caring, and physically accessible seem particularly important.

The teenager who more often had a delivery without medical intervention also perceived the birth experience more negatively than older women did. Although the overall length of labor did not vary, nor the first stage of labor, the teenager had a shorter second stage of labor. The more negative perceptions could be related to expectations, lack of preparation for the experience, or the absence of previous painful events in the adolescent's life. The teenager more often reported that she was afraid during labor. She was less likely to attend antepartum classes where she might have had some misconceptions clarified. Careful planning and thought are required in preparing the teenager for the birth experience. Group classes developed especially for teenagers are important. Fewer teens have mates to attend classes with them, and they are hesitant to ask questions with older women present. Individual sessions are too threatening for the early and middle adolescent, who responds best to interactions within her peer group. Visual aids and concrete examples are important for illustrating events of labor. A uterine contraction may be described more accurately as resembling a muscle cramp because many may not have experienced menstrual cramps.

The pride in their accomplishments during labor and delivery was evident in the comments by both Alma and Alison, however. Alison spoke of her willpower. Amy, in contrast, noted that they had "vacuumed her baby out." This comment suggests that she sees the vacuum extraction as comparable to a vacuum cleaner with which she is familiar. Her early response to her infant is along the same lines that she seems to feel about herself, "He's skinny—hopeless." Deutscher (1970) suggested that women view the birth experience as their first act of mothering, and as such it has long-lasting effects on their mothering behaviors.

There was a significant, positive correlation with the perception of the birth experience and observed mothering behaviors during the first year among the teenage group (Mercer, 1985b). The correlations were .35 at 1 month, .32 at 4 months, .45 at 8 months, and .47 at 12 months. An important part of nursing intervention is to praise the young woman's accomplishments during labor and to give on-the-spot positive feedback after her hard work. The young woman may need help in separating out the difficult, painful events as distinct from the potential joys of the baby or of mothering. The older woman verbalized these differences well (see discussion following).

Cultural beliefs influence how new mothers respond to their newborn infants. The accepted positive attachment behaviors for white, middle-class women may not reflect attachment in other cultural groups; two thirds of the teenagers were from non-Caucasian cultural groups. Learning something about the cultural groups' beliefs are important in order to plan meaningful antepartum and postpartum care. Amy's disappointment in a skinny baby who seemed hopeless may have reflected cultural values of a preference for plump babies. For example, Brown and associates (1975) reported that black women vocalized to and stimulated large male infants more so than female or smaller male infants, indicating a cultural preference for large male infants. The skinny baby, on the other hand, may have been a lack of fit with her expectations of the larger "Gerber Baby" image that women tend to have, rather than that of a newborn infant.

Care of Women in Their Twenties

Almost one third of this age group reported nausea and vomiting during early pregnancy. Betty couldn't enjoy her pregnancy because everyone was so worried about her fetus being so small. Barbara saw her pregnancy as wonderful; she did mention that toward the end her increased size interfered with comfortable sleeping. Bonnie, like Amy, noted the restrictiveness during later pregnancy:"I could hardly walk the last month." This group of women as a whole were more ready for pregnancy than the teenage group, and this may have permitted them to be more tuned in to early symptoms. Just over three-fourths (77%) attended prenatal classes, compared with half (51%) of the teenagers.

This group of women had a more positive perception of their childbirth experience than did the younger and older groups. Their cesarean birth rate was similar to that expected for the general population, and three-fourths of them had attended antepartal classes. Their better preparation and higher personality integration (compared with the teenagers) yet lower cesarean rate than that of the older women probably contributed to their more favorable perceptions.

Both groups of older women articulated an awe for the child that they had had a part in producing. Bea's "high" during the early postpartum period and her viewing of motherhood as "a new path of life" indicates some of the excitement of making this transition.

The importance of reinforcement for hard work during labor is dramatized by Bonnie, who remembered that she was brave during labor and delivery. It was important to her that a nursing instructor had told her students that Bonnie was very brave. This helped offset the fact that she had to have a forceps delivery that tore her in five places and led her to say, "I'm just destroyed."

The correlations of the perception of the birth experience and later mothering behavior were somewhat weaker in Group 2 than among teenagers but were significant at each test period except 8 months—.32 at 1 month, .27 at 4 months, .18 at 8 months, and .26 at 12 months. Sensitive, personal care during labor and delivery that enables feelings about self, apprises the woman of her good performance, and provides informational support is critical. Providing the new mother with an opportunity to review her labor and delivery experience may help her to separate unavoidable external events so that they are not attributed to her inadequacies. A positive self-concept is central to mothering.

Nursing Care for the Women 30 Years and Older

Women in Group 3 indicated more overall readiness for the pregnancy and also prepared in greater numbers for the transition—92% attended prenatal classes. Attending classes may have been a more natural or common way of preparing for the unknown for this more highly educated group of women, almost two-thirds (63%) of whom had a baccalaureate or higher degree.

The older women with longer life histories had to resolve earlier losses; Cathryn was superstitious about letting anyone know that she was pregnant because she had had a stillbirth 6 years earlier. Carmen was worried during early pregnancy because she had had a miscarriage 5 years previously. The complexity of life situations may be greater for this older group who are unmarried than for unmarried teenage women. A teenager, for example, has not had to relinquish a 7-year relationship; thus, she may not experience the extent of grief that an older woman may have to deal with. Therefore, an important part of nursing intervention may be counseling in regard to resolving earlier losses or making appropriate referrals for counseling.

The older, more educated woman may intellectualize her mother-infant interactions more so than a younger woman. Note Carrie's comment about "bonding this morning because it was unavailable to me yesterday."

Disappointment in the type of birth experience was an additional loss that occurred more frequently in this older group; 31% had cesarean births. Cathryn spoke of such anger during labor that she cursed the baby inside, yet she delivered vaginally. Cynthia and Carmen both expressed disappointment at progressing to complete dilation and then having to have cesarean births. Carmen had not wanted to have epidural anesthesia, but the length of the labor was so exhausting, she made the decision to have it.

Interestingly, among this older group of women there was never a significant relationship between their perceptions of the birth experience and their observed maternal behavior (Mercer, 1985b). Motherhood was viewed as a peak experience despite disappointment with their birth experience. Cathryn articulated this bipolar emotional response quite well—from anger and hopelessness to ecstasy and feeling beyond words to express her feeelings. Cathryn described the mother-child interaction as discovery and as acquaintance with a totally new person; however, she described the interactional capacity of her son as one might portray a new boyfriend.

Nursing intervention during pregnancy should be directed at helping the older woman view the childbirth more realistically. A desire for a natural birth experience without medication is not congruent with the realistic outcome for most women. Dealing with the loss of her expectations for the birth experience may take time for the woman who has succeeded in a career and in everything else that she has done. Referral to a self-help cesarean support group provides an opportunity to work through feelings that may require as long as a year to be resolved (Tilden & Lipson, 1981; Lipson & Tilden, 1980; Lipson, 1981; Lipson, 1982). Cesarean support groups provide a safe milieu in which women may resolve negative feelings about their birth experiences and plan for more positive birth experiences in the future.

CHAPTER 4

The Infants

The infants who were a part of this study had a gestational age of 37 weeks or more and had no diagnosed anomaly at birth. There were five sets of twins, two in each of the two younger groups, and one set in the older age group. Overall, the infants were rather evenly distributed by gender; 49% were male, and 51% were female. Teenagers had male infants significantly more often than older women; 62% of the teenagers had a male infant, compared with 39% of Group 2 and 54% of Group 3.

Following an overview of infant competencies, growth, and development, the infants' general health status and growth and development over the year are presented; in subsequent chapters these variables are related to other mothering variables. Change in the infants' schedules, their feedings, crying, and the stimulation, safe environment, and discipline their mothers provided for them are discussed. Maternal perceptions of the neonate, profile of a good baby at 4 and 8 months, the infants' temperaments, and the relationship of the infant's temperament to maternal temperament follow, with implications for nursing intervention concluding the chapter.

INFANT COMPETENCIES

Infants are born with a wide range of competencies that help to assure their survival. Immediately after delivery, infants experience a period of alertness that probably results from the stimulation received during labor and delivery and from their new environment. This initial alert period coincides with a period of euphoria that newly delivered mothers experience. Thus, as mothers examine their new infants with much excitement and curiosity, their infants are in an alert state to maintain eye contact and provide positive feedback that increases the meaning of these early interactions.

Immediately following birth infants turns their heads toward and are alert to the human voice; they prefer rhythmic and continuous sound from a female or higher-pitched voice (Brazelton, 1979). Infants prefer the human face over other objects. They prefer complex patterns such as checkerboard or bull's-eye to simple patterns, moving objects to stable ones, black and white contrast to monochromes, and also bright colors and contour changes (Blackburn, 1983). Infants ranging from less than 1 hr to 71 hr old imitate adult facial gestures of mouth opening and tongue protrusion (Meltzoff & Moore, 1983). Infants recognize milk odors over water odors at birth, and when just a few days old, they recognize their mothers' odor and indicate a preference for her breast pad (Porter, Cernoch, & Perry, 1983).

Both the infant's physical appearance and helpless thrashing movements serve as initiators of adult care-giving behaviors (Bell, 1974). Infants are able to maintain these care-giving behaviors through their cues that indicate their conditions, their sensory and fatigue limits, and their protest behaviors (Bell, 1974). Through these behaviors infants exert considerable control over their mothers.

Following the period of alertness, Brazelton (1979) reported that infants experience a 24- to 48-hr period of depression and disorganization if their birth experience was uncomplicated and if they have no medication aftereffects. A recovery of optimal functioning then occurs after several days that represents the infant's neurological and integrative capacities (Brazelton, 1979).

Infants must first achieve control over their physiological system, including breathing, heart rate, and temperature control; full-term infants have less difficulty with this than preterm or at-risk infants (Brazelton & Als, 1979). After the infant achieves control over basic physiological demands, she begins to gain control over the motor system as it affects the range, smoothness, and complexity of movement. When the infant has integrated the control over physiological and motor systems, she is able to achieve control over transition of her states of consciousness (Brazelton & Als, 1979).

State of Arousal

States of consciousness or arousal range from deep sleep, light sleep, awake/drowsy, quiet alert, and active alert to crying. Importantly, infants adapt their mobility and state behavior to a sensitive environment that meets their needs (Brazelton, 1979); this usually occurs during the first month. Infants use their state of consciousness to control the quantity and type of input received from the environment. The infant's state is recognizable by a group of characteristics regularly occurring together—body activity, eye movements, facial movements, breathing pattern, and level of response to both external and internal stimuli (Blackburn, 1983). Variability of an infant's state indicates her capacity for self-organization; this adequacy is determined by the ability to quiet herself as well as her need for stimulation (Brazelton, 1979). Infants' optimal response to the environment occurs when they are in the quiet alert state, at which time they interact more enthusiastically with others.

If the environment stimulation becomes fatiguing, infants close out stimulation by averting their gaze and discontinuing eye contact. Gaze aversion seems to be greater with either minimally active or excessively active partners (Field, 1981). Caretakers can help infants in their organization of state by expanding the quiet, alert, and sleep states and by helping infants regulate the transitions between states (Brazelton & Als, 1979).

Temperament

Temperament is defined as the individual's emotional reactivity or behavioral style in interacting with the environment; temperament describes how an individual behaves rather than what the individual can do or why she does it (Carey, 1981). Infant temperament contributes significantly to both the environment and to infant interactions with the environment. Temperament appears to have a constitutional basis, to continue from infancy with relative continuity, and is affected by the environment (Bates, 1980).

Carey (1981) classified categories of easy, slow-to-warm-up, and difficult infants, based on clusters of temperament responses. Infants with difficult temperaments appear to induce different caregiving behaviors than infants with easy temperaments. A difficult temperament is characterized by arrhythmic behaviors, low approach and adaptability, intenseness, and a predominantly negative mood (Carey, 1981). The easy infant is rhythmic, approaching, adaptable, mild, and has a positive mood (Carey, 1981). The slow-to-warm-up infant is low in activity, approach, and adaptability, negative but variable in rhythmicity, and mild in intensity (Carey, 1981). Bates (1980) argued that the concept of a difficult temperament has little empirical evidence and that it might more accurately be thought of as a social perception. However, since temperament exerts its main effect on relevant outcome through a process of transaction between the child and the social environment, it makes sense to measure temperament as it is perceived by those important persons in the child's life. However, a careful critique of 26 temperament instruments concluded that there are psychometric and reliability problems with current measures (Hubert, Wachs, Peters-Martin, & Gandour, 1982). Of more practical help to new parents is Brazelton's (1969) approach in describing the range of normal behavior in infants, using the categories of quiet, average, and active infants to illustrate different patterns of behavior and development over the first year.

Maternal response to difficult or irritable infants may be mediated by other infant characteristics and the mother's support system. Mothers in one study responded more often to highly irritable female infants than to highly irritable males (Crockenberg & Smith, 1982). Infant alertness at 1 month was a strong predictor of involved maternal contact at 3 months; female infants were more alert than males, which could have contributed to mothers responding more frequently to females. Fussing and crying were not associated with neonatal irritability but with mothers' unresponsive attitudes and behavior. At 1 year maternal social support was related to the infant's secure attachment; social support was especially important for mothers with irritable infants (Crockenberg, 1981).

GROWTH AND DEVELOPMENT

Infants influence maternal behaviors through their unique responses and also may reflect the quality of mothering care they receive through their growth and development. Well-nurtured infants show remarkable growth and social and motor development during the first year of life.

Infants double their birth weight as early as 4 months, and bottle-fed infants doubled their birth weight in 113 days, compared with breast-fed infants who took 124 days (Neumann & Alpaugh, 1976). Boys doubled their birth weights in 111 days, compared with girls who did so in 129 days. Solid foods were fed to bottle-fed infants at an average age of 1.9 months and to breast-fed infants at an average age of 3.9 months, which may account for some of the differences in weight gain.

At birth the newly born infant lifts her head and has strong grasp and hand-to-mouth reflexes. By 2 months infants make thrashing, crawling movements and are able to suck their fingers and circle one hand around the other. They smile at pleasant situations and are gaining increasing interest in the environment. By 4 months infants enjoy being pulled to a standing position and may enjoy splashing in their bath. When propped up, they hold their heads steady. They reach for toys, play with their fingers, and are able to grab one hand with another. When on their abdomens, they hold their heads high, supporting the upper body with straightened arms (Brazelton, 1969).

By 8 months infants can crawl and pull themselves to a standing position by holding onto furniture. They can pull tablecloths off tables and pick up tiny objects between the thumb and forefinger as they enjoy exploring the world. They enjoy playing with their food and may scream loudly when something displeases them. They prefer their mothers to others for security and for caretaking at this age. The 8-month-old is a great imitator.

At 12 months the infant may be able to walk with legs wide apart but crawls if she is in a hurry to get somewhere. She climbs into laps very easily. Finger foods are a delight, and untying shoes is interesting. The 1-year-old has a growing vocabulary and may be able to tell you what she wants (Brazelton, 1969). She also rewards her mother with hugs and kisses.

As infants age they initiate more interactions while mothers initiate more games, terminating or redirecting activities, and verbal requests, and they perform fewer caretaking or repositioning activities (Green, Gustafson, & West, 1980). Infants' locomotor abilities relate to many of the changes in maternal behaviors, and their social environment is in part determined by their developmental status.

The Development of Self

Sander (1962) observed five time segments of early ego development during the first 18 months of life. The first 2½ months of life, or period of initial adaptation, corresponds to the undifferentiated phase of ego development when responses from the mother are important in stimulating and meeting the infant's needs. A period of reciprocal exchange from 2½ to 5 months is one of the most pleasurable of the early phases because of the reciprocal interaction that occurs as the mother and infant alternate back and forth in stimulating exchange. A period of early directed activity by the infant occurs from 5 to 9 months, when the infant takes the initiative in interacting with the mother and learns to anticipate the mother's response. The period of focalization on the mother from 9 to 15 months is a time when the child learns to manipulate the mother. The infant's demands are intense and unrelenting, and she prefers her mother to meet her needs. The infant's increased mobility assures self-confidence when the mother is secure enough to continue reciprocity and allow the infant freedom to explore. From 12 to 18 months a period of self-assertion emerges in which negative behaviors and responses begin. The child struggles for assurance of the mother's availability while struggling to assert herself against her mother.

Brazelton and Als (1979) also described four clear stages of infant development paralleling ego development: the infant's achievement of control over input and output systems; the infant's ability to attend to and use social cues to prolong states of attention and to incorporate more complex messages; the mutual reciprocal feedback system between infant and parent push the infant to her capacity, with the parent allowing the infant to withdraw and incorporate new experiences; and the infant's opportunity and ability to demonstrate and incorporate a sense of autonomy.

Stechler and Kaplan's (1980) three stages in the psychological development of self extend the ideas of Sander (1962) and Brazelton and Als (1979). They see the first stage as a preself stage encompassing Sander's periods of initial adaptation and reciprocal exchange from birth through 5 months. The preself coalesces out of early physiological states with the help of good nurturance and reciprocal interactions and has the capacity to regulate her own states.

Stage two, the preawareness of self, is a transitional period, during which the infant develops the capacity to take the initiative, to sort out options, and to determine and achieve goals. The infant's experience of self is enhanced through her joy of repetitiveness in practicing her skills and being an active doer. The infant begins to accept prohibitions during this period and to inhibit actively her own behavior, developing her capacity for self-regulation. This corresponds to Sander's period of early directed activity from 5 to 9 months.

At stage three the self emerges, as the child displays a capacity for self-restraint in response to prohibition. At this phase the child has a self defined as a doer and a knower, a self defined as object with contradictory wishes that must be resolved, and a self as a locus within which the experience is located. The capacity to create a totally new behavior in a solution to a conflict leads to mastery. This stage begins at approximately 1 year or older.

The first year of life is a period of great change in all realms for the infant. The transactions between the developing infant and her mother result in growth for both. The infants in this study are viewed within this context.

THE INFANTS' GROWTH AND DEVELOPMENT

Infant Growth over the Year

Although the teenagers' infants weighed significantly less at birth than infants in groups 2 and 3, they overcame this difference at 1 month; and at 8 and 12 months they weighed significantly more than Group 2 infants. Group 3 infants at 8 and 12 months did not differ significantly from either Group 1 or Group 2 infants by weight. At 1 year the distribution of the total sample of infants did not differ significantly from the expected national percentile intervals by weight. More of Group 1 infants (60%), compared with 48% of Group 2 and 40% of Group 3 infants, were *above* the 50th percentile.

Infant weights at birth, 1, 4, 8, and 12 months by grams were, respectively, as follows: Group 1, 3,265, 4,468, 6,829, 9,032, and 10,445; Group 2, 3,462, 4,379, 6,773, 8,592, and 9,821; and Group 3, 3,460, 4,226, 6,762, 8,840, and 9,944.

Other research found no significant differences in the birth weights of infants of teenagers less than 16 years of age and women aged 20 to 24 years, even though teenagers' infants had a shorter gestational age (Horon et al., 1983). Maternal weight gain was more predictive of infant birth weight among teenagers, and race and gender were more predictive among the 20-to-24-year-olds. The findings at 1 year are in contrast to earlier research that reported 62% of teenagers' infants' weights below the 50th percentile (Osofsky & Osofsky, 1970).

The distribution of infants' lengths in this sample indicated that more were longer than expected in the national percentiles. Infants never differed significantly in length by age group. Infant lengths at birth, 1, 4, 8, and 12 months by centimeters were, respectively, as follows: Group 1, 49.8, 54.7, 63.6, 71.1, and 76.8; Group 2, 50.4, 54.9, 64.1, 70.9, and 75.5; and Group 3, 50.7, 55.1, 64.0, 70.9, and 75.4.

The head circumference data could not be compared to the national population distribution because the measurements were not made to tenths of centimeters. Infants' head circumferences never differed significantly by age group. Infants' mean head circumferences at 1, 4, 8, and 12 months by centimeters were, respectively, as follows: Group 1, 37.6, 41.6, 45.6, and 46.4; Group 2, 37.4, 41.9, 44.8, and 46.4; and Group 3, 37.9, 41.5, 45.5, and 46.7.

Infant Development over the Year

Maternal age was no handicap to the infants' development over the first year. Teenagers' infants who were ahead in both motor and social development at 1 and 4 months began to lose this advantage by 8 months, although they compared favorably with other infants.

At 1 month Group 1 infants scored significantly higher than Group 2 infants in motor development, with Group 3 infants scoring in between and not differing significantly from either. At 4 months Group 1 infants were significantly ahead of both groups 2 and 3 infants in motor development. At 8 and 12 months there were no significant differences by age group in motor development.

At 1 month groups 1 and 3 infants were significantly ahead of Group 2 infants in social development, but by 4 months Group 1 infants were ahead of both groups 2 and 3 infants. At 8 months no significant group differences were observed, and by 1 year Group 2 infants surpassed both groups 1 and 3 infants in social development.

More of the teenagers reported help from their mothers, and their infants may have been receiving more stimulation from two mother figures during the early months. Teenagers' help from their mothers decreased at both 8 and 12 months, and this also could have contributed to their infants not staying ahead in social and motor development (Mercer, Hackley, & Bostrom, 1984b). An alternative explanation for Group 1 scoring higher in motor development is that 70% of the teenagers were non-Caucasians, with 41% being black. Others have reported black superiority in gross motor development during infancy controlling for socioeconomic status (SES) (Walters, 1967).

Group 1 infants' loss of their developmental advantage at 8 months may be explained another way. Other researchers reported that it is not until the eighth or twelfth month that the mothers' psychosocial assets, especially stress from life events, begin to affect their ability to interact sensitively and constructively with their infants (Barnard & Eyres, 1979). Group 1 mothers were at a disadvantage psychosocially (see Chapter 2), and if their ability to interact with their infants was affected, this could have affected their infants' development.

GENERAL HEALTH STATUS OVER THE YEAR

Infant Health

At birth there were no significant group differences in newborn health status as measured by spontaneous respiration and by 1- and 5-min Apgar scores. However, health problems were evident at the time of the hospital interview when mothers expressed concern about their infants' status. These problems increased in number as the infants aged, but at this early interview hyperbilirubinemia and fever were the most frequently identified problems.

Teenagers' infants had a poorer health status the first month following birth. In Group 1, 26% of the infants remained in the hospital following their mothers' discharge, contrasted with 22% of the infants in Group 2 and 10% of the infants in Group 3. The primary reason for the infants' extended stay in the hospital was treatment for hyperbilirubinemia. Treatment for infections was the second greatest reason for infants remaining in the hospital after their mothers' discharge. Teenagers' reports rated their infants' overall health as poorer than groups 2 and 3. There were no significant group differences in the number of infant illnesses reported. Infections, hyperbilirubinemia, and colds and/or congestion were the most frequently reported illnesses, in that order.

At 4 months the health status of groups 1 and 2 infants did not differ; Group 3 infants had significantly fewer reported illnesses than the infants from the two younger groups from 1 month of age. Over one-third of all mothers (36%) reported their infants had had colds, flu, or croup (24%, 50%, 22%, respectively). Twelve percent reported that their infants had eye, ear, and throat infections (8%, 18%, 5%, respectively).

Almost two-thirds (62%) of the infants were seen by physicians for routine checkups only between 1 and 4 months; one infant was seen by the public health nurse only. One-third of the infants were treated by physicians for health problems; 3% of these were seen in the hospital emergency room. Nine of the infants (3%) were hospitalized: three for 1 day; four for 3 to 7 days; and two for 2 weeks.

Five infants (2%) had surgery: pyloric stenosis (two), hernia repair (two), and an obstructed bile duct (one).

The number of reported infant illnesses from 4 to 8 months did not differ significantly by age group. Colds, flu, or a virus were the most frequently mentioned (57%); 25% had eye, ear, nose or throat infections. Three birth defects were reported—hemangioma, double kidney, and cross-eyes. Eight percent had a fever, 8% had either a rash or eczema, 6% had diarrhea, 5% had croup or pneumonia, and 4% had roseola.

From 4 to 8 months 46% were seen by a physician for routine checkup only, and 44% were seen for illnesses. Four percent were seen in the emergency room, and six (2%) were hospitalized—five for 1 to 3 days and one for over 1 week.

At 1 year there were no significant group differences in the number of infant illnesses since 8 months. Infant colds, coughs, and flu were reported most frequently (56%); croup and bronchitis were reported by 48%; and ear infections were reported by 32%. Thirteen percent reported a fever, and 11% reported diarrhea. Two infants had surgery (strabismus and a herniorrhaphy). Two infants had their feet casted.

During the 8- to 12-month period, one third of the infants were seen by a physician for regular checkups only; 54% were treated for illnesses. Nineteen (8%) were treated in the emergency room, and seven (3%) were hospitalized from 2 to 7 days.

Infant Accidents

At four months 10% of the mothers reported infant accidents. The reported accidents included falls from bed/sofa, burns from cooking or a cigarette, and bumps, none of which required a physician's care. There were two accidents in which parents took the infant to the emergency room—a burn and a fall down the stairs. Of the 68 reported accidents, 9% were reported by the teenagers, 47% by Group 2, and 44% by Group 3.

A question may be raised whether teenagers' infants experienced fewer accidents or whether the teenagers felt less comfortable reporting accidents. Accidents for which a mother feels the blame are very difficult to report. A woman from Group 3 put a decongestant in her 3-week-old baby's nose rather than giving it orally; the infant stopped breathing, and the paramedics and pediatrician had

to be called. This mother was unable to report the accident at 1
month; it was not until 4 months that she was able to talk about it
with others. Other researchers have reported increased accidents
during the child's first 5 years among teenagers' children, but attributed the increased incidence to SES, environmental factors, and
lack of experience (Taylor, Wadsworth, & Butler, 1983).

The infant's increased motor ability at 8 months was reflected in
an increased number of accidents reported (28%). Falls and bumps
that did not require a physician's attention were the most frequent
types of accidents reported (22%). Four percent of the accidents
required medical attention: falls or bumps (3%), ingestion of noxious
substances and burns (1%).

At 1 year the number of infants experiencing accidents was similar to that at 8 months (29%). Falls and bumps that did not require
medical care were the most frequently reported infant accident
(17%). Infant burns that did not require medical care were reported
by 4%. Accidents that required medical care included falls (4%),
dog bites (1%), swallowing noxious substances (1%), fingers pinched
in the door (1%), and vaginal lacerations of one Group 2 infant that
were allegedly caused by the mate who was not the father of the infant. A referral was made to the Children's Protective Services in
the latter situation.

INFANT SCHEDULES OVER THE YEAR

At the end of the first month the majority of the infants (61%)
still had an irregular and unpredictable schedule. This meant that
their mothers were unable to plan time for themselves and had many
sleep interruptions. The younger the mother, the more likely the
schedule was reported as regular (67%, 40%, and 19%).[1] One-fourth
of the women described their infants' behaviors as erratic, without
any kind of schedule. These findings are congruent with Grossman
et al. (1980), who reported that most infants in their study were
not on a regular schedule at 2 months postpartum.

However, almost one-fifth of the mothers (19%) expressed relief

[1] Series of three figures in parentheses indicates percentages for the three groups
from the youngest to the oldest, respectively.

that they had 5 to 6 hr of uninterrupted sleep at night at 1 month. Almost half of the women reported that their infants' schedules included three night or early morning feedings: 10:00 or 11:00 p.m., again at 2:00 or 3:00 a.m., and at 6:00 or 7:00 a.m. Although more of the teenagers (60%, 36%, and 55%) reported a regular schedule for their infants, they were less likely to be satisfied with the infants' schedule (18%, 35%, and 51%). Part of this dissatisfaction may stem from the three night/early morning feedings. The older the woman, the more likely she was to be pleased with her infant's schedule.

Barnard and Eyres (1979) reported that infants had more regular day sleep and fewer night awakenings at 4 months. Three-fourths of the women reported that their infants had a regular, predictable schedule at 4 months. Six percent noted that the infant's schedule was changing; the infant appeared to be sleeping less. Ten percent reported that their infants had no schedule and that their infants' behavior was totally unpredictable. The two older age groups tended to report infants as having a more regular schedule, a change from 1 month when more teenagers reported that their infants had regular schedules.

By 8 months almost all of the infants (88%) had regular, predictable schedules. The others reported that their infants had erratic behavior, except for three women who were unaware of their infants' schedules (two were working, and one grandmother had informal custody of her infant). Almost half (48%) of the infants were sleeping through the night; 18% reported their infants had slept through the night earlier but now awakened occasionally because of teething. Seventeen percent of the infants were waking once a night, and 11% were still waking twice a night. Mothers considered a 5:00 a.m. or 6:00 a.m. feeding as a night feeding. Barnard and Eyres (1979) reported that infants in their sample tended to have more regular night sleep at 1 and 8 months.

Just over half (58%) of the women were pleased with their infants' schedules at 8 months. One-fifth of the women worked their schedules around their infants. Fifteen percent of the women reported some difficulty with their infants' schedules and wished the schedules were different. The infants' schedules remained less than ideal for 42% of the women at 8 months.

By 1 year most of the infants were sleeping through the night (85%). The number of mothers pleased with their year-old-infant's schedule (60%) did not differ greatly from 8 months. Schedules were described as either flexible or easily adjusted to fit their own. One-fourth of the women viewed their infants' schedules as difficult or demanding at 1 year.

INFANT FEEDINGS

The majority of women elected to breast-feed their infants initially. The older the infant's mother, the more likely the infant was being breast-fed. The percentage of women breastfeeding at postpartum hospitalization, 1, 4, 8, and 12 months were, respectively, as follows: Group 1, 62, 34, 21, 16, and 5; Group 2, 82, 76, 56, 36, and 23; and Group 3, 93, 91, 74, 58, and 28.

At 1 month 14% of the women were giving their infants foods other than breast milk or formula. One-third of the teenagers, 11% of Group 2, and 2% of Group 3 were giving their infants cereal at 1 month. Teenagers said that their mothers had told them to put cereal in the bottle so that their infants would sleep through the night. However, as noted by the schedules described above, this did not seem to work. Whether this difference in diet contributed to the teenagers' infants' greater weight gain is conjectural. Two of the teenagers also were giving their infants orange juice; two of Group 3 were giving their infants tea. The tendency of teenagers to act on advice from their mothers rather than physicians is in agreement with the findings of Zuckerman, Winsmore, and Alpert (1979).

Recommendations are that healthy infants are not given solid foods before 5 months (Foman, Filer, Anderson, & Ziegler, 1979). Others reported that 41% of 120 women 18 to 32 years were feeding their infants solids at 1 month and that another 16% were doing so by 2 months (Entwisle & Doering, 1981). Mothers' reasons for introducing solid foods early were that the infant could go longer between feedings or sleep through the night; however, similarly to the infants in this study, solid feedings did not have this effect.

Three-fourths of the mothers reported that the infant feedings went well, with no problems at 1 month. The remaining one-fourth reported that feedings were a hassle; burping was a problem; and breast-feeding problems such as sore nipples, milk not letting down, or running out of milk caused much anguish.

Mothers spent a large portion of their time in infant feeding during the first month. Teenagers spent less time feeding their infants; they more often reported that their infants ate in 15 to 20 min (48%, 30%, and 18%). The most frequently mentioned time required for infant feeding reported by one-third of the women was 25 to 30 min. Ten percent reported spending 50 to 60 min in feeding, and 7% reported spending 1 hr to 1½ hr in feeding. Most of the women reported that they held their infants to feed them (84%, 94%, and 98%). Barnard and Eyres (1979) observed that more highly educated women tended to feed their infants more often at 1 month; although that was not true with this sample, the more highly educated the woman, the more time she spent in feeding her infant.

By 4 months only one-third of the women were feeding their infants milk only. Fifty-six percent were feeding their infants cereal, 41% were feeding their infants fruit, 27% were feeding vegetables, and 11% were feeding meat. Significantly more teenagers were feeding fruit, vegetables, and meat than the two older groups.

Feedings were going great for 81% at 4 months, with no problems noted. Those who reported problems said that the infant was eating less, was less interested or more playful, was spitting up, or was struggling with the breast.

By 8 months three-fourths of the infants were eating strained/junior baby foods, 66% were eating finger foods such as crackers and fruit, and 62% were eating table foods. Five women from the two younger groups said they fed junk food such as colas, potato chips, and pickles to their infants.

The 8-month-old's feedings overall (79%) were not problematic for their mothers; they ate well. Other mothers reported their infants were displaying more specific dislikes, were more picky, were refusing solids, or were drinking less milk.

By 1 year three-fourths of the infants were eating table foods, 20% were eating strained or junior baby foods, one infant was eating premasticated table food, and one infant was totally breast-fed. Almost three-fourths (71%) reported that infant feedings were going well; the teenagers reported that feedings were going well significantly more often than did the older women (78%, 69%, and 52%). The other women noted that their infants ate less, were more picky, or occasionally were difficult to feed.

INFANT BATHS

As expected developmentally, by 4 months the majority (87%) of the infants were enjoying their baths. Only two women reported that they were not giving their infants tub baths; 7% reported that the infant was bathing with either the mother or the father. Seven percent of the infants cried, screamed, clutched the tub, and in general did not like their baths; another 5% were indifferent—they tolerated the bath quietly without smiling or crying.

By 8 months practically all of the infants (96%) were enjoying bath time; 14% were bathing with a parent. Four of the 4% who did not enjoy or were afraid of their baths had eczema and hated the washcloth; it probably was painful to them. Most infants were bathed daily, 3% were reportedly bathed one to two times a week and 2% were bathed every other day.

INFANT CRYING

Infant crying signals alarm to the mother. During the first month, when the mother is learning to read infant cues, crying is especially disturbing. With experience, the mother learns to meet her infant's needs and to distinguish between different types of cries.

At 1 month the majority (55%) reported that their infant's crying was distressing. However, 41% noted that the infant had a reason for crying and that they tried to determine the reason. The teenage mother was less likely than the older women to feel the infant had a reason for crying (20%, 47%, and 47%). A few of the women (7%) reported that they felt sad and helpless or that they cried when the baby cried; 4% noted that they felt guilty or frightened when the infant cried. Three percent reported that they felt angry or annoyed when their infants cried, and 1% said that the crying was funny or cute. Nineteen percent stated that crying was good for the infant. The mother's feeling very bothered by crying during the postpartum period to the extent that she feels hopeless, helpless, or like crying herself has been cited as a warning sign of difficulty with later parenting (Gray, Cutler, Dean, & Kempe, 1980).

How the mothers responded at 1 month to their infant's crying varied: 59% said that it depended on the type of cry; 2% let the infant cry; 23% never let the infant cry; and 7% let the infant cry if he was fed and dry. The 1-month-old infant's cry held many meanings for the women. More than half (58%) noted that crying was the infant's way of communicating a need; teenagers less often held this view (30%, 68%, and 63%) and more often said that crying meant the infant was spoiled or being mean (13%, 2%, and 3%). Over one-fourth (27%) noted that the infant wanted to be held or cuddled, was bored or unhappy when he cried. One-third noted that crying indicated the infant was hungry or wet; significantly more of the teenagers gave this response (51%, 35%, and 27%). One-fifth felt crying indicated the infant was hurting or uncomfortable.

Women responded differently to daytime and nighttime crying; only 28% reported that they responded the same regardless of the time. Twenty-seven percent did not let the infant cry at night; 7% moved the infants into their beds when they cried. Eight percent noted that they played with the infant when she cried during the daytime but not at night.

By 4 months mothers reported changes in their infants' crying; 45% noted that the infant cried less often. More women in Group 3 reported less frequent crying (38%, 39%, and 56%). One-fourth of the women noted that the cries were louder, deeper, and stronger in general; over half observed that the cries were more expressive, and different types of cries were evident.

Mothers' overall response to infant crying at 4 months was to feed the infants if they seemed hungry or try to determine the cause of the crying (84% but with significant group differences—64%, 91%, and 88%). A few of the teenagers gave vague responses ranging from picking the infant up to slapping, giving medicine, or ignoring. Group 3 women responded more quickly to an angry cry (average 1.53 min, compared with 3.88 min for teenagers and 3.23 minutes for 20-year-olds). Mothers responded less quickly to a sleepy cry (group average of 5 to 7 min). An infant is learning to trust that her needs will be met during the first year; the Group 3 infants who cried less may have been having their needs met more quickly, so they did not have to cry as much.

The assertive 8-month-old communicated more clearly with her cries; 42% of the mothers described their infants' crying as more specific than it had been at 4 months. The crying was described as louder by 36%, as occurring less often by 28%, and as being whiny by 16%.

The 1-year-old's cry overall was described as more specific, louder, and more demanding or more spoiled than the 8-month-old's. This change in cry is congruent with the infant's development of self in which she has learned that she can manipulate the environment somewhat. Almost one-fifth (17%) of the mothers observed that cries were less frequent than at earlier ages.

Overall, infants did not have to wait to have their hunger cries responded to by 1 year. One third of the women said they anticipated their infant's hunger or that the infant ate three meals and did not cry for food; half noted that they responded immediately to their infant's hungry cry. Twelve percent stated they responded within 5 min, and 3% stated they responded within 10 to 24 min to a hungry cry.

Sleepy cries did not command as immediate a response as hunger cries. Fifty percent of the mothers reported they responded immediately to a sleepy cry, 20% responded within 5 min, 11% responded in 10 to 15 min, and 2% responded in 20 to 30 min.

Mothers were less patient with the demanding 1-year-old's angry cry. Over one-third (36%) reported that they ignored their infants' angry cries, but 28% responded immediately, 15% responded within 5 min, and 7% responded in 10 to 15 min. Nine percent of the mothers reported that they responded to an angry cry by swatting, spanking, or yelling.

INFANT STIMULATION

As infants develop, they demand and require novel and interesting stimuli. Mothers responded to these developmental needs in a variety of ways.

At 4 months mothers were using a variety of creative approaches in helping their infants to learn new things. They were teaching their infants the following: to talk, 69%; motor skills or coordination, 67%; to play, 47%; to identify objects through visual stimulation, pointing out and naming things, 45%; sounds, music, 16%; social interaction, 14%; to appreciate reading, 11%; touch, 10%; to entertain self, 8%; training (responding to commands, toilet training, feeding self), 5%; swimming/water skills, 3%; trust, 3%. The only significant age group difference was in teaching the infant to talk; Group 3 women mentioned this more often (65%, 66%, and 80%).

The 4-month-olds' increased capacity for social interactions was evidenced by the activities that the mothers said their infants enjoyed the most with them: motion activities (carry, jump, dance, swing, bounce), 71%; auditory (talk, sing, music, laugh), 71%; affection (kiss, hug, cuddle, rock, hold), 49%; and outings 34%. The teenagers less often described their infants as liking affection (23%, 60%, and 51%).

At 4 months 41% of the mothers stated they spent 3 to 4 hr daily interacting with their infants apart from caretaking activities; 22% spent 1 to 2 hr, 22% spent 5 to 6 hr, and 13% spent 7 or more hr. Three women from groups 2 and 3 stated they spent from 30 to 60 min a day interacting with their infants in non-caretaking activities.

At 8 months mothers were beginning to teach the infant to become independent. Mothers reported that they were teaching their infants the following: vocalizations, 58%; identification of objects, 40%; motor skills, 38%; to play with toys, 31%; socialization to environment, 28%; social games, 19%; to enjoy reading, 19%; music/singing, 14%; discipline, 12%; cognitive skills (counting, ABCs, shapes), 20%; feed self/brush teeth, 10%; to swim, 6%; and to watch television, 2%. Mothers in groups 2 and 3 more often reported they were teaching their infants to play with toys (11%, 37%, and 33%); and the older the woman, the more often she reported that she was socializing the infant to the environment (11%, 24%, and 42%).

At 8 months almost three-fourths of the women reported that the activity their infants enjoyed most was playing with them—patty-cake, tickle, and peek-a-boo. More than half stated that their infants liked to have them to play with their toys with them. Half stated that their infants enjoyed body contact such as holding, dancing, cuddling, or kissing. Rough play, such as tossing the infant in the air or chasing her, was reported by 42%. Thirty-seven percent reported their infants enjoyed vocalizing such as counting, nursery rhymes, and reading. Forty percent enjoyed outings, and 30% enjoyed singing, whistling, or music. One-fifth noted that their infants enjoyed their help in crawling or walking. There were no significant group differences for any of these activities or in the amount of time the mother spent with her infant in such activities.

When asked what they were teaching their 1-year-olds, mothers responded as follows: to identify objects, 59%; to talk, 44%; reading, books, 41%; to play with toys, 30%; discipline, self-control, 19%; colors, shapes, textures, 16%; to feed self or other self-help, 15%; counting, ABCs, spelling, 14%; to watch television/*Sesame Street,* 7%; gentleness with animals, 5%; toilet training, 4%; self-respect and confidence, 1%. These mothers were either consciously or unconsciously fostering the 1-year-old's development of self in their teaching of self-control, feeding or other self-help, self-respect and confidence.

Play and physical and social types of interactions were the activities that infants enjoyed most with their mothers at 1 year. Reported activities included games with the mother (hide-and-seek, peek-a-boo, horsey, tickle, see-saw), 75%; play with toys, 69%; outings and social interactions with others, 60%; physical games (chase, catch, dance, roughhouse), 57%; reading books, 39%; swimming, 15%. Other activities named to a lesser extent included television, eating, kissing, and motor skills. The older the mother, the more emphasis placed on reading books (18%, 38%, and 51%) and outings (28%, 40%, and 52%).

There were no significant group differences in the amount of time the women spent in these activities with their infants at 1 year. One-third of the women stated they spent 2 to 3 hr daily in other than caretaking activities; one-fourth spent from 4 to 8 hr; and 8% spent 1 hr or less. One-third said that the time spent varied from day to day because of their work schedules; working mothers in general spent more time in play activities and outings on weekends than on weekdays.

Father's Involvement

Father involvement in infant play and stimulation gradually increased over the year. As suggested by other researchers, fathers tended to differ somewhat in their play by introducing more physical and more creative types of play.

Fathers also were involved in teaching infants by 4 months. Over half of the women said that their mates were not teaching the infants anything different from what they were teaching; however, one-fourth noted that their mates engaged in rougher, more active physical play. Six percent stated that their mates were more adult, more formal, or quieter, and 6% stated mates were more creative and imaginative in the kinds of stimulation they provided for the infant.

Fathers continued to teach rougher, more physical, or more playful and fun things to the toddler at 1 year, as reported by 33% of the mothers. Another 16% of the women reported that fathers were teaching more creative things, such as animal sounds or a second language.

Freedom of Movement

The developing infant needs freedom and space to explore and experiment with newly developing motor skills. Most of the mothers were sensitive to the growing infant's increasing need for mobility.

At 4 months the infant had a wide range of places where she was allowed to play. The older the mother, the more likely she responded that she took the baby with her wherever she went in the house (55% of total, 30%, 41%, and 62% by age group). Fifty-five percent allowed the infant to play on the floor; 38% put the infant in an infant seat or an infant swing. One-fifth (21%) listed the mother's bed or the sofa as a play area, which was also the greatest source of infant accidents (falls from bed or sofa) at this time. Teenagers listed the bed or sofa more frequently (38%, 11%, and 13%). Nine percent of the infants were restricted to their cribs for play.

By 8 months the majority of the women reported that their infants were allowed to play all over the house (52%). One-third reported that infants played in walkers, playpens, or chairs. Only 14% of the women continued to restrict the infant to the crib or to one room in the house (22%, 18%, and 7%) at this time.

Over three-fourths (78%) let their infants play all over the house at 1 year; 12% were restricted to two rooms that were safer; and 10% were restricted to one room and playpen or crib. Group 1 infants were more restricted to a playpen or one or two rooms, which may be one reason that their infants did not stay ahead in motor and social development.

INFANT SAFETY

Infant safety has two components: the mother provides a safe environment for the infant to explore, and she teaches the infant what is safe and unsafe.

At 4 months, although 10% of the infants had experienced accidents, almost three-fourths of the women (72%) reported that safety had not come up as something to teach their infants yet; groups 2 and 3 responded that way most often (57%, 77%, and 76%). One-fourth said that they kept the infant away from unsafe situations; 16% responded they said no. Four women used tactics such as letting the infant fall in their arms from the table and putting the infant down harder and harder, and letting the infant feel a lukewarm coffee cup. Only 7% of the women were using physical means to teach unsafeness, but the teenager was more likely to say she hit, tapped, or patted the infant's hand when she reached for something unsafe (9%, 2%, and 2%).

By 8 months, when asked how they were teaching the infant that something was unsafe, only 8% said that the situation had not occurred yet. Sixty percent were saying no, with the younger women using this response significantly more often (78%, 66%, and 47%).

Removing the infant or the object was reported by 45% of the women. One-fourth of the women reported slapping the infant's hand, arm, or bottom, with teenagers using this method most frequently (49%, 26%, and 17%). One-fifth of the women were saying, "ouch," "hot," or "bad" to discourage the infant, with the older women using vocalization significantly more often (11%, 16%, and 27%). Eight percent reported using distraction, and 6% reported maintaining a safe environment.

Efforts to provide a safe environment were evident at 8-month home visits for interviews. Many mothers had covered electrical outlets, placed safety latches on kitchen cabinets, and put up gates across stairways to create a safer environment for the active, mobile 8-month-old. Other homes had many attractive nuisances such as plants, whatnots, and other types of clutter within easy reach of the exploring infant.

When asked how they were teaching their 1-year-olds that something was unsafe, only 2% stated that this had not happened, that their home was childproofed. The most frequent responses (37%) were to say no and distract or remove the infant from the situation, or to say no and act out, scold, or explain ("hot"). One-fourth of the mothers reported they spanked the infant's hand along with saying no.

Teaching and Discipline

Maternal attitudes about physical punishment were congruent with mothers' reports of what they were doing. As discussed in Chapter 2, the older the woman, the less likely she was to favor physical punishment. Younger mothers were using more physical punishment to discipline their infants.

When asked how they were disciplining their 1-year-olds, the women replied as follows: slapping, spanking, or swatting, 66%; moving or distracting, 55%; saying no and explaining why, 31%; had not disciplined, 7%; harsh vocalization, 5%; isolation, 5%. A very socially isolated Group 1 mother said she whipped her daughter with a riding crop; she was relieved to be referred to a social worker from Children's Protective Services who could help her. The younger the mother, the more often she reported slapping, spanking, or swatting (43%, 18%, and 17%) and the less often she reported using distraction (5%, 24%, and 28%). This finding indicates that maternal attitudes about discipline are translated into maternal behavior, and it is congruent with the teenagers' more strict disciplinarian attitudes.

Although 61% of the women reported they had been talked to as a form of discipline, only half were using that method; 52% reported they had been spanked, and 66% were spanking their children. Eight percent reported receiving harsh reprimands, and 5% were using that method; 24% had been isolated, and 5% were placing their children in a playpen as punishment. Differences may be expected because the women were reporting the types of discipline they remembered receiving, and discipline as an older child or as a teenager would be quite different from that for a 1-year-old. For example, talking to a 1-year-old will result in little immediate change in behavior, but removing the child to a different situation or using some form of distraction will remedy the undesired behavior at the moment.

Areas in which the women reported disagreeing with their mates regarding discipline included the following: mate more strict, lets cry, 29%; mate more protective or lenient, 29%; mate more inconsistent, 10%; and mate uses more physical punishment, 7%. More infrequent responses included mate teases, is a sexist, or has cultural differences. Overall, there seemed to be a balance in partner relationships; there were as many who viewed their mates as more strict as viewed their mates as more lenient.

FUTURE PLANS FOR THE CHILD

Mothers' future plans for their child were quite diverse. Future plans ranged from more immediate plans to enroll the child in a play group to far future plans regarding college years or the presidency. Responses included the following: nursery school/kindergarten, 23%; good school/education, 23%; take to parks, zoos, camping, 17%; singing/piano/music, 14%; private school, 12%; to be a good person, happy, worthwhile, 12%; travel, 12%; better environment/move, 12%; swim class, 11%; sports, 10%; play groups/interactions with other children, 7%; ballet/dance, 6%; creative outlets, 6%; a specific profession, 5%. Three saw their child as being a future president, three mentioned bank accounts, and three mentioned toilet training.

The only categories in which group differences were observed were in wanting the child to attend private school (28%, 14%, and 5%) and plans to enroll the child in play groups/interactions with other children (0%, 6%, and 13%). The teenager's desire for her child to attend a private school indicates that her school experience was less than optimal. Several teenagers mentioned that they didn't ever want their children to experience the pain that they had experienced.

MATERNAL PERCEPTIONS OF THE NEONATE

Maternal Perceptions of Neonate at Birth and at One Month

Maternal perceptions of the neonate may provide data for intervention. Infants rated as average or less than average at 1 month had more emotional problems at 4 and 10 to 11 years than infants who had been rated as better than average at 1 month (Broussard, 1976; Broussard & Hartner, 1970). To derive maternal perception of her neonate, the mother rated her infant on Broussard and Hartner's (1971) Neonatal Perception Inventories (NPI) on the behaviors of crying, feeding, spitting up or vomiting, bowel movements, and a predictable pattern of eating and sleeping; she then rated an average infant on these same behaviors. The total score for her baby is subtracted from the total score of the average baby form. A positive score indicates that a woman perceives her infant more favorably on these behaviors than she perceives an average infant.

At the initial test period the first 2 days after birth there were no significant age group differences in maternal perception of the neonate. Eighty percent of the teenagers, 76% of Group 2, and 70% of Group 3 rated their infants more positively than an average infant. Three-fourths of the total sample rated their infants positively, which is similar to Barnard and Eyres' (1979) findings that 79% did so. At 1 month 75% of the women again rated their infants more positively than the average infant; 66% of the teenagers, 76% of the 20-to-29-year-olds, and 80% of those 30 years and older. Similarly, 77% of the women in Barnard and Eyres' (1979) study rated their infants positively.

Fifty-seven percent of the group rated their infants more positively than an average infant at both early postpartum and 1 month (48%, 60%, and 58%). Eighteen percent who rated their infants positively during the early postpartum, rated their infants negatively at 1 month (30%, 17%, and 12%). Eighteen percent who rated their infants negatively at early postpartum rated their infants positively at 1 month (18%, 16%, and 21%). Seven percent of the women rated their infants negatively at both test periods (5%, 7%, and 8%).

Maternal Perceptions of the Neonate and Later Maternal Behavior

Differences were observed in maternal behaviors at 8 months following birth based on perceptions at both the early postpartum and 1-month test periods. Four groups were tested: those who rated their infants as above average at both test periods; those who rated their infants as above average at early postpartum and below average at 1 month; those who rated infants as below average at early postpartum and as above average at 1 month; and those who rated their infants as average or below at both early postpartum and 1 month.

Women whose infants were rated as above average at both early postpartum and 1 month or above average at early postpartum and average or below at 1 month reported significantly more gratification in the mothering role at 8 months than women whose infants were rated as average or below at *both* test periods. Women who rated infants as average or below at early postpartum and as above average at 1 month had gratification scores that were in between those two groups and did not differ significantly from either.

Women reported higher feelings of love for infants who were rated as above average at both early postpartum and 1 month than did those who had rated their infants as average or below at both test periods. Women who changed their ratings either way for the two test periods scored in between the two groups and did not differ significantly from either.

Observer-rated maternal behaviors were higher in the group who rated their infants as above average at both test periods than in those who changed from above average to below or average and those who rated infants as average or below at both test periods. Those who changed from average or below average to above average had scores that were in between and did not differ from either of the two groups. Observers (research assistants) were totally blind to the women's NPI scores.

There were no significant differences among the four groups for self-reported ways of handling irritating child behaviors at 8 months.

However, a more favorable score was observed in the group of women who had changed their ratings from average or below average
to above average at 1 month.

There were no significant differences in infant growth and development by the women's ratings of infants at the two test periods.
However, infants who were rated as above average at both test
periods had the highest scores, and infants who were rated as average
or below average at both times had the lowest scores.

An infant rated as above average at both postpartum and at 1
month was the beneficiary of higher feelings of love, more adaptable
or competent maternal behavior, and her mother's greater gratification in mothering at 8 months. The mother's gratification in the role
at 8 months may in part relate to her perceptions of her neonate, or
a common variable such as her view of motherhood may relate to
her satisfaction in the role and her perceptions of the neonate.
Realistically, the infant who is below average on items on the NPI
is more difficult to care for (cries more, spits up or vomits more,
and is less predictable for sleeping and eating). It may be easier to
develop feelings of love for an infant who is above average in these
categories during the first month. The more competent or adaptable
maternal behaviors for above-average infants at early postpartum and
1 month and infants who changed from average or below to above
average at 1 month indicates that less difficult infants are easier to
learn to care for.

At 1 year differences in all maternal role behaviors were tested
between mothers who had rated their infants as above average at 1
month and those who had rated their infants as average or below.
There were no significant differences in mothers' maternal role behaviors in any of the age groups or the total sample. In this sample of
mothers, initial perceptions of the neonate along with the 1-month
perceptions appeared to have greater potential for identifying later
differences. Long-term follow-up would be necessary to determine
whether infants who were rated as average or below average would
have the same incidence of emotional problems reported by Broussard (1976; Broussard & Hartner, 1970).

Degree of Infant Bother

There were no significant group differences for scores on the Degree
of Bother Inventory (Broussard & Hartner, 1971), which allowed the
mother to rate how much the infant's behaviors (crying, feeding,

spitting up or vomiting, sleeping, bowel movements, and predictable pattern) bothered her. When each of the behaviors was viewed separately, the only behavior in which age group differences was found was crying. The older woman's scores indicated that the infant's crying bothered them significantly more than was the case with the two younger groups of women.

PROFILE OF A GOOD BABY

Learning how a woman views a good baby provides guidelines for whether her expectations are realistic and whether her infant seems to fit her idea of a good baby. The infants' sleeping patterns and pleasant social interactive personality were important to the mothers.

Four Months

When women were asked to list five behaviors of a good 4-month-old, the most popular response was smiles/laughs a lot, is happy or has a good temperament (56%), and the next most frequent response was sleeps at night/naps well (43%). Teenagers most often noted that a good baby cries very little or is not fussy (58%, 36%, and 35%); 40% of the total sample gave this response. Thirty-nine percent stated that a good infant responds to or is vocal to the mother; the older the mother, the more frequently she gave this response (15%, 39%, and 54%). One-third were concerned that the infant eat well, and one-third were concerned that the infant entertain herself. Eleven percent noted that a good baby is affectionate and loves her mother or makes her laugh.

Eight Months

When asked to list five behaviors characteristic of a good infant, the most frequent response was sleeps well (48%); 46% stated the good infant smiles/is happy/has a good temperament. Thirty-seven percent noted that the good infant eats well; 35% reported she entertains self; and 32% reported that she responds, talks, and interacts. Other responses included the following: cries very little, 24%; is curious, alert, smart, inquisitive, 19%; is playful, 16%; is affectionate, 16%; adapts easily, is patient, 12%; is healthy, 11%. Fifteen percent stated that nothing that a baby did was bad, that everything a baby did was good.

The older the woman, the more likely she was to respond that a good infant smiles, is happy, or has a good temperament (34%, 43%, and 57%), or adapts easily, is patient (3%, 11%, and 18%). Group 2 women more often listed that a good infant is affectionate (3%, 21%, and 16%).

INFANT TEMPERAMENT

Unique responses from birth have supported the idea that there are innate differences in an individual's responses to stimuli and to life in general (Buss & Plomin, 1975; Thomas & Chess, 1977, 1980). Nine categories of infant temperament were measured—activity level, rhythmicity, approach-withdrawal, adaptability, intensity, mood, persistence, distractibility, and threshold to stimulus—at 4 and 8 months.

The 4-month findings regarding infant temperament must be viewed with caution because the reliabilities for intensity, persistence, distractibility, and threshold to stimulus were very low, ranging from .06 to .49. At 8 months reliabilities were acceptable for all temperament categories. It is difficult to know whether mothers were more objective or sensitive to their infants' behaviors at 8 months to contribute to the increased reliabilities.

Four Months

There were no significant age group differences in the categories of activity level, mood, and distractibility. The teenagers' infants were scored as being less rhythmic than Group 2 infants, and Group 3 infants scored in between the two younger groups. The younger the age group, the greater their infants tended toward withdrawal as opposed to approach in new situations.

Group 3 infants were scored as more adaptable than the two younger groups of infants. Both of the younger groups' infants were scored higher on intensity than Group 3 infants. Group 1 infants were scored higher on persistence than Group 3 infants, with Group 2 infants scoring in between and not differing significantly from either. Group 3 infants had a higher threshold to stimulus than

Group 2 infants, but Group 1 infants scored in between without differing significantly from either.

In general, the teenagers' infants were scored by their mothers as more arrhythmic, more withdrawn, less adaptable, and higher in intensity than infants of older mothers. Group 3 tended to score their infants lower in persistence and intensity and higher in threshold to stimulus, approach to new objects, and adaptability.

The infants were then classified into five diagnostic clusters: easy, intermediate low, slow to warm up, intermediate high, and difficult. Easy, slow-to-warm-up, and difficult clusters were defined earlier in the chapter; the intermediate clusters included all others who did not fit into the three major clusters.

More than three-fourths of the infants (77%) were rated as easy (70%, 76%, and 83%) 9% were rated as intermediate low (15%, 11%, and 3%), 7% were rated as slow to warm up (8%, 9%, and 5%), 2% as intermediate high (0%, 1%, and 6%), and 4% as difficult (8%, 3%, and 3%).

Correlations with Maternal Temperament at 4 Months Because individual differences in mothers (such as attitudes) rather than differences in infants, may contribute to early ratings of temperament (Sameroff, Seifer, & Elias, 1982; Vaughn et al., 1981), correlations between maternal and infant temperaments were done by age group. In the teenage group there was a significant positive relationship between maternal and infant adaptability only (r = -.36). In Group 2 there were significant positive relationships between maternal and infant rhythmicity (r = -.26), adaptability ($\bar{r}$ = -.27), quality of mood (r = -.34), persistence (r = -.23), and distractability (r = -.19). In Group 3 there were significant positive relationships between maternal and infant rhythmicity (r = -.23), persistence (r = -.24), and threshold to stimulus (r = -.26). (Because high infant scores reflect low or negative on each trait, and high maternal scores reflect high for each trait, the negative correlations indicate positive relationships.)

Eight Months

There were significant group differences in only two of the temperament categories at 8 months. Group 3 scored their infants significantly higher on approach behaviors than the two groups of younger women. The two groups of older women scored their infants' behaviors significantly higher in adaptability than did the teenage group.

By diagnostic cluster, 70% of the women rated their infants as easy (74%, 71%, and 67%), 10% as intermediate low (2%, 10%, and 14%), 5% as slow to warm up (5%, 7%, and 3%), 10% as intermediate high (7%, 8%, and 12%), and 5% as difficult (12%, 4%, and 3%). Overall, fewer infants were in the easy cluster at 8 months (70%) than at 4 months (77%). Twelve infants who had been categorized as easy at 4 months were categorized as difficult at 8 months. A few more Group 1 infants were in the easy cluster at 8 months than at 4 months (74%, compared with 70%).

The overall percentage of infants in the difficult cluster varied little from 4 to 8 months. More Group 1 infants were in the difficult cluster at 8 months than at 4 months (12%, compared with 8%). The more difficult infant may have contributed to their declining gratification in the mothering role. Ten of the 14 subjects who withdrew from the study at 8 months had infants who were categorized as difficult at 4 months.

There were no gender differences by diagnostic cluster. Maternal role strain was not greater for mothers of infants in any one cluster.

Correlation between Maternal and Infant Temperament at Eight Months Significant positive relationships were observed in the teenage group for maternal and infant temperament categories of adaptability (r = -.30) and quality of mood state (r = -.35). In the Group 2 positive significant relationships were observed between adaptability (r = -.38), quality of mood state (r = -.36), intensity (r = -.25), and persistence (r = -.22). In Group 3 significant positive correlations were observed only for the category of intensity (r = -.23). (Again, the negative correlations indicate positive relationships.)

Whether the older, more mature women in Group 3 rated their infants' behavior more objectively is conjectural. There were fewer relationships between the mother's own temperament and that of her infant.

The Relationship of Temperament Variables to Mothering Behaviors

Because infant temperament has been linked with later mothering behaviors (Campbell, 1979; Simonds & Simonds, 1981), infants were grouped by the five temperament clusters to determine whether their mothers' maternal behaviors differed at 8 months. There were no significant differences in gratification in the maternal role, observed maternal behavior, of self-reported ways of handling irritating child behaviors by infant cluster. This finding differed from that of Feiring (1976), who observed that mothers with difficult infants had greater difficulty adapting to the maternal role.

Women who had difficult or slow-to-warm-up infants had significantly lower feelings of love for their infants, however. Simonds and Simonds (1981) observed that mothers of difficult and slow-to-warm-up preschoolers tended to use detachment and distancing as a way of controlling their infants. The finding that mothers of 8-month-old difficult and slow-to-warm-up infants scored their feelings of love lower than mothers of infants in other temperament clusters raises the question of whether these feelings may continue on through preschool years to reflect behaviors observed by Simonds and Simonds. The difficult or slow-to-warm-up infant's behaviors apparently do not elicit feelings of attachment to the extent that infants in other temperament clusters do.

IMPLICATIONS FOR NURSING INTERVENTION

The growth and development of these infants during the first year following birth agree with other research in which evidence was lacking that young maternal age contributes to poorer health and developmental outcome for their infants (Mercer, 1984; Merritt et al., 1980; Roosa et al., 1982a, 1982b; Rothenberg & Varga, 1981). However, subtle differences appeared throughout to suggest that in some areas of teaching, infant stimulation, and discipline older women focus on different kinds of behaviors (cognitive and socialization skills) and provide an environment with less physical punishment. These subtle differences in maternal behavior may not influence infant behavior during the first year but may have long-range effects. For example, more older women reported that they read to their infants, and that activity was recently associated with higher intellectual and social development at 5 years of age (Squires, 1985).

By 4 months three-fourths of the infants were on a predictable schedule and cried less, and four-fifths ate well. However, a source of accidents was falls from sofas or beds where one-fifth of the women reported they put their 4-month-old to play. Safety in relationship to the developing infant is a very important area to stress;

the 4- to 5-month-old is just learning to roll over and can easily roll off the bed or sofa, much to the surprise of mothers who are accustomed to an infant staying where she is placed. All women would benefit from learning more about infant competencies and the types of auditory, visual, and motor stimulation that are safe and that infants prefer.

Introduction of Solid Foods in Infant Diet

Sixty percent of the teenagers' infants, 48% of Group 2 infants, and 40% of Group 3 infants were above the 50th percentile for weight at 1 year (Mercer, 1984). The larger weight gain of the teenagers' infants raises several questions. Teenagers introduced solid foods earlier, and fewer breast-fed over the year. Do teenagers overfeed their infants and establish a pattern for later obesity and hypertension? Is feeding a concrete mothering act in which teenagers feel more secure? Neuman and Alpaugh's (1976) findings indicate that early introduction of solid foods contributes to more rapid weight gain during the first year. Mothers of lower SES had less knowledge about nutrition, and both they and their children had a greater incidence of adiposity than middle-class mothers in a recent study (Saltzer & Golden, 1985). There is indication that the trend toward greater obesity in lower-SES groups begin. very early because lower-SES children and mothers are alike in adiposity, whereas this relationship was not found for middle-class children. More teenagers were in a lower SES than those in groups 2 and 3.

The myth that early introduction to solid foods leads to the infant's sleeping through the night or going for longer intervals between feedings needs to be dispelled. Findings in this study and in Entwisle and Doering's study (1981) indicate that early introduction of solid foods does not affect infants' sleep patterns.

When teaching that infants should not have solid foods introduced before they are 5 months old, it is important to include the teenagers' mothers because they are the major information source for this group of women. The major objection to introduction of foods other than milk before 5 months is that it may interfere with establishing sound eating habits and contributes to overfeeding (Foman et al., 1979). Until the infant is able to sit alone and has good neuromuscular control of her head and neck, she cannot indicate a desire for food by opening her mouth and leaning forward or indicate lack of interest or satiety by leaning back and turning away (Foman et al., 1979). Early feeding of solids may be linked to forced feeding and/ or overfeeding.

Infant Schedules during the First Year

The greatest change in the number of infants with a regular schedule occurred from the first to the fourth month with little change there-after (39% at 1 month, 75% at 4 months, 88% at 8 months, 75% at 12 months). Mothers need to know that the majority of infants just do not have a regular schedule before 4 months.

Mothers may not think about the amount of time required for feeding the infant when they think of schedules. It takes an average of 25 to 30 min to feed an infant. Each infant develops her own pace, but mothers need to know the general range of time to expect to spend in infant feeding. With feedings every 3 to 4 hr this trans-lates to a minimum of 3 to 4 hr per day spent in feeding the infant; that does not include the time spent in changing diapers before and after feedings.

Infant feedings become easier from 1 to 4 months, then become more difficult after 8 months; 75% of the mothers said feedings went well at 1 month and 81% at 4 months, but by 12 months only 71% reported that feedings were going well. The infant's rapid growth spurt is slowing by 1 year, and her need to eat less may not be recognized by mothers. A 1-year-old prefers foods that she can eat by herself, probably a reflection of her developing autonomy.

Teaching Safety Needs of Infant

The socialization of the infant during the first year of life changes as motor and cognitive skills develop over the year. For example, teaching the infant that something was unsafe had not come up for 72% of the mothers at 4 months, for 8% at 8 months, but for less than 2% at 12 months. Teaching how to provide a protective environ-ment is a very important part of counseling during the first year of life. Accidents occur among infants of mothers of all ages.

The use of infant car seats when driving with the infant is critical from birth and mandatory by law in many states. Before the infant begins to crawl, mothers should be encouraged to inventory all areas of their homes and to write down a list of childproofing that must be done. Large tablecloths may look lovely, but if a curious infant pulls a bowl of fruit down on her head, then the grief outweighs any temporary enjoyment of beauty. Burns from pulling cords of electric coffeepots or from reaching for hot cups of coffee are common. Ingestion of poisonous dishwashing detergents and other caustic agents may be prevented. Covering electrical sockets, putting safety latches on cabinet doors, and placing harmful detergents on high shelves help provide a safe environment for the exploring infant.

Discipline

The lack of parental agreement about discipline was not expected for many. There are really *six* persons negotiating about how the child should be disciplined—the mother, the father, the mother's parents, and the father's parents. Even if the grandparents are deceased or live thousands of miles away, their imprints on the mother and father are present to be negotiated between the mother and father.

Teenagers will benefit by role-modeling behaviors that distract the exploring infant. Fewer teenagers reported using distraction in disciplining their infant. With concrete examples to show how easily an infant can be distracted to a novel object or sound, these young women might adopt these behaviors and use less physical punishment.

Infant Crying

Counseling about infant crying is an important area for intervention because it is evident there is a wide array of attitudes about infant crying. Almost one-fifth of the women in this sample felt that crying is good for the month-old infant; however, Bell and Ainsworth (1972) found that early maternal responsiveness to infant crying was associated with secure attachment after the eighth month. Infants whose mothers had responded to them promptly also cried less and had a wider range of communication than other infants.

Newton (1983) outlined several helpful suggestions for parents regarding crying: encourage parents to rethink their attitudes about infant crying; help parents find factual information about crying; explain that responding promptly and lovingly has not been related to reinforcing crying or leading to a demanding child; explain that responding does not always mean holding—changing the infant's location, offering stimulation, talking to, or taking on an outing are all alternatives; and explain that infants sense the parents' emotional state and continue to cry when anxiety or tenseness is sensed. The teenager in particular can benefit by learning that crying is not spoiled or "mean" behavior during the first half of the first year.

Group 3 women who expressed frustration and feelings of incompetence at infant crying may need additional assurance. Group 3 was bothered more by infant crying than groups 1 and 2 at 1 month; the crying infant perhaps dramatizes a situation for which they have no ready solution. Pickens (1982) observed that career women over 30 experienced role inadequacy as mothers and as career women the first 3 to 4 months following birth.

Maternal Perceptions of Infant Responses/Temperament

The lone significant correlation between persistence in maternal and infant temperaments in Group 3 at 8 months indicates that this older group of women may be making more objective assessments of their infants. In groups 1 and 2 women's temperament categories of adaptability and quality of mood were significantly related to their infants' adaptability and quality of mood. It is impossible to know whether mothers tended to rate their infants similarly to themselves, or whether there was more of a fit between mother and infant for temperament categories in these age groups. Vaughn and associates (1981) reported that in their sample, the Carey Infant Temperament Questionnaire was an assessment of maternal characteristics as well as maternal perceptions of infant temperament.

Regardless of whether maternal perceptions about infant behavior reflect maternal characteristics, these perceptions were associated with how mothers felt about thier infants at 8 months. Mothers' perceptions of their neonates as measured by Broussard and Hartner's (1971) inventory during the first days of life and at 1 month were related to their reported feelings about the mothering role and about their infants. Women who perceived their infants as average or below average at early postpartum and 1 month derived less gratification in the mothering role, had lower feelings of love for their infants, and were less competent in mothering behaviors at 8 months postpartum. Women whose infants were classified in difficult and slow-to-warm-up diagnostic clusters at 8 months also reported lower feelings of love for their infants.

The nurse's careful listening to a mother's perception of her infant's behavior is important. If a particular type of behavior is bothersome to the mother, this needs to be discussed in regard to the infant's development, any change that can be expected to occur, and possible strategies for coping with the behavior.

Ranges of normal behavior and expectations need to be stressed rather than established norms. Terms such as *active, persistent,* and *easily upset* are good terms to use in describing a difficult infant to a mother. Demonstrations on how the infant who is high on withdrawal and irritability temperament traits can be coaxed during quiet alert states, cuddled, or maybe made comfortable and left to quiet alone can be the most helpful to new mothers. A modified Brazelton newborn assessment done by the nurse while the mother observes oftens highlights infant competencies and infant capabilities and abilities of which the mother is unaware, and it can greatly relieve her. Even if she has a highly irritable, withdrawn infant, a mother is pleased to see that her infant can raise her head away from confining positions and brush a cloth from her face. The behaviors demonstrate culturally valued aspects of independence or of being a fighter for many.

Social Support

When the nurse identifies a more difficult infant, it is helpful to determine who will be helping the mother when she goes home. When a mother has high social support, irritable infants are less distressing. Additional social support in the form of reassurance in their mothering role, available respite situations, and 24-hr phone lines that provide information and encouragement are important to women who doubt their infants' capacities or their abilities to care for their infants.

CHAPTER 5

First Month: Pervasive Fatigue and Frustration

The first month of motherhood was a period of much change in routines and household schedules, as well as within the personal lives of the women. The lack of a predictable schedule for the majority of the infants meant that plans could not be made and that sleep was frequently interrupted. Mothers had not recuperated from childbirth and continued to experience health problems over the month. This milieu contributed to feelings of frustration and inadequacy, although teenagers less often described these feelings. The 20- to 29-year-old women were quite open about expressing their feelings of frustration in dealing with motherhood:

- A week ago, I really preferred not to even have her; I felt like bouncing her off the wall.
- I get so frustrated I want to shake my baby; I don't do it, but the feeling is there.
- Sometimes I want to hit him, but I know I can't.
- The first week I felt I didn't want her; I didn't feel free to do anything, and I still haven't gotten over it.

The group of mothers 30 years and older expressed frustrations and also questioned their decision to have an infant:

- This surely is different; I have never undertaken anything that I felt more incompetent in. I have the feeling that I don't know what I'm doing.
- When I was first home I thought I must be crazy. What did I want to do this for?

- I cried all of the way home from the hospital. I felt that I had crossed a threshold and could never go back. I never thought about what having a baby would be like. It was a mourning period.

The latter statement typifies the grief work described by Rubin (1967a) in achieving the maternal identity. This mother is grieving the loss of her earlier life-style. She realizes that she can never return to her earlier non-mother self.

At the first-month-postpartum interview 276 mothers partici- pated; 61 mothers aged 15 to 19 years in Group 1, 126 aged 20 to 29 years in Group 2, and 89 aged 30 to 42 years in Group 3. Their responses to the challenges of motherhood during this period follow an overview of research about the first month postpartum. The vig- nettes depicting the personal experiences of the 12 women whose childbirth and early postpartum experiences were described in Chap- ter 3 are continued, with proposed nursing interventions for the first month postpartum concluding the chapter.

TASKS OF THE FIRST POSTPARTUM MONTH

The first postpartum month is particularly trying for first-time parents who are making many adjustments in the transition to parenthood. Multiple tasks face the new mother during this post- partum period. She has to identify and place her infant within her family context; this involves identifying the infant's physical charac- teristics and behaviors and relating these observations to family mem- bers and events (Gottlieb, 1978; Mercer, 1981b; Rubin, 1984). As she studies her infant's behavior, she sensitizes herself to the in- fant's cues and learns to meet the infant's needs.

Acceptance of the infant by other family members is of critical importance. The new mother works hard at assimilating the infant into the family unit and learning to manage the infant's care along with managing the household (Boss, 1980). She redefines her roles in relation to her mate, her infant, her parents, her career, and other roles (Sheehan, 1981). The grief work illustrated above indicates that the transition to motherhood, while highly anticipated, creates disequilibrium as new relationships are developed.

Mothers face these tasks handicapped by fatigue and emotional tension created by the postpartum adjustment and recuperation from the birth process (Grossman et al., 1980; Gordon, Kapostins,

& Gordon, 1965). More physical symptoms are reported by women during the first postpartum month than at any time during pregnancy (Leifer, 1977).

MATERNAL CONCERNS

Lack of an opportunity to review the events that occurred during labor (Carlson, 1976) or to make sense of gaps in memory of the birth process (Affonso, 1977) may contribute to feelings of lower self-esteem and lead the mother to question her ability to be a good mother. Many emotional concerns about herself, her baby, husband, family, and others persist during the early hospitalization period and her first week at home (Bull, 1981). The new mother's concerns about her infant are intense and constant during the first week at home.

Special programs of intervention during the postpartum period have provided support in some areas, but have not reduced the number of concerns that the inexperienced mother faces. Home visits by a public health nurse helped alleviate mothers' concerns about infant feeding, but those who were visited reported a greater number and more intense concerns about infant crying than those who had no visit (Brown, 1967). Infant crying raised anxiety and feelings of helplessness, as was discussed in Chapter 4. When a mother is unable to stop the cry, she feels helpless and that she is failing to meet her infant's needs. One explanation for the greater number of concerns expressed by mothers visited by a public health nurse is that they were encouraged to express their concerns, and with this encouragement were more comfortable expressing them.

Women who participated in family-centered care during the first 2 months postpartum also reported more physical and psychological problems than women receiving traditional care (Jordan, 1973a, 1973b, 1973c). Unless special interest is displayed or permission is granted for voicing concerns (inquiry is made and time allotted to discuss them), women may be hesitant to admit that they need help. Mothers found information provided during postpartum hospitalization about the infant's physical care and feeding particularly helpful but expressed a desire for more information about infant behavior (Bull & Lawrence, 1985). In some situations, there is a maternal need during the first six weeks postpartum for validation that they were doing the right thing for their infants, rather than instructions about infant care (Sumner & Fritsch, 1977).

Those who enroll in special classes or programs usually receive encouragement to explore their concerns in classes; however, such persons may have higher anxiety or greater concerns than those who don't enroll in such classes (Fillmore & Taylor, 1976). Similar to findings in the studies cited above, the amount of in-hospital demonstration, home assistance, and advice were all positively related to concern scores (Fillmore & Taylor, 1976). Breast-feeding, modal age for having first child (20–24 years), extent of reading about child and infant care, years of education, experience with infant and child care, amount of in-hospital demonstrations of infant care, amount of assistance at home with the infant, and number of sources of advice on infant care problems predicted 53% of the variance in the crying concern score. Predicted variance in other concerns included routine care, 47%; feeding, 45%; elimination, 35%; sleeping, 31%; bathing, 29%; and all concerns, 45%.

Breast-feeding mothers had lower average concern scores than bottle-feeding mothers (Fillmore & Taylor, 1976). The modal-age first-time mothers (20–24 years) had higher concern scores than women aged 15 to 19 and 25 to 38 years in every category except crying. Women with more years of education and experience with infant and child care had lower concern scores. Infant crying was the greatest concern to all mothers, with elimination and routine care the next greatest concerns; this is in contrast to earlier findings by Adams (1963) that caretaking activities were mothers' greatest concerns. There are two important components in concern—interest and anxiety (Fillmore & Taylor, 1976). Interest in learning about the infant plays a positive role in the mother–child relationship. A certain amount of anxiety also has been associated with commitment to the care of the infant and in providing good mothering care (Robertson, 1962).

POSTPARTUM DEPRESSION

High anxiety during the postpartum transition period may contribute to depression (Paykel et al., 1980). Mild clinical depression was observed in 20% of 120 mothers at 6 weeks postpartum by Paykel and associates (1980). Recent stressful life events were most strongly related to depression, with previous history of psychiatric disorder, younger age, early postpartum blues, a poor marital relationship, and lack of support having a lesser influence. Lower incidences of postpartum depression have been reported by others—10 to 14% on the third day postpartum (Manly, McMahon, & Bradley, & David-

son, 1982) and 12% during the first 9 weeks (O'Hara, Ne
Zekoski, 1984). In contrast, Brown (1978) reported very l
partum depression among teenagers but rather an emotio
she also noted that the majority of the teenage mothers had much
support at home. Hostility peaked and feelings of deprivation were
high at 1 month among mothers in another study, although depression was not noted (Mercer, 1980).

Other maternal age differences in depression have been suggested.
A significantly greater number of women 27 years and older were
depressed postpartum than those aged 18 to 26 years (Uddenberg,
1974). Many factors are thought to contribute to postpartum depression: feelings of incompetence in the role, fatigue, body image,
and conflict with the maternal role. Fatigue and the lack of any personal time appears to be a critical problem; women reported less time
for husbands, household tasks, and for themselves during the first
month postpartum (Grubb, 1980). Conflict over the mothering role
was a major stressor contributing to postpartum depression (Melges,
1968).

Dissatisfaction with her body image also contributes to the new
mother's feelings about herself and to depression, particularly when
her bodily functioning is not yet up to par (Rubin, 1984). The unmet expectation that the expanded body size of pregnancy will
have returned to the prepregnancy size can cause much concern
(Gruis, 1977). At 4 weeks many women expect that they can wear
prepregnancy clothes and are distressed with flabby abdomens and
excess weight. By contrast, only 6% of the total responses of teenage
mothers related to body image concerns (Mercer, 1980). A more
attractive appearance and better hygiene was observed among teenagers than among older women postpartum (Brown, 1978). Multiparous mothers felt better about their body image than primiparous
mothers at 2 and 6 weeks postpartum (Strang & Sullivan, 1985),
which may indicate that they did not expect their bodies to have returned to prepregnancy conditions or that they had less time to
focus on themselves.

SELF-CONFIDENCE AND MOTHERING

The woman's personality characteristics of ego strength, self-confidence and nurturant qualities have been identified as basic determinants of her capacity as a mother (Shereshefsky et al., 1973; Wise &
Grossman, 1980). Mothers who do not trust themselves or their
caretakers during the early postpartum period have difficulty trusting

their infants to respond positively to them (Kennedy, 1973). Mothers who expressed negative feelings also were more outwardly aggressive toward their 2-week-old infants with behaviors such as shaking them or yelling at them (Kennedy, 1973).

When there are difficulties with postpartum adaptation, the mother's self-confidence and concept are affected. Mothers who had greater difficulty adapting during the postpartum had a decrease in self-concept scores at 3 months (Curry, 1983). Arnold (1980) found a positive relationship between self-concept and maternal self-confidence among teenagers who had previous mothering skills.

MOTHER-INFANT INTERACTIONS

The process of mother-infant attachment that began during pregnancy, continues postpartum (Cranley, 1981b; Leifer, 1977). Extensive research during the postpartum period has focused on the process of mother-infant attachment and early interactions that enhance the process. Effects of early contact on maternal-infant bonding have not been consistently supported (Lamb, 1982, 1983). Although short-term effects of early contact on maternal attachment have been observed, no enduring outcomes have been found. Special at-risk groups of women may benefit more from early contact—those with less social support (Ainsfeld & Lipper, 1983); or from special teaching—teenagers with less support, education, and ego development (Levine, Coll, & Oh, 1985).

Maternal Age Differences

Postpartum observations comparing early mother-infant interactions by maternal age group have differed. The possibility of a critical age for maternal readiness was suggested (Jones et al., 1980). Findings by Hardman (1975) that teenage mothers 13 to 15 years old had fewer positive and more negative responses to their infants than a group who were 16 to 17 years old indicate that a certain level of maturity facilitates transition to the maternal role.

Older women in a sample 17 to 30 years old were more competent in caretaking and mothering (Ragozin et al., 1982). Older and better educated women also tend to prepare more for the mothering role through classes (Pickens, 1982). For example, a survey of 611 couples in childbirth classes identified that 45% were 26 years or older, 68% had 1 or more years of college, and 76% planned to breast-feed (Watson, 1977); these characteristics differ from the general pregnant population. As was discussed above, interest and a certain level of anxiety seem to accompany a commitment to motherhood; indications are that the commitment to motherhood may increase with increasing age.

Cultural Variations

Many cultural variations in mother–infant interaction have been observed. A different sequence of attachment behavior events were reported among black low-income women (15–24 years) from those reported for other groups, which were characteristic for that cultural group (Bampton, Jones, & Mancini, 1981). Japanese mothers talk to their infants more when they are crying, and American mothers talk to their infants more when they are in a happy state (Caudill & Weinstein, 1969). American mothers also have a livelier approach to infants, whereas Japanese mothers seem to have a more quieting, soothing approach. Egyptian mothers' behavior toward their newborns is directed toward drawing the infant into the family circle; the desire to make him a family member is stronger than the desire to identify him as an individual (Govaerts & Patino, 1981). American mothers spend significantly more time in evaluating and delineating their infants' behaviors and functioning than Chinese mothers (Chao, 1983).

In summary, all reports agree that the postpartum period is a difficult transition period for first-time mothers. Research thus far has been able to account for one-third to over one-half of the sources of maternal concern postpartum. Depression has been reported as accompanying early mothering in 10 to 20% of samples. Data are lacking about variables affecting the adaptation to motherhood the first month postpartum, particularly for the woman who is 30 years or older. Responses of women in this study indicate maternal age differences in several areas.

MOTHER'S OVERALL FEELINGS: PHYSICAL AND EMOTIONAL

There appears to be a close relationship between the mothers' physical and emotional feelings. Their bodily function had not returned to prepregnancy status. They were experiencing pain and soreness from surgical incisions and engorged breasts, and they encountered several physical problems during the first month. This physical state, along with the situation of an infant who had not yet achieved a predictable schedule, contributed to a state of pervasive fatigue and over half of the women feeling blue or depressed at 1 month.

Physical Feelings and Problems

Physical Feelings The mothers used a variety of colorful terms to describe their physical feelings; several feelings were described by some. The pervasive, overall feeling reported by the majority of the women (55%) at 1 month was fatigue; they never felt rested. The older the woman, the more likely that she reported fatigue (43%, 57%, and 62%).[1]

When assessing their health status, a majority (61%) were somewhat hesitant in admitting their feelings and used more neutral terms such as, "things are going all right," "oh, better," "so-so," or "a little improved." Less than one-fourth (22%) reported that their overall feelings were either lousy, rough, "the pits," or strange (10%, 30%, and 20%). Ten women who described feeling strange noted that they felt stupid, unstable, or lacking in confidence; no teenager described such a feeling of strangeness.

Only 7% of the women described their overall feeling state as great, fantastic, happy, or terrific. There were no significant group differences.

Specific Physical Problems Almost half of the mothers reported a physical problem during the first month following birth. Significantly fewer teenagers reported a physical problem (21%, 48%, and 49%). The most common physical complaint was the soreness, numbness, or pain in either the episiotomy or cesarean birth incisions; 22% described this problem, and the older women did so significantly more often than the teenagers (9%, 23%, and 30%).

Thirteen percent of the women had gynecological problems that included vaginal bleeding with clots and cramps, and infections of the endometrium, fallopian tubes, breasts, or perineum, e.g., stitches ripping out. None of the teenagers reported vaginal bleeding prob-

---

[1] Series of three figues in parentheses indicates percentages for the three groups from the youngest to the oldest, respectively.

lems. Seven of the women had been hospitalized to treat a problem during their first postpartum month, four from Group 1 and three from Group 2.

Twelve percent of the women reported a variety of problems such as hemorrhoids, backache, skin problems, edema, and engorged or sore breasts (3%, 15%, and 15%). Colds, viruses, flu, or other upper respiratory infections had been problematic to 7% of the women (no group differences). Two women in each of the two older groups reported chronic health problems such as diabetes or myasthenia gravis.

Teenagers scored significantly more favorably than both of the older groups on maternal health status factor that was derived from overall feelings during the first month and the number of problems described. Fewer cesarean births among teenagers probably contributed to this difference. The more youthful body had a greater resiliency in healing postpartum, and this study supports the conclusion of Merritt and associates (1980) that from a medical viewpoint 16 to 19 years was an ideal age for childbirth if women have prenatal care. Differences between groups 2 and 3 were not notable.

Emotional Responses

Just under one-fourth of the mothers (24%) described a "high," a feeling of excitement or of feeling good with no blues or depression. More teenagers expressed positive emotional feelings than the two older groups (39%, 18%, and 22%). This finding agrees with the Brown's (1978) observations that more teenagers than older women experienced an emotional high postpartally.

Almost one-third of the women (30%) reported that they had had the blues or were depressed earlier but that they were now feeling better. Eight (3%) identified the depression as occurring after their mothers or other relative who had been helping them left. Although there was still some tenseness or anxiety felt, their current feelings were improved over those experienced earlier. Only 1% of the women in the study reported more neutral emotional feelings during the first month postpartum.

Just over half (53%) of the women reported that they were still blue, depressed, cried easily, felt deprived or on edge, up and down, or sad at 1 month postpartum. Significantly more of the two older groups reported these feelings (23%, 61%, and 61%). Again, differences between teenagers and groups 2 and 3 were significant, supporting Brown's (1978) observations that fewer teenagers experienced depression.

Isolated feelings of loneliness or of being ostracized by friends were described. A few reported that they were working out feelings about their birth experience and were depressed about that.

Although the depression described by the women was not categorized in any clinical manner, four-fifths of the women were blue or upset to some extent during their first postpartum month. Fatigue and the felt responsibility in mothering both seemed to play a large part in these feelings. It is important that the differences in the physical status of the age groups be kept in mind. Group 1 had fewer operative interventions for delivery and felt better physically the first month; their bodily functioning must be kept in mind. Rubin (1984) stressed that until a woman recuperates from childbirth and feels whole, she feels inadequate to the task of mothering; this may account for more reported depression in the two older groups.

MAJOR CONCERNS ARISING DURING THE FIRST MONTH POSTPARTUM

Major concerns identified by the women at this time are listed in the order of their reported frequency: infant, $n = 438$; mothering, $n = 258$; career, $n = 112$; husband/mate relationships, $n = 55$; and body image, $n = 43$. These findings are in agreement with others about the infant and mothering the infant being major sources of concern during the first month (Adams, 1963; Fillmore & Taylor, 1976; Sumner & Fritsch, 1977) but in disagreement with Gruis (1977), who reported body image a major concern. The large number voicing concern about career or returning to work at 1 month is a new finding but is probably indicative of the national economy changes and the higher cost of living.

Concerns about the Infant

The great majority (87%) of the women listed from one to three concerns about their infants (30% listed one, 30% listed two, and 23% listed three concerns). There were no significant group differences in number of concerns listed or in the numbers reporting specific concerns about the infant, with one exception, which suggests that the level of interest in and anxiety about mothering was similar among all ages at this time.

Almost half of the women (47%) were concerned about their infant's health in some way. There was concern about potential sickness, colic or spitting up, and the infant's response to innoculations.

Over one-third of the women were concerned about their infant's future (29%, 39%, and 36%). Thirty-nine (14%) were concerned about the far future such as the year 2000, the infant's leaving home, and a savings account for the infant's education. Other future-oriented women did not go beyond the high school years, but they wanted to be sure their children would be happy, went to good schools, had good study habits, had a religious upbringing, were popular, and had friends. A couple of the teenagers' statements indicated much personal pain as they described wanting something less painful for their child than they had. One teenager wondered whether she should have relinquished her infant for adoption.

Just over one-fifth (22%) were concerned about more immediate decisions in infant care. These included such things as when to move the infant out of their bedroom, whether the infant was getting enough to eat, what to do in an emergency, and the correct temperature of the room.

Their infant's growth and development was a concern for 16% of the women. Concern was expressed about physical and emotional growth, weight loss, and infant behavior.

Fifteen percent of the women had concerns about their infants' skin or hair. Rashes, peeling skin, and hair falling out raised questions. One infant had a hemangioma diagnosed during this time. Nine percent of the women worried about their infant's breathing pattern; a few were afraid of crib death. A television program on sudden infant death syndrome (SIDS) during this period seemed to have contributed to some of the women's anxiety. Seven percent worried about the infant's bowel movements, particularly constipation, irregularity, and difficulty in having a movement. Seven percent also worried about the possibility of accidental injury to the infant—a car accident, the infant's rolling off the bed, or choking in the event he spit up.

The occurrence of accidents was the *only* area of infant concern in which significant age differences occurred; the older the woman, the more likely she was to worry about an accident involving the infant (2%, 4%, and 16%). Group 3 women seemed a little more tuned in to the possibility of accidents.

Concerns about Mothering

Over one-third of the women (37%) voiced concern about the quality of their mothering. They wished to be good mothers and were fearful of doing "something wrong" or "warping" the infant in some way. All ages were similarly concerned about their mothering.

One-third (35%) were concerned about their lack of time and difficulty in scheduling time for self, housework, husband, and the baby. "The baby takes over your whole life" was a common remark. The older the woman, the more likely she was to report this concern (18%, 28%, and 56%). More of the teenagers were living with family; therefore, they had less responsibility for a household. The women in Group 3, who had been accustomed to maintaining schedules and managing time efficiently in their careers, had more difficulty with this.

Seventeen percent of the women described the first few days after returning home from the hospital as overwhelming. They stated that they had been afraid of the baby and had compulsively checked on the baby every hour. Group differences were not significant, but fewer teenagers mentioned this.

Infant crying aroused feelings of incompetency in 17% of the mothers. They felt that the baby's needs were not being met and worried that something was wrong with the infant. Group differences were not significant, but fewer teenagers were bothered by the infant's crying. When women were asked specifically about their responses to infant crying later in the interview, a higher percentage were bothered by the crying (see Chapter 4). However, the order in which women voiced their total concerns does not indicate that in this sample crying was a major concern, as others have reported.

Fifteen percent were concerned about their overprotectiveness, caution in safety of the baby, concern about the baby's well-being, or their feelings of possessiveness. Significantly fewer teenagers had this concern (3%, 21%, and 13%).

Six percent of the women were worried about discipline or how to cope with the infant's behavior. These mothers were concerned that their infants not experience the trauma they had experienced as children, they were afraid they would spoil the infant, or they worried about their ability to maintain patience and control of self.

Concerns about Career or Employment Role

One-fourth of the women were concerned about making the decision to go back to work or were ambivalent about going back to work. These mothers anticipated difficulty in returning to work and voiced sadness at the potential of missing important developmental milestones such as their infant's first word or first step. Significantly fewer teenagers reported this concern (5%, 21%, and 18%), which is a reflection of fewer teenagers planning to return to outside employment.

Significantly more of Group 3 women voiced concern about balancing the mother and career roles (3%, 2%, and 9%). Finding quality child care was a major concern for 5% of the women. This probably indicates Group 3's stronger commitment to a career role, as well as their awareness of the demands of a career.

Concerns about the Husband/Mate Relationship

There were no significant age differences among the women (20%) reporting concerns about the relationship with their mates. Thirteen women (5%) reported very negative kinds of relationships, such as the mate acting as if he were single, lacking dependability, or being in jail. Most of the women reporting such negative relationships were separated already. Thirteen described a deterioration in mate relationships in which there were more arguments, things just were not the same, the mate was jealous of the baby, or he was a perfectionist. Twelve women expressed a general lack of time for their mates, found it hard to cook dinner and to meet the needs of both mate and infant. Two teenagers said that their husbands were jealous of the baby.

Various concerns that the mate relationship would change, that the husband would get bored, that they couldn't go out with their mates, or that it was harder to be a wife than a mother were described by 3%. Three percent reported difficulties around the issue of sexual intercourse—it was either painful due to soreness, or the women didn't want to have intercourse and their husbands did.

Body Image Concerns

There were no age differences among the 16% of the women who expressed concern about their body image. Losing weight was a major concern for 6% of the women. Four percent were concerned about being flabby and out of shape; 4% were concerned that they couldn't fit into their clothes. These women may not have been less concerned about body image than the women in Gruis's (1977) sample but may have had other concerns that overshadowed body image concerns. A more recent study indicates that the postpartum body image is somewhat more positive than body image during pregnancy (Strang & Sullivan, 1985).

WORK TOWARD MATERNAL ROLE ATTAINMENT

Several women were quite articulate about the challenge that the maternal role presented for them. In addition to the feelings of frustration and grief that were presented at the beginning of the chapter, Group 3 were quite open about their feelings of incompetency.

- It's illusory.
- I have never undertaken anything that I felt more incompetent in; I have a feeling that I don't know what I'm doing. I read books and they all say different things. Law is more precise.
- It doesn't register that I am a mother, but it doesn't really register that she [baby] is here to stay.
- I'm amazed at myself. I used to plan conventions and meetings for over 200 people at a time, and yet a simple thing like getting ready to take her to the doctor throws me into a tizzy.
- You have to develop and learn the role — different than I thought. I thought it would come naturally as a result of giving birth. I'm still trying to adjust but don't have it refined yet.

Statements such as these are not easily made by those who don't have a strong ego and much self-confidence. There were no comments of this type from Group 1.

Overall Feelings toward Motherhood

The majority of the women (59%) spoke in warm, positive tones about their overall feelings in the mothering role. They used words like *great, wonderful, nice, fun, exciting, neat, fulfilling,* and *enjoy.* Although the differences were not significant, fewer teenagers spoke this positively at 1 month.

One-third of the women spoke of motherhood as an overall change requiring adaptation, getting organized, different, or a time of learning new things. There were no age group differences regarding change.

One-third described the overall role as hard, challenging work. The work was described as important but weighted with responsibility and with ups and downs.

Ten percent of the women saw the role overall as isolating, confining, or boring. The restrictions of not being able to do as they pleased were felt by all age groups similarly.

The overall response to what motherhood was like was flat among 8%; words such as *OK, all right, same,* or *not much change* were used. Significantly more teenagers responded flatly (20%, 2%, and 7%). Teenagers were less animated in their responses than groups 2 and 3 in general, but in this instance they may have been hesitant to share their true feelings of uncertainty. Six percent described motherhood as frustrating or nerve-wracking. Some expressed a wish sometimes for "things to stop." Five percent found the role scary, strange, or worrisome. There were no group differences in those who viewed motherhood either as frustrating or as scary.

Most Difficult Things about Mothering at One Month

When asked what was the most difficult for them in the mothering role, the lack of time and the extreme pressure posed by this lack of time was a central issue the first month following birth. The lack of time to go on outings with the baby caused the women to feel tied down and isolated. Erratic infant schedules made it difficult to plan time and interfered with time that might otherwise be available for taking a bath or reading a book. Women commented that there was no time for caring for themselves just as Grubb (1980) reported earlier.

Time deprivation was a difficulty cited by 61% of the women. Significantly fewer teenagers noted this difficulty (62%, 92%, and

92%). The lack of enough hours in the day was most keenly felt by the older groups.

Feelings of incompetence were viewed by almost half (46%) as the most difficult thing about mothering. There were no significant group differences in reported inability to determine the cause of the infant's cry, read cues, or to keep the infant happy. Women felt challenged in "keeping their cool," in being patient and able to cope.

Sleep deprivation was quite difficult for one-third of the women; more teenagers than older women reported this difficulty (44%, 27%, and 35%). Women stated they were exhausted because of little or interrupted sleep and from getting up at night with the baby.

Just over one-third of the women (35%) described the difficulty of the constant responsibility in the mothering role. Always considering the baby first and having to get advice to be sure things were done right were felt more keenly by Group 2 (11%, 33%, and 22%). One would expect that the teenager might feel these difficulties more so than older women; however, their situation of living with parents or other adults may have provided them with some relief. They did not escape sleep deprivation, however.

Eight percent of the women cited breast-feeding problems as most difficult. Problems included having an inadequate milk supply, leaking, sore nipples, and nursing difficulties.

Teenagers were more likely to deny that there was anything difficult about motherhood (13%, 1%, and 6%); 5% of the women maintained that nothing about motherhood was difficult. The teenagers who reported this may have done so because of reliance on family members for help, or they may have been less comfortable in admitting that motherhood was difficult.

The Easiest Things about Motherhood

Two fifths of the women described the functional tasks of mothering as the easiest thing about motherhood. Changing, feeding, and caring for the infant were specific acts in which they felt skillful.

One-fifth of the women maintained that there wasn't anything about motherhood that was easy. Almost one-fifth (17%) described cuddling, loving, rocking, nurturing, or other affectionate activities as the easiest thing about mothering. Twelve percent said that playing with the infant or otherwise enjoying her was the easiest. Twelve percent described having a good, mellow, easy, healthy, or happy baby, or having things go smoothly as the easiest thing about mothering. There were no significant age differences in areas that were viewed as easiest by the mothers.

Maternal Role Attainment Behaviors at One Month

Maternal role attainment behaviors included feelings about the baby, perception of their baby as compared to an average baby, identification behaviors, infant growth and development, gratification in the role, observed maternal behavior, and self-reported ways of handling irritating child behavior. When determining the predictors of each of the maternal behaviors, the variables of race, education, and marital status were forced into the regression models at the first step because the three groups differed significantly in these three areas.

Feelings of Love for the Infant From a possible score of 10 to 40, the range of scores were 25.5 to 40, with a mean score of 35.2 and a standard deviation of 2.67. There were no significant group differences in these self-rated feelings of love for their infant.

Personal characteristics outweighed infant characteristics in predicting maternal feelings of love at 1 month, which were 27.5% predictable. Predictive variables included race, education, and marital status, 1.0%; child-rearing attitudes, 12.6%; infant-related stress, 8.7%; positive life events, 3.6%; and self-concept, 1.6%. The extent of stress that the infant caused in the household during the first month was the second greatest predictor, however, indicating that emotional affiliation moves more cautiously with partners who are more disruptive of a person's familiar life-style.

Perception of Their Neonates As was the case at early postpartum, there were no significant group differences in perception of the neonate at 1 month. The range of scores was from –10 to 11, with a mean of 1.96 and standard deviation of 2.98. A negative or 0 score suggests an at-risk situation according to Broussard and Hartner's (1971) sample and indicates that the mother rated her infant the same as or less favorably than an average infant. More of the women

(75%) viewed their own infants more positively than an average infant, which is higher than Broussard and Hartner's Pittsburgh sample (61%) but in agreement with Barnard and Eyres' (1979) Seattle population (77%).

Perceptions of the neonate were 21.3% predictable. Predictive variables included race, education, and marital status, 1.3%; bother from infant behaviors, 10.5%; infant health status, 6.2%; easy infant, 1.8%; and infant coming home from the hospital with the mother, 1.5%. Practically all of the variance accounted for related to their infants' behavior or health status. This finding indicates that the perception of the neonate is an objective measure of infant behavior and status more than an indicator of emotional feeling. However, when parents estimate their infant's behavior incorrectly, it is usually more positive or better than the child is (Barnard & Eyres, 1979).

Identification Behaviors The women checked a list of characteristics, such as eyes, hair, and skin, in which their infants resembled themselves or a family member. This measure was to indicate a component of attachment and work at the maternal task of placing their infant within the family context. The range of the number of identifying traits with family members for the total sample was from 2 to 28, with a mean of 9.05 and a standard deviation of 2.90. Group 2 identified significantly more infant traits with family members (range, 4-28; mean, 9.39) than Group 3 (range, 2-16; mean, 8.47), but the teenagers scored in between the two groups without differing significantly from either (range, 4-13; mean, 9.18). Group 3 women, because of their older age, may have had fewer family members nearby to encourage this sort of identification.

Identifying behaviors were only 12.4% predictable. Predictive variables included race, education, and marital status, 1.6%; positive life events, 4.5%; maternal perinatal health status, 1.9%; negative life events, 2.4%; and child-rearing attitudes, 2.0%.

Infant Growth and Development Growth and development were considered a measure of mothering because the infant's progress in these areas reflects his care. The teenagers' infants gained significantly more weight over the first month (mean, 1,214 g) than infants in groups 2 (mean, 946 g) and 3 (mean, 987 g), who did not differ significantly. However, as noted in Chapter 4, infant weights at 1 month did not differ significantly, nor was there a difference in length. Group 1 infants scored higher than Group 2 infants in motor development, with Group 3 infants scoring in between. However, both Groups 1 and 3 infants scored significantly higher than Group 2 infants in social development and on the growth and development factor derived from weight gain, length, and motor and social development.

Variables predicting the infant growth and development factor included race, education, and marital status, 6.1%; infant-related stress, 3.0%; general stress, 4.1%; and informational support, 3%. A total of 16.2% of the variance in infant growth and development was accounted for at 1 month. However, the forced variables indicate that the greatest predictor is either genetic factors or cultural practices related to the mother's race (race was the only forced variable that was significant). Maternal stress, however, had significant negative effects on infant growth and development the first month, and informational support had positive effects.

Gratification in the Mothering Role Both Groups 1 (range, 38-68; mean, 55.6) and 2 (range, 36-70; mean, 54.3) scored significantly higher on gratification in the mothering role than Group 3 (range, 34-68; mean, 51.8). This difference could be due to overall health status because fewer in the younger groups had had a cesarean birth. However, this finding is in agreement with Russell (1974) and Steffensmeier (1982), who reported that parents with more education derived less gratification in parenting. An alternative hypothesis is that the older group of women were more self-actualized women before giving birth. Many commented that they never felt bored and felt fulfilled prior to the birth; less boredom since the birth and greater fulfillment are two items on the measure.

Gratification in the maternal role was 22.2% predictable at 1 month. Predictive variables included race, education, and marital status, 9.6%; positive life events, 7.8%; physical support from mate, 2.7%; and self-concept, 2.1%. Educational level appeared to be the major predictor because it was the only one of the forced variables that reached a level of significance.

Maternal Behavior Significant group differences occurred in observed maternal competency behaviors. The two older groups scored significantly higher (Group 2 range, 22-39, mean, 33.7; Group 3 range, 26-39; mean, 34.4) than Group 1 (range, 18-39; mean, 31.6).

Maternal behavior was predicted by the following variables: race, education, and marital status, 6.9%; perception of the birth experience, 6.6%; easy infant, 3.6%; infant health status, 3.3%; child-rearing attitudes, 2.9%; self-concept, 2.1%; and physical support by mate, 1.8%, accounting for 27.2% of the variance. Race was the only forced variable that was significant and was the major predictor of maternal behavior at 1 month. The perception of the birth experience was the second largest predictor, supporting the conclusion that women's feelings about their initial mothering act were influential in their mothering the first month.

Ways of Handling Irritating Behavior Group 1 scored significantly less favorably (higher score is less favorable) (range, 5-11; mean, 8.4) on the self-rated ways they handled irritating child behavior than Group 3 (range, 3-11; mean, 7.5). Group 2 (range, 1-14; mean, 7.9) did not differ significantly from either.

Only 9.8% of the variance in ways of handling irritating child behavior could be accounted for at 1 month. Predictor variables included race, education, and marital status, 6.0%; and infant-related stress, 3.8%. Both race and educational level entered the model at a significant level, so these two variables were major predictors.

COPING STRATEGIES, RESOURCES FOR MOTHERING AT ONE MONTH

Coping

The mothers' physical and emotional status influenced their coping abilities; fatigue from lack of sleep and rest also reduced their ability to cope. The situation was almost overwhelming for some as they wondered if things would ever get better.

Talking with people who were sympathetic or sensitive to their situation was the strategy utilized by the majority of the women (60%) in coping with motherhood. Group 3 reported this method of coping significantly more often than the two younger groups (57%, 52%, and 73%). Legitimation of feelings is an important strategy in dealing with any role transition, especially from a peer who has had a similar experience (Silverman, 1982).

The two younger groups stated that they asked questions as a method of coping significantly more often than the older group (34%, 37%, and 20%); almost one-third (31%) of the mothers reported asking questions. Seeking and obtaining information is also important in adapting to transitions (Silverman, 1982). The two

older groups stated they read books as a method of coping significantly more often (3%, 21%, and 18%); 16% of the women reported
reading.

Fifteen percent reported that they usually kept concerns to themselves, lived with them, tried to forget them, or put them out of their
minds. There were no age differences in those reporting this method
of coping.

Eleven percent reported they took some action to remedy the situation as a way of coping. There were no group differences among
those who reported seeking a babysitter or going out to relieve stress.
Nine percent of the women reported they used inner strengths
within themselves in coping, such as prayer, meditation, talking to
themselves, and positive thinking.

Teenagers tended to seek information, whereas Group 2 tended
to talk with those who understood what they were experiencing,
to seek information, and to read books, and Group 3 tended to seek
persons to talk with and to read books. The teenager's repertoire
of seeking help is not as sophisticated as that of women in groups
2 and 3.

Resources for Coping

The mate was the most frequently identified resource to help cope
with mothering; he was named by 36% of the women. Significantly
fewer teenagers listed the mate (23%, 41%, and 35%).

Parents were listed as a source of help with coping by 30% of the
women (36%, 32%, and 24%). A woman in Group 3 stated, "My
mother and I were never close until recently. Not only did she help
with housework, but she helped me psychologically. She admitted
her feelings of inadequacy and lack of confidence when she raised
us. I never knew that." A woman from Group 2 noted, "It is more
meaningful to get praise from Mother. She *knows* what I'm going
through." This is another example of how the legitimation of feelings from a person who has experienced a similar transition is very
helpful in adapting to a role transition.

Just over one-fourth (27%) named friends as a source of help
with coping. One-fourth reported that their pediatricians or doctors
were a major source of help in coping with motherhood. One-fifth
of the women named the nurse at the well-child clinic, hospital nursery, clinic, advice line, midwife, or social worker as a major source

for help with coping. Just less than one-fourth (23%) named a family member who was helpful—sister, sister-in-law, cousin, brother, aunt, or mother-in-law. There were no age differences in naming health care providers or family members.

One-fifth listed other mothers or friends with children as sources of support. They noted that only mothers with young children could really understand their feelings and know what they were experiencing, another illustration of the importance of the legitimation of feelings by an experienced individual. The older the woman, the more often she named women with children as support in coping (10%, 17%, and 31%).

Group 1 more frequently relied on the mother to help with coping (which may be classified as emotional support), whereas Group 2 tended to rely on both their mates and mothers more often, compared with Group 3, who relied on other women with children and mates. Because of their older age, Group 3 women may have had fewer mothers available for emotional support. Group 2's coping network is the most intimate of the three groups and has greater potential for providing more extensive emotional support.

Resources for Social Support in Overall Mothering Role

The women's major source of help with the mothering role was their mates; in most cases this was also the mates' initial transition to the father role and they were as inexperienced as the mothers. Two-thirds of groups 2 and 3 reported that their mates were the most helpful to them in the day-to-day mothering, contrasted with one third of Group 1. Half of Group 1 named their mothers, mothers-in-law, or grandmothers as more helpful, compared with one-third of groups 2 and 3. These differences in support the first month reflect the percentage married in each group, with mates named as first source of help for the married couples. The person with whom the mother lives is available 24 hr per day, compared with friends or others whom the mother would hesitate to call at 2:00 a.m.

When the women listed the persons who were helpful to them, there were no significant differences in the *size* of the support networks. There was, however, a difference in the type of help that mothers described receiving. Group 1 more often received informational support than did Group 3 (36% and 21%), but those in Group 2 were in between (32%) and did not differ significantly from either. Both Groups 1 and 2 reported they sought information more often as a way of coping with mothering. Each older age group had significantly more emotional support than the group younger than they (39%, 75%, and 89%).

All three age groups received comparable physical support during the first month, and this was the most frequent type of help reported by 86% of the women. There were no significant group differences in ratings of whether the help received had been as much as was needed or in the two factors for social support variables—mate physical support and general physical support.

The teenage support group, made up largely of mothers or mother-figures, tended to offer what the teenager described as information-al (gave advice, answered questions, understood infant behavior, showed me how to do things) rather than emotional support (attentive, concerned about me, made me rest, gave me time, understanding, emotionally being there, confidant). Mates, the major support persons in groups 2 and 3, were viewed as giving emotional support more than informational support. This makes sense because the father has less informational support to supply; however, both types of support are important in role transitions. The father can, however, legitimate the mother's feelings to foster her coping with the maternal role; but he needs the same sort of legitimation of his feelings, and it is questionable whether the woman can provide this to the extent the father needs because of her physical and emotional state the first month postpartum.

MATE'S ROLE IN CARETAKING ACTIVITIES

Because the mate was most often named as the person who helped with both coping and day-to-day mothering, the extent of his involvement in infant care is of interest. Women rated the extent of their mates' involvement in the care of their infant; 85% of the fathers were involved in a minimum of what the woman considered a moderate amount. The ratings of the extent of father involvement were as follows: 8%, none; 7%, very little; 30%, a moderate amount; 29%, a good bit; and 25%, a great deal. Well over half of the fathers appeared to be very actively involved in child care. Father involvement did not differ significantly by age group.

Father involvement in the infant's care included the full range of care activities: play with, 83%; changes diapers, 78%; feeds, 50% (72%, 41%, and 46%—fewer teenagers breast-feeding); bathes, 42%; soothes, comforts, rocks, puts to sleep, 37% (21%, 40%, and 44%);

holds, 21%; burps, 11%; and dresses, 3% (8%, 2%, 0%). Although the Group 1 fathers had more opportunities to feed their infants because fewer were breast-fed, only half as many Group 1 as groups 2 and 3 fathers soothed, comforted, rocked, or put their infants to sleep. Feeding may have met the Group 1 fathers' need to nurture or comfort their infants.

Decision Making in Infant Care

When asked who made routine decisions regarding the baby's feeding and sleeping routines, and the like, the responses were as follows: Joint, 18%; mother, 67%; varies, 4%; and the baby, 10%. Mothers elaborated that the baby fussed when hungry or gave cues when sleepy, and that was the reason for saying the baby decided routine things like feeding and sleeping. Bell (1974) reported that the infant initiates approximately 50% of all mother-child interactions. One teenager said that her mother made routine decisions. The difference in who made routine decisions was not significant by age group; the major difference was that Group 3 mothers made more routine decisions jointly (15%, 17%, and 25%) and fewer of these decisions alone (77%, 71%, and 55%). This could be a reflection of their longer length of time in relationships in which a pattern of joint decision making has been established.

More important decisions, such as calling the doctor or deciding on a babysitter were reported as being made jointly, 60%; by the mother, 32%; by the father, 3%; and variable, 3%. One teenager reported that her mother made more important decisions about the baby.

Two-thirds of the women reported that they felt good about the decision-making process in their home; the older the woman, the more likely she was to be satisfied with the decision-making process (57%, 65%, and 72%). One-fifth noted that the decision-making process in their families was fair, and they were comfortable with it. One-tenth stated that they talked things out and went through a process of agreeing and disagreeing. Teenagers tended to be less satisfied with the decision-making process; more often than older women they related that either both parties were stubborn or that they were dissatisfied with their mates' decisions.

HOW THE INFANT HAD CHANGED THE
WOMEN'S LIFE-STYLES

There were significant group differences in the womens' rating of the change in their life-styles, from none to a great deal. Groups 2 and 3 tended to rate a great deal of life-style change more often than the teenagers (43%, 60%, and 62%).

When asked to describe how the infants had changed their life-styles, mothers' answers clustered in areas of schedules for eating and sleeping, 34%; mobility/social life, 34%; maintenance of household, 30%; time/always there, 28%; relationship with mate, 13%; and relationships with others, 16%. Seventeen noted their lives were brighter and more pleasurable and that they were more mature, patient individuals. The older the age group, the greater the likelihood that schedules (14%, 25%, and 67%), household maintenance (15%, 16%, 64%), time/always there (17%, 28%, and 37%), and mate relationships (3%, 16%, 15%) were reported changed. Because teenagers more often lived with other adults, they did not have responsibility for managing the household; however, the infants' eating during the night, causing their sleep disruptions, were changes. Teenagers either did not perceive the changes as life-style changes or were unable to articulate them to the same extent that older women were.

Scores on the checklist of bothersome factors indicating infant-related stress did not differ significantly by age group. From a possible range of 23 (no bother at all) to 115 (very much bother), the total sample scores ranged from 23 to 84 (mean, 52; SD, 12.28). Although the mothers felt bad and were fatigued as a result of accommodating to the infant, these life changes were rated in the midrange of bother. One reason for this may be that such changes were anticipated.

ADVICE MOTHERS WOULD GIVE TO OTHER
MOTHERS OF ONE-MONTH-OLD INFANTS

Because the women noted that other mothers were more sensitive to their feelings and knew what they were experiencing, their own advice to other mothers was interesting. The low response to this last question at the end of the interview and the women's fatigue level may have contributed to the fact that several said they had no advice.

Twelve percent said that they would tell other mothers that motherhood is all-consuming, hard, takes a lot of time and responsibility, and that a mother gets fatigued from little rest. Eleven percent stated that patience, flexibility, ability to take one day at a time as they come, or an open mind were important. Seven percent stated they would stress the importance of a support system, someone around, or family as important to talk with. Another 7% would tell mothers that motherhood is rewarding, fun, or maturing. Seven percent would caution mothers to listen to others but to take advice with a grain of salt. Six women stated that an individual should be really sure she is ready to mother.

Although the women were hesitant to give advice, the more frequent agreement about what kind of advice to give centered around the difficulty of the mothering role, the flexibility needed for the role, and the importance of having someone to talk with.

SELECTED WOMEN'S EXPERIENCES
THE FIRST MONTH

All women whose names begin with *A* are in Group 1, *B* in Group 2, and *C* in Group 3. The first two in each group reported that they were unmarried at the time of birth of their infant.

Alma

Alma, a single 16-year-old, was living with the father of the baby and his mother. Although she appeared tired, she was dressed neatly in slacks and a comfortable top. Alma asserted that she had been fine during the past month but had had less sleep than she had needed. She reported a cold that lasted a day but no depression. The lack of sleep was mentioned in her answer to several questions.

> It's fun being a mother. Everything is fine except for no sleep. It is getter better because he now has a schedule and I can sleep.
>
> The kind of things that worry me are illness—cold or flu. I was afraid he'd get my cold. I call the hospital if I'm worried.
>
> He doesn't cry much—not very hard or long. He wants attention, someone to talk to him. I spend about an hour a day talking to him, holding his toys up for him to see. I sing to him and walk around with him to show him things and tell him the names of things. The baby's

father has been the most helpful to me. He amuses the baby, helps with him, and praises me.

I stay home more and sleep less. I do think about going back to school and who is going to take care of the baby. My aunt will probably babysit.

Alison

Alison stated that she had been OK with no physical problems since the birth. However, she had stayed upset and crying because of disagreements with her boyfriend (father of baby). She appeared rested but pale. She looked much younger than 18 years, although she was about 40 lb overweight.

I like being a mother; I just have to get used to giving all my time to someone else. It makes me feel more responsible. It was hard waking up during the night to feed him, but now he sleeps straight through the night.

I don't worry about anything. If something was wrong, I'd call the doctor. He's a good baby and doesn't cry except when he's hungry.

My mother has been the most helpful. She watches the baby for me to go out, and if I'm really tired, she'll watch him while I sleep.

I spend several hours a day picking him up and talking to him. I'm concerned if he is getting enough to eat. I don't know what his father's primary concerns are.

Alice

Alice, 19 years old, noted that she had been fine except for being tired. She had not been sleeping during the day, and her son was up a lot at night. She and her husband were living with her mother. She was very neat, well-groomed, articulate, and relaxed during the interview. Her baby was happy, clean, and well dressed.

I felt I needed more help the first few days. I was up all night. Everyone worked, and I felt I had to do it myself.

Motherhood is still a shock. I was expecting a girl. I look into his eyes and I see my own. I think he is so much like me. He looks like me. He doesn't want to go to sleep, and he'll eat anything. I'm not sure about what I'm doing. I'm just learning. Now I can tell if he's hungry or tired; the cries don't all sound the same now. I can see a lot of what I used to do in him now. He knows who his mother is. He quiets when I hold him and looks into my eyes.

The first week at home he spit up blood, and I rushed to the emergency room. He had sucked blood from my cracked nipple. He has gas and colic and constipation. I give him syrup for that. He may have a dislocated hip; he has to wear double diapers.

Now I talk to my mother and stepmother and my friend about what to do for the baby. My friend wanted the baby more than I did. She calls often and invites us up to see her. She is really being involved.

I don't like to hear him cry. He sounds so sad. I assume it's his way of letting me know something is ailing him. I can feel him growing. I'm pleased about that. He seems to be content, feels secure, snores like his daddy. I see so much of us in him. I think it is so fascinating now he can be so much like us. I wonder what more will come out. I talk and sing to him several hours a day. He likes to be picked up and comforted.

Things have changed quite a bit. I can't come and go as I please. My education is interrupted. My major concern is to get an apartment—have our own home, settle into our own environment—and to help my husband get more money. I plan to get a part-time job when I go back to school. My husband doesn't worry much. My parents are letting us stay here; it's OK, and we are comfortable. When someone tells you it's hard, believe them.

Amy

Amy, a married 18-year-old who was living with her family, said she had been OK since leaving the hospital. She did not mention her husband during the interview. Her appearance was rather disheveled, and she remained quite obese from weight gained during pregnancy. A public health nurse had been making biweekly visits. Amy was concerned about her baby's spitting up. When asked about what motherhood was like, her description fulfilled the apathetic projection of what she had anticipated at birth (a lot of worries and responsibility).

It's hard and tiring. It makes you mad sometimes. Sometimes I can't take it when he cries. Sometimes I hand him over to my mom. Having to wake up at night and having to do everything for him makes it hard to get rest. Nothing is easy now. I can't do what I did before, like shopping. It's not the same anymore. I don't know what he wants when he cries.

My mother has been the most helpful. She washes his clothes when I am sleeping and washes his bottles. But it is a lot less help than I have needed. [During her postpartum hospitalization Amy had said she had "nobody" to help her.]

I hold him several hours a day. But it's hard—hard work. It's hard work if you don't have no help.

Betty

Betty described the first month as pretty good, except for a couple of nights when the baby had gas and she got panicky. She also said she had some depression—cried for no reason. Her son had had to stay in the hospital 2 weeks after she came home because of an infection; worry about this and the chore of pumping her breasts added to her fatigue and depression. This 22-year-old, single women lived in a cluttered, run-down house with her parents; however Betty was well-groomed and quite attractively dressed in slacks and matching top. When asked what motherhood was like, she said:

I love it. It's what I've always wanted. I feel like I want to go out. There are times when I miss that, but I still love it. It's hard because you are always tied up with the baby. You don't want to leave them; you have them with you always.

His umbilical cord is still wet—leaking. He has gas and cries, and I don't know what's wrong. I go to my mother for help. I've called the nursery twice. He doesn't cry unless something is bothering him. That bothers me because I know something is wrong; he is a quiet baby.

My mate has been the person most helpful to me. He makes me feel good and talks to me a lot. If it wasn't for him, I'd really be in a spot. He compliments and comforts me. We're living with my parents the past 2 months.

He is an alert baby. He looks at things and watches me more. I play with him, tickle and talk to him, walk him, rock him, and hold him about an hour and a half a day.

I'm concerned where we'll eventually live. Where we'll be bringing him up. I want to bring him up in a good neighborhood. My mate is concerned about finances, but he doesn't want me to go back to work.

You've got to have a lot of patience and be as calm, cool, and collected as possible.

Barbara

Barbara, a single 26-year-old, also noted that she had been tired the past month but that she was doing rather well overall. She noted that her career had prepared her for stress and long stretches of working hard. Her stitches had been sore, and she was somewhat disturbed that her cat was not handling having a new baby around at all well. She spoke of motherhood in glowing terms as she had a few days following her daughter's birth:

> It's been wonderful. I'm enjoying it. I really wanted a child and I'm glad I did it. I wanted her to be healthy more than anything and she was. She has her own personality definitely. I really feel blessed. It's a wonderful responsibility. It does require a lot of time, and you need to be ready for it. I'm loving giving the patience.

> Since I've become a mother, I've become more cautious about everything. I really want to protect her, and I almost get scared for her wellbeing at times. To deal with my concerns I talk about my feelings, and that helps a lot. I also meditate and concentrate on what my concerns are and then deal with it and face it. For example, I had to work through taking a bus with her.

> When she cries, I feel concerned because sometimes I can't tell what's wrong. She really has a set of lungs. It can be very trying, but I haven't felt any anger or that I couldn't handle it. I know she is trying to communicate and to express herself.

> My mate has been the most helpful to me. He's been here and willing to do anything for her. He talks to her, changes her, et cetera.

> She is wonderful, has a very good personality, very distinct. She is going to be a very strong person. She definitely has a temper. I tend to spoil her because she is very precious. I talk to her, sing to her, walk with her, and play with her toys according to her attention span.

> My major concerns are keeping it together—myself healthy, her healthy, and our house normal. My mate's primary conerns are money and providing.

Bea

Twenty-one-year-old Bea was dressed neatly in slacks and a blouse and was quite receptive to the interviewer. The sparsely furnished home was neat and clean. She noted that she had felt fine emotionally, but physically she felt only "so-so." She described a 1-day depression when she realized that her body was a wreck.

> I'm fat and my body is all stretched out. I have a lot of work to get in shape.

> Motherhood is enjoyable. I have a lot of fun with my baby, but it is tiring too. I feel good about it. It is difficult getting up in the middle of the night. It's hard to see my husband snoring while I'm feeding her in the middle of the night. It's also a chore to go out; it takes a lot of time. The rest is easy. Nothing worries me about being a mother.

> The baby's cry is normal. I don't run to pick him up all the time. If he's fussy, I'll let him fuss for awhile. He has a mad cry that bothers me. I'll let him cry it out. I'll change him and feed him, and if he still cries, I have to let him cry. I have things to do.

> My husband has been the most helpful to me the past month. He has been supportive.

> He's getting so big already. He's going to be a month old tomorrow. It's amazing. I wish time would have gone this fast during my pregnancy. I spend several hours a day doing things with him. I talk to him. He likes noises, voices, and to be around people.

> I don't have any concerns right now. My husband's major concern is his work.

Bonnie

Twenty-eight-year-old Bonnie was nicely groomed and appeared to be in excellent health. She seemed eager and happy to talk about her feelings, herself, her baby, and her husband. She held her child comfortably during the interview. She said she was just beginning to feel better, however. She noted that she was still bleeding, and her chronic hemorrhoids were getting better. She reported that she was being tutored 2 hr per day and attributed her improved emotional state to that. When asked about motherhood she said:

> I'm still getting used to being a mother. The whole idea of being a mother is strange. The responsibilities I have—I feel a better human being. I was so free before—I was bored. Everything is more meaningful. Sometimes I really feel stupid. I had a lot of expectations. Sometimes I'd like for things to stop, but it's like a clock. I'm learning to take each day at a time. Fear is the only thing that is hard—fear of what I am going to do if

she gets a cold. And then I realize that everybody gets a cold. Fear of her getting constipated, fear of leaving home. The easiest thing is to give love and to feel her love me back.

Setting a good example in front of her is a concern. I pray about it. I don't like for her to cry. I try to prevent her from crying, but I realize she has to cry at times, so I let her cry some, but it pierces me. She wants me to hold her and take care of her when she cries.

My husband, mother, sister, a friend, and a baby care course have been the most helpful to me the past month. They've given me encouragement and support.

She is a good baby. She has eye contact. She likes to be left alone aside from cuddling. She likes to be independent, secure. I spend about an hour a day talking to her, cuddling, watching television, looking outside, and listening to music.

My primary concerns at this time are to maintain a level of independence for myself and to pursue a career for myself. I can be so involved with her. I want to continue with grad school. My husband's major concerns are his baby and making enough money to take care of her and his wife. At this point I don't feel secure enough—a proficient mother. I don't feel like I'm a bad mother, but just that I can't speak on it enough.

Carrie

Thirty-three-year-old Carrie was very attractively and fashionably dressed when interviewed. Since she separated from her husband, she had been living with a woman who has a 13-year-old daughter. Carrie had to leave her daughter in the hospital for 3 days after she was discharged because of jaundice. Her episiotomy had been so sore that she took three sitz baths a day. She described that she had felt unbalanced in her body and had been trying to balance herself. When asked what motherhood was like, she said:

> It was emotional to think I'd had the baby, and the baby was mine—the realization that I've had her. It's a lot of things—very strong rewarding feelings to having a baby, a lot of responsibility, a lot of work, and a new direction of my energy. I have to take care of her first or else she'll continue to fuss. I feel good about it. I feel that it's lovely, I think that it really enhances a woman. It is difficult; I have to reorganize a lot of things. My dad has been here for a week, really helping me. I know if I had a husband I could team up and it'd make things easier. The easiest thing is the closeness you feel with the baby, a very deep level of intimacy—another level of intimacy with a man. A baby gives you a lot of pleasure.

I'm worried about her skin—if it's going to clear up. I am filing for a divorce, and the financial settlement and stress of resolving the situation with my husband is hard. I worry that the separation from her father will have a negative effect on her. I talk to people to get different perspectives.

She doesn't cry a lot. Once in a while she is colicky. She is talking to me—telling me that she needs something; I think she has gas pains. She makes faces, and I'll rock her and soothe her. My friend has been the most helpful to me the past month. She called every three days to see how I was doing—unconditional support. She was with me during delivery, a real smart lady.

She is following people with her eyes. She smiles and is becoming a lot more affectionate. She seems like more of a person to me now; she is more secure, can wait for me to prepare myself to nurse her. I spend several hours a day talking to her, taking her for walks, taking her to socialize with people. She likes to be part of things.

My major concerns are to keep myself in a good place—unstressed—so that I am good for her.

Cathryn

Cathryn, a 36-year-old single mother, was living with her parents in a well-furnished, comfortable home. She had her makeup on and was neatly dressed in warm-up pants and a tee shirt. She stated that she felt good at 1 month postpartum, although she was not "too clear in my head." and "About two days a week I feel real emotional. I know it's just hormones, but I can't control it." Cathryn's response to what motherhood was like at 1 month was much less rosy than at early postpartum:

Everything feels new. At the hospital everything felt new. And now every waking moment I'm aware of something else. I feel good about motherhood. I don't think of it as good or bad; it just feels different. I get very possessive about Albert. I get jealous of my parents if they show extra affection to Albert. I feel more mature—a certain security. It feels like a great achievement to have a baby. The most difficult thing is my sleep pattern; because I don't feel rested I'm at a loss, like with Albert crying. I could be more rested if I'd go to bed early, but I've never gone to bed early before. It is easy getting to know him and seeing him respond to certain things that you've figured out.

It worries me that he won't like me [laughs], or that I'm not paying enough attention to his needs or that I might allow him to get sick. I handle this by getting to know him by spending as much time as I can with him.

His crying tears me up, but I know that he should be crying—he's releasing tension. My parents want to console him always. I have to stop them sometimes.

My mother has been the person most helpful to me over the past month. She is so completely helpful with both physical and emotional help. I've had more help than I've needed, but I don't complain. I'm having it easy.

Albert's getting very strong and expressing himself. He's not limp anymore. He's looking at things very intensely. I'm sure that he's hearing things a lot more sharply. I spend several hours a day talking to him, playing with him, and just cuddling him.

He has changed my life-style a great deal. I usually move around and go out a lot. My primary concern is my relationship with the baby's father; that's completely unsure. The second thing is work. It's really important to have someone help you. It could be overwhelming. I considered doing it on my own, but I think that I'd be overwhelmed. Even though I'm appreciative of my parents, I don't feel I'm experiencing enough of an individual relationship with my baby. I'd advise anyone to have her income worked out ahead of time so she wouldn't have to think about that for awhile.

Cynthia

Cynthia, a 40-year-old married mother, looked tired and somewhat depressed although she stated she felt fine at 1 month but hadn't been able to get too much done. She said that being a nurse made not knowing all of the answers in mothering situations hard. Her house was spotless, neat, and well furnished. She nursed her baby during the interview but did not talk to or smile at her baby. She seemed more concerned with details of caretaking and unable just to enjoy the baby, although she was very attentive and gentle. Cynthia described her feelings about motherhood with little enthusiasm, in much the same way that she had shortly following birth:

I just go from day to day. I still don't accomplish as much as I think I should. I also feel it's important to spend time with the baby. I talk to myself.

I can't think of anything particularly difficult about mothering. Taking care of him is the easiest. What worries me most now is returning to work in three months. We've arranged for a day-care center. I'll be having a long day, taking the baby back and forth.

He doesn't cry excessively. He cries when he's hungry. He's either wet or hungry when he cries—has unmet needs. My husband has been the most helpful person to me with emotional support and helping take care of the baby. My mother was helpful the first two weeks.

He's established a good pattern of eating and sleeping. He's alert, looks around, and focuses. I spend about an hour a day holding him, talking to him, or rocking him.

He has changed my life-style a good bit. I'm not as independent. I'm not missing work because it is only temporary that I'm away. I don't know of any major concerns now. My husband's concerns are finances after I go back to work and expenses for child care, clothes, baby equipment, et cetera.

Carmen

Carmen, a 31-year-old Hispanic, was proud of her husband's pride in their baby and his attentiveness to them. However, she was missing her work environment and the stimulation that she had enjoyed in her job. Carmen's home was very neat and clean, and she was attractively dressed for the interview. She still lacked confidence in caring for her baby. She described the first postpartum month as "rough." Because of jaundice, her son was kept in the hospital 2 days after she went home. The earlier mood swings she had were now fewer. She described motherhood:

It's interesting. The only problem is when he cries and I don't know what's wrong. I don't have experience. That's the hardest. Getting opinions from everyone, so I follow the doctor's instructions. Everyone disagrees. It's easy to stay with the baby all day.

I worry about managing the baby's care. I check on him a lot. I am afraid to drive with him. I am afraid to bathe the baby. My sister-in-law, who is staying with us, helps bathe the baby. It takes three hours to do it.

It makes me nervous when he cries and I don't know why. I am concerned that he is hurting. My husband won't let him cry. I know he is spoiled. Everyone holds him even when he's not crying. He needs something when he cries. A friend who calls and gives me advice has been the most helpful during the past month.

He likes to listen to you. He follows bright colors and follows you. He loves to look around, he's curious. I talk to him a few minutes every day. My husband picks him up and brings him to our bed and turns on the radio.

My life-style has changed a great deal. The daily routine is changed. I forget about eating. I used to be real hungry. The baby takes my attention, and the day goes by fast. I don't have any major concerns about anything. My husband is concerned with the baby. He goes right to the baby when he comes home. Now he thinks about his own father, how his father felt as a father.

ANALYSIS AND IMPLICATIONS FOR NURSING INTERVENTION

The major concerns of mothers during their first month of motherhood centered around their infants, their ability to mother the infant adequately, their careers, and their relationships with their mates. The common, pervasive theme among mothers was that of fatigue, regardless of age. The fatigue was related to sleep deprivation, contributed to their frustrations, and taxed their coping abilities. Four-fifths of the women had felt blue or depressed at some time during the first month, although typically the mood was of brief duration.

Implications for intervention will focus first on sleep deprivation and fatigue, social support, and the mothers' major concerns. Difficulties experienced during the first month postpartum were not age-specific; therefore, needs during this period are addressed by topic with focus on age where appropriate.

Sleep Deprivation and Fatigue

During this first month, when sleep deprivation due to nighttime feeding and care was high, the mother's feelings of love for the baby, gratification in the mothering role, and both observed and self-reported maternal behaviors were lowest (Mercer, 1985a). Frequent feedings every 3 to 4 hr during the night and day meant that the usual rhythm of sleep was interrupted. Deprivation of sleep or alteration of the circadian rhythm of habitual sleep interferes with perceptual and cognitive performance and mood state (Hayter, 1980; Killien, 1985; Taub & Berger, 1974). However, women tended to attribute mood swings and altered perceptual and cognitive functioning to hormonal imbalance more often than to lack of sleep. An important area of intervention would seem to be in planning for help to permit a mother to experience cycles of deep and rapid-eye-movement (REM) sleep each night for several reasons.

Lack of sleep—hence, impaired perceptual and cognitive functioning—has potential to make it more difficult for the mother to learn appropriate responses to meet her infant's needs or to interpret infant cues. Sleep deprivation no doubt contributes not only to fatigue but also to the postpartum blues or depression that is commonly reported during the postpartum (Hopkins, Marcus, & Campbell, 1984); however, critical reviews of research do not cite this as a possibility, although a changed cognitive style of perceiving and processing information is noted (Affonso & Domino, 1984; Arizmendi & Affonso, 1984). More teenagers voiced dissatisfaction with their sleep time than did older women; however, fewer teenagers reported being blue or depressed or having physical symptoms, and none described weird or strange cognitive functioning. This observation refutes the above argument, but teenagers may have been more comfortable describing their lack of sleep than other feelings. Since more teenagers lived with their mothers during this time, they may have had some nighttime help that was unavailable to older women.

Following birth, most women are exhausted. As soon as the danger from hemorrhage from a relaxed uterus is past, the postpartum nurse should take special care that the new mother's rest or sleep is *not* disturbed except for a very good reason. Many women have not had a restful night's sleep for the month prior to birth and have an extensive need for deep sleep.

Mothers need to be reminded of the interruptions that they will experience in all activities, including their usual patterns of sleep. They need instructions to ignore a household chore when a free moment arises and should be encouraged to nap during the day when the infant naps. Live-in help for a few weeks may provide valuable relief if this is possible. However, breast-feeding women have no alternative but to be awakened for feedings.

Social Support

The source and nature of social support during the postpartum period is also important for new mothers. A serious question is raised, however, about the kind and extent of support that women need following birth. Does the women who is more anxious seek out greater support systems (hospital demonstrations, more home assistance, and more advice from others), or is there a point at which too much information too soon raises anxiety rather than decreases it? One cannot generalize that only the teenage mother relies heavily on her mother for help. Cathryn, the single 36-year-old, lived with her mother and depended on her mother's help. The Group 2 mothers randomly selected for the vignettes all noted that the mate or husband had been the most helpful during the first month. Overall, two-thirds of the older women and one-third of the teenagers named their mates as the most helpful person.

Mates need encouragement to talk to other fathers so that they get some legitimation for their feelings in their new father roles. Because they are the major source of support for the mothers, it is critical that they have the support they need.

Although there was no significant difference among the three age groups in the number of persons available to help the women, the kind of help they described receiving differed significantly. The teenager, who more often received support from her mother, reported more informational support. Teenagers also received less support from mates and reported less emotional support. Support from both mates and mothers seems critical. The risk of maternal rejection of the child is greater when young mothers are isolated from a supportive social environment (Colletta, 1981).

Smith (1983) identified that families incorporate the adolescent mother and child by either role sharing, role blocking, or role binding. In role blocking the adolescent either abdicates the mothering role, the role is usurped by family members, or there is a combination of abdication and reusurpation. In role binding the responsibilities and tasks are delegated and performed by the adolescent mother alone. In role sharing, the family unit becomes involved in identifying tasks and functions to meet the need of the infant in addition to the needs of other family members. Alison, Alice, and Amy seem to be in role-sharing families, although Amy tends to perceive hers as somewhat role-binding.

Of interest was the finding that the older woman tended to utilize talking with friends and reading books for personal coping resources more often than teenagers. The teenager not only more often lacked a mate as a major source of support, but her friends also were less often reported as helpful. However, teenagers also reported having fewer friends and social interactions (Chapter 2). Curtis (1974) found that pregnant teenagers more often than nonpregnant teenagers reported spending time in solitary activities (watching television, sleeping) rather than in sports and social activities; although this may be a factor contributing to her pregnancy, it may also represent an established pattern that needs to be changed. The teenager lacks the confidantes who can legitimate her feelings and allow her to express her anxieties in making the transition to the maternal role. Earlier research verified why friends may not have been utilized by teenagers (Mercer, 1980); friends were described as talking about dates, parties, and what they were going to wear. Their callous remarks, such as "Why is his skin so red?", were upsetting.

Pertinent clinical concerns for the nurse are to determine who is available in the teenager's (or other woman's) network. Who does the teenager have for support? How much support will the listed persons be able to provide? How does the nurse help the teenager to establish peer contacts and begin to become more socially interactive with others.

Major Concerns

The Infant's Care The women in this study raised many concerns about their infants that ranged from immediate health, growth, and development to the far future when the infant becomes an adult. Perhaps the large number of future-oriented concerns result from the social reality of the possibility of nuclear war, environmental pollutants, and greater difficulty in finding and keeping gainful employment. Overall, the mothers' major concern was their ability to recognize and respond appropriately to signs and symptoms of their infants' illness. Another study established that teenage mothers' priorities were learning how to take the baby's temperature and identifying the signs and symptoms of infant illness (Davis & Eyer, 1984). Others found that mothers would like information on infant behavior in addition to physical care of the infant and infant feeding (Bull & Lawrence, 1985). These areas should be major priorities for teaching.

Many counseling and teaching strategies have been suggested for teaching about infant care and infant development. These strategies would be useful in providing information about all concerns.

Pridham's (1981) approach to teaching problem-solving is one way of incorporating knowledge and applying it in a number of useful ways. Part of problem-solving to recognize signs and symptoms of infant illness would include taking the infant's temperature. Learning basic healthy signs such as skin turgor, skin color, sleep

and eating patterns, and expected growth and developmental milestones help prepare the mother to problem-solve to deal with a wide
range of situations, rather than in one specific crisis that may not
occur.

Programs of teaching need to be carefully planned so that they
are not limited to teaching parents practical tasks only, and parents
are helped to problem-solve so that they are not overwhelmed in
situations that are ambiguous or unclear (Pridham, 1981). Learning
to problem-solve is important because no parent can be taught about
all possible variations to all infant responses.

In an attempt to prescribe methods of preparing mothers for the
postpartum transition period, programs of anticipatory guidance
have been tested. Teaching about infant behavior during the early
postpartum (infant crying, feeding, spitting up and vomiting, sleeping, elimination, and predictability) had a positive influence on
mother's perceptions of their infants at 1 month (Hall, 1980).
Teaching how to recognize infant illness also would be helpful during
the early postpartum. However, with shorter postpartum hospitalization periods, teaching time is quite limited. With more patients
electing early discharge, 12 to 24 hr following birth, creative approaches need to be tried, such as bimonthly afternoon or evening
classes that both parents could attend.

Demonstrations and other valuable information may be put on
audiovisual cassette tapes that parents could borrow from the hospital unit to watch at home. Important information needs to be repeated, especially if instructions were sandwiched in when the mother was packing and/or talking with the physician, and the staff from
records was getting information for the birth certificate. Many hospitals have their own instruction pamphlets; however, the younger
mother does not tend to read for her sources of information.

Field and associates (1982) demonstrated two effective training
programs for teenage mothers, biweekly home instructions in care
giving and sensorimotor and interaction exercises, and training as a
paid teacher's aide in an infant nursery. Growth and development
of infants in both groups was superior to infants whose mothers
had not received any instruction; infants of mothers in the paid
groups did somewhat better.

The highest rate of telephone inquiries by mothers occurred
during the first 3 weeks postpartum when health care support is
less available (Sumner & Fritsch, 1977). In some situations, referral
to the public health nurse or visiting nurses' association may be the
best resource for meeting teaching and counseling needs. Planned

programs of home visits have had positive outcomes such as reducing infant accident rates, higher scores on assessments of the home environment and maternal behavior, fewer problems and fewer nonparticipating fathers, but *only* when an antepartal home visit had been made during the seventh month of pregnancy (Larson, 1980).

Mothering When mothers are helped with increasing their knowledge and skills to meet their infant's needs, this also addresses their second area of greatest concern—mothering competencies. In addition to problem-solving in order to assess the infant's health status, discussions about organization of infant equipment, time, and flexibility are in order. Carmen's comment about taking 3 hours to bathe her baby needed to be explored. Not only was there potential for the infant's being chilled, with possibility for hypoglycemia, but the resulting fatigue for Carmen in a task that requires that length of time warrants exploration to determine how the time could be decreased. Did they assemble the necessary supplies? Did they put the infant in the tub and quickly sponge the infant, then lay him on a dry towel that was open on a nearby surface?

The change in household schedules and household maintenance following the baby's birth is particularly problematic for the older mother; as one mother stated, "There is no schedule." The older first-time mother will benefit from anticipatory guidance about these changes and about the need to seek household help if these kinds of changes are particularly problematic for her. Few infants (39%) had any kind of a predictable schedule during the first month. It is well for parents to think ahead that their infant will probably *not* have a schedule for the first month or so, and for them to plan accordingly.

The idea that very young infants may be spoiled needs to be dispelled. Role-play in how to try to stop infant crying, and the expression of frustrating feelings while attempting to quiet the baby, help relieve tension. Infant crying is a great source of maternal tension (Newton, 1983).

The fewer concerns expressed by the teenagers about lack of time, changes in household schedules, and infant crying may be interpreted two ways. First, Zuckerman et al. (1979) observed that teenagers tended to go to their mothers with concerns rather than to health professionals. Realistically, if the teenager is in a role-sharing family (as described above), these areas may not be problematic for her. The teenagers also had more experience in caring for infants than did older women, and they may have felt more competent because of this earlier experience.

Telephone follow-up from the postpartum unit has proved beneficial. All women need permission to voice concerns that "don't seem important enough to call the doctor for." Referral to public health nurses or visiting nurse associations can provide welcome information and reassurance for many mothers.

Employment Concerns about going back to work, finding competent child care, and missing developmental milestones were foremost at 1 month. Since there is no longer an option for many women to remain home with their young infants, community action needs to be taken to help alleviate the concern about quality of child care. Sexual and other forms of child abuse have been widely publicized, and this has increased anxiety among working mothers who must leave children in day care.

Lists of persons in the community with good references for child care should be made available. Support groups with other working mothers allows an opportunity to share ideas about organization of time, spending quality time with their infants, and how to deal with guilt feelings about employment outside the home.

Mate Relationship Satisfaction with the mate relationship has been associated with less strain (Leifer, 1980) and better performance during the postpartum period (Grossman et al., 1980). One-fifth of the women reported concern about changes in their relationships with their mates. This is particularly problematic because two-thirds of groups 2 and 3 and one-third of Group 1 list their mates as the person most helpful to them with mothering.

Alma's boyfriend supported her by helping with the baby and praising her—the latter being important role affirmation that she was doing a good job. In contrast, Alison reported that the father of her baby worried her and kept her upset. This lack of consistency in relationships may be one reason only one third of the teenagers listed their mates as most helpful. Nakashima and Camp (1984) reported that marital conflict was lower in situations when men 20 years or older were paired with adolescents, in contrast to those fathers who were 19 years and younger. A group of fathers 20 years and older married to older women were functioning at the postconformity level of ego development, whereas fathers 20 years and older married to adolescents were functioning at the conformity level, and fathers 19 years and younger were functioning at the pre-conformity level, as were most of the adolescent mothers. If this pattern of mate selection is true in other populations, teenagers tend to have less mature mates, regardless of the mate's age.

Maintaining a confidential, respectful relationship with the adolescent mother will promote her acceptance of advice to seek counseling for both the young woman and her mate. One of the teenagers in this sample reported physical abuse by her mate, and others worried about erratic behavior of the mates toward their infants. Realizing the possible developmental level of both the young woman and her mate, along with the high divorce rate for this group, group sessions in which incidents can be role-played with acceptable solutions worked out may be a promising method of help.

Counseling with both the mother and father is important for all ages, beginning during pregnancy, about the impact of the infant on their life-style. Couples need to have the lack of time, lack of privacy, and change in household schedules that will occur with the infant's arrival spelled out. It is important to talk about the impact of fatigue on both partners but particularly on the mother, who is also recuperating physically from the birth. The irritability that occurs with sleep deprivation needs to be addressed. By discussing these changes in advance, parents may be able to view the changes less personally when they occur.

Planning for special time alone is necessary. With lack of privacy and loss of spontaneity in deciding to do things on the spur of the moment, deliberate plans must be made if a couple is to be able to have time alone. Couples who can afford it would benefit by having a relative come in and spend the night while they have dinner and a restful night's sleep at a local motel. Breast-feeding mothers may leave bottles of breast milk that has been pumped in advance for night feedings in such cases.

Body Image Women need to be encouraged during pregnancy to think ahead to the first month postpartum regarding planning for meals, time for hot baths, and for rest. Many women commented that they did not have time to eat all day. Menus for nutritious easy meals, frozen meals, and quick nutritious snacks should be planned in advance, so that the busy mother will not become shaky from hypoglycemia. In a fatigued state, it is difficult for a mother to determine whether she is shaky because she is weak or nervous or from lack of food. A good diet is essential for her adequate body functioning, and ability to function is intrinsic to her body image. The majority of women were breast-feeding (81%) at early postpartum, but this had dropped to 71% by 1 month. The breast-feeding mother needs diet counseling to assure she consumes around 2,500 to 2,600 calories daily to meet her energy needs; teenagers need 100 to 200 additional calories.

Discussion of how the body gradually expands over a 9-month period, and will take a few months to return to prepregnancy or near prepregnancy size is critical. Caution to set aside clothes with expandable waistbands, wrap-around styles, and clothes that are easy to take on and off is important. Frank acknowledgment that it will be impossible to wear prepregnancy clothes right away will help prevent disappointment for the great majority who can't.

The usual recuperation of the body during postpartum needs to be addressed. If a woman has hemorrhoids during pregnancy, she will have hemorrhoids for awhile postpartum. They will be more uncomfortable when her perineum is sore from the episiotomy. Hints to take a mild analgesic and sit in the tub prior to attempting to nurse or do other things will increase her ability to enjoy activities.

SUMMARY

The first month postpartum is the most difficult period during the transition to motherhood, characterized by maternal fatigue, frustration, depression, and concern about the infant and about the ability to mother. Despite help from others, women encountered uncertain situations and worried that they would harm their infants because of their inexperience. Their physical recuperation from the birth experience and their social support system affected their feelings about motherhood and themselves.

CHAPTER **6**

Four Months Following Birth: A Turning Point

At 4 months postpartum an identifiable adaptation phase in mothering was evident. Almost two-thirds of the women reported that they were comfortable with the maternal role and felt it had become internalized as part of their identity. The infant's increased ability to communicate and to sleep for longer periods during the night and the more predictable schedule were signals to the mother that she was competent and doing the right things. Mothers described their infants more positively than at 1 month, were more aware of infants' needs, and had much improved timing and sensitivity toward them. Teenagers poignantly reported positive aspects about their infants:

- I'm proud of him; I don't have nothing else in the world.
- Now I have a live baby doll who does everything.
- She's a great little kid; I think she might be kind of fun to keep for awhile.

Group 2 women also reported positive change:

- She's so responsive, a functioning member of the family, not a lump. I used to feel that she was a burden.
- We are really and truly deeply in love with him, and we have a mutual love now. A response that wasn't there before.
- She's more responsive—more of a person. I get feedback from her, and I get a lot of fulfillment from that.
- Having her love me totally, no matter what I do is the greatest reward.

Group 3 comments included:

- When she smiles at me, that lets me know that she knows I'm her mother. It's sort of a mutual bonding.
- Before two months, he was just another person; now I really enjoy him when I'm feeding him.
- He stops feeding for something interesting to look at.
- He has a definite personality. He is very serious and very responsive and curious.
- It's much easier now, he's on a routine.

Barnard and Eyres (1979) also observed that by 4 months families were more settled and better adjusted to their infants.

The 264 women's responses to motherhood at 4 months postpartum (53 in Group 1, 122 in Group 2, and 89 in Group 3) are the focus of this chapter. Following a presentation of their responses, perspectives of the 12 selected women are presented. Proposed nursing interventions conclude the chapter.

OVERALL FEELINGS: PHYSICAL AND EMOTIONAL

Physical Feelings and Problems

Although women were more rested at 4 months, they reported more health problems than at 1 month postpartum. Two-thirds of the women reported a health problem at 4 months postpartum; 44% reported one problem, and 22% reported two problems. The most frequent health problems reported by 25% of the women were colds, flu, or other upper respiratory infections. This is similar to the 22% of mothers reporting colds or other upper respiratory infections in Barnard and Eyres' (1979) Seattle sample at 4 months.

Their weight was a major health concern, with 14% concerned about being overweight and 10% concerned about weight loss. Three percent of the women reported excessive vaginal bleeding; they had experienced either a dilation and curettage, polyp removal, or biopsy for dysplasia. One teenager reported having had a therapeutic abortion.

Other health problems reported included reproductive tract infections, 6%; chronic illness or condition, 5%; gastrointestinal prob-

lems, 4%; breast problems or infections, 4%; joint or muscle problems, 4%; emotional tension or headaches, 3%; hair falling out, 2%;
anemia, 1%; injuries/accidents, 1%. Three women had been hospitalized during the period from 1 to 4 months. Four women (all
in their twenties) were pregnant at 4 months postpartum.

Although there were no significant group differences in the health
problems reported, the older the woman, the more favorably she
tended to rate her health. The factor used to measure maternal
health status at 4 months did not show significant differences by age
group.

Emotional Responses

Although physical problems had increased, the women's overall
emotional response was more positive. This may have related to their
increased feelings of competency in mothering, diminished fatigue,
and their infants' increased social responsiveness to them.

By the fourth month, over half of the women (53%) reported
feeling good, all right, healthy, or great. One-fifth of the women
reported that they felt much better. The extreme fatigue experienced
during the first month postpartum had declined for the majority;
only 14% reported feeling tired. However, 12% reported feeling
hectic or experiencing emotional disequilibrium. There were no significant differences by age group. The disequilibrium experienced by
these women indicates that not all women had adapted to motherhood at this time.

MAJOR CONCERNS AT FOUR MONTHS POSTPARTUM

The mother's primary concerns at 4 months were similar to concerns
at 1 month, except that mothers reported fewer concerns. This was
probably a reflection of their greater feelings of competency in
mothering. By 4 months mothers had observed other infants of similar age and were making comparisons with their own infant. These
comparisons, along with pediatricians' assessments, were reassuring;
the majority of the mothers had no concerns about their infants'
growth and development.

Concerns about the Infant's Growth and Development

One-third of the women in groups 1 and 2 expressed concerns about
their infants' growth and development at 4 months, contrasted to a
only one-fourth of the women in Group 3. Mothers' concerns did not
differ significantly by age group.

Their infants' growth was the concern most frequently cited
(11%). Mothers feared that their infant was either overweight, underweight, growing too fast, or too small for 4 months.

Concerns about social and motor development indicated women
did not have a sound knowledge base about the range of expected
infant behaviors. The infant's social development was an area of concern identified by 8%; possible overstimulation of the infant, anxiety
toward strangers, fear of the infant being a "mama's baby," and the
infant's not talking or smiling were major social interaction concerns.
The infant's possible delayed motor development was of concern to
4%; their infants were either not crawling, rolling over, or using
their hands.

Five percent were concerned about their infants' physical appearance: eyes too close together or too far apart, blinking unevenly,
weak or crossed eyes, birthmarks; inverted nipples; and either bowed
legs or the feet turning out. Birth defects had been identified in 2%
of the infants by the fourth month; narrow ear canals, tibial torsion,
thyroid problems, tumor in the bile duct, and a kidney problem.
Miscellaneous concerns cited by one or two women included crib
death, not wanting the baby to be like her, allergies, flaky scalp,
spitting up, and constipation.

Primary Concerns Reported

A major concern at 4 months was the additional role of career or
employment outside the home; 41% of the mothers were employed
at this time. It is not surprising that the concern cited most often
(34%) focused on role conflict; balancing the mothering role with
one or more other roles was very difficult. Half of those with role
conflict were attempting to resolve issues in relation to their life's
goals; these issues related to concern about balancing work or school
with motherhood roles. Significantly more of Group 3 were concerned about balancing career and motherhood roles (0%, 6%, and

23%).[1] The other half of the women experiencing role conflict reported their primary concern was balancing mate and motherhood role.

Their competency or mothering ability was a primary concern for one-fifth of the women. Mothers questioned the adequacy of their own mothering and whether the child care they had sought while they worked was optimal. Employment outside the home permeated the women's major concerns through role conflict, guilt about leaving a child, or the child care provided.

Ten percent of the women reported their infants' health or the possibility of sudden infant death syndrome (SIDS) as a primary concern. Eight percent of the women had concerns about their personal health. Three women were concerned about their unmarried status at this time, and three were concerned about family planning.

Except for concern about balancing work and motherhood roles, there were no significant group differences in primary concerns. Group 3's greater concern in this area may reflect either a greater commitment to a career role, greater insight into requirements for advancing in a career that might take additional time from mothering, or a greater need to achieve excellence in both roles.

WORK TOWARD MATERNAL ROLE ATTAINMENT

Mothers expressed an overall feeling of accomplishment at 4 months postpartum. This seemed to be a result of both their feeling of greater competency and the infant's increasing social responsivity. Comments by the women illustrate this well:

- I'm proud of myself to be able to mother her—to give her what she needs.
- Things are balancing out now.
- Things are better—more of a schedule.
- It gives you a good feeling that you could make a baby so perfect. I take him out and people will stop and say how cute he is, and then he smiles and they go crazy.

---

[1] Series of three figures in parentheses indicate percentages for the three groups from the youngest to the oldest, respectively.

Overall Feelings about Motherhood

The majority of the women (63%) responded positively in describing what motherhood was like for them at 4 months. By this time, many of the women in Group 3 had reorganized their lives and were more accepting of the infant as a permanent part of their lives; groups 1 and 2 did not seem to have made quite as much progress in this direction. One-third of the women were very enthusiastic about motherhood; they "liked it a lot," "enjoyed it," or described it as "great." Group 3 responded with this kind of enthusiasm significantly more often (28%, 20%, and 44%). Almost one-fifth (17%) focused on how the infant had changed, making mothering more fun; 13% described mothering as being much easier at this time, or as allowing them more freedom.

Overall, approximately one-third were continuing to have difficulty in adapting to motherhood. One-fifth of the mothers described it as harder or busier (25%, 26%, and 12%) at 4 months than it had been when "the infant just lay there and slept." Eleven percent focused on their ambivalence about pursuing work or school and the mothering role. Others responded rather flatly with an OK and a few stressed that they liked being needed.

Both rewards and costs of mothering were evident as mothers described their feelings. Teenagers' comments included the following:

- Now I'm a mom. I'm grown up now. No time for games; I ain't as fast as I used to be.
- It's almost the same as when he wasn't here, but now I have more responsibility. I used to play more with people. Sometimes I can't do what I want to do. I used to think more about the future, but now I don't. I just think more about each day.

Group 2 comments reflecting their feelings included the following:

- I own something just for me now.
- I miss the time alone with my husband. I don't think I was ready for this.
- Motherhood definitely pushes you over the generation line. You're not just a "kid" to your parents. You have a changed role in your family as an adult.

Group 3 responses included the following:

- Six weeks was the turning point. After that I still got tired, but I could go out and participate in a normal fashion.
- When the baby was two and a half months old, I went out with friends, a turning point. There is life after birth.
- On good days we talk and play. On bad days, I want to work and sleep; I want to put her in a closet and bring her out the next day. I want to do something else. There is a conflict over her and my needs.
- He's attached to my mother. He thinks she's his mom. That's depressing. I'd rather not work. He's used to her all day. He's fussy with me. His face lights up when she comes in.

The last mother's comment indicates that her son was more attached to the primary caretaker during his waking hours (his grandmother) than to his mother. This was an additional problem for the employed mother to deal with. The women's other comments reflected their pleasure with their new status as a mother and feelings of responsibility that seemed to contribute to their maturation.

Feelings about Self as a Result of Motherhood

Motherhood represented an accomplishment that was very fulfilling for more than half (53%). Women described more positive feelings about themselves in several areas; they liked themselves better, felt more mature, confident, unselfish, enriched, or were more responsible and unselfish.

One-fourth of the women denied that motherhood had any effect on how they felt about themselves; they maintained that they felt the same as ever about themselves. Overall, one-fifth (22%) saw motherhood as having a negative effect on how they felt about themselves; they were self-censuring about their appearance or behavior or dwelled on stressors. Some described emotional changes that ranged from being less outgoing, less womanly, to being more maternal. There were no significant differences by age group for any of these feelings.

Challenges at Four Months

There tended to be general agreement across age groups about which were the easiest and most difficult tasks of motherhood at 4 months. The numbers of women reporting the difficult tasks had diminished considerably by 4 months, another indication that the majority had adapted to motherhood. However, time remained elusive for the majority; no free time was available.

Easiest Mothering Tasks As was the case at 1 month, caretaking tasks continued to be listed more frequently as the easiest task (27%). Playing with the 4-month-old was listed by 26%; they reported much fun in the infant's smiling at them and enjoying the play. Tickling the infant was a frequently named form of play. Loving the baby was the easiest thing for 14%, and 8% said that everything about mothering was easy at this time. Five percent appreciated the infant's good mood.

Seven percent noted that nothing was easy about mothering. There were no significant differences by maternal age for any of the easiest tasks.

Most Difficult Mothering Tasks Major challenges or demands on the women's resources at 4 months were similar to those at 1 month; however, fewer women reported them. For example, sleep deprivation was reported by only 5% as problematic at 4 months, compared with 33% at 1 month. Teenagers more often mentioned sleep deprivation (13%, 2%, and 4%). Well over half (59%) of the women reported their infants slept through the night, and another 6% noted that their infants rarely awakened during the night, so that roughly two-thirds of the women were having a full night's sleep.

Fewer (9%) reported role incompetency as the most difficult at 4 months, compared with the 27% reporting this as the most difficult at 1 month. Only 8% reported role responsibilities as the most difficult, compared with 35% who reported this as the most difficult at 1 month.

The time required by the role continued to make its demands throughout this period; 58% reported the time requirements as most difficult at 4 months, compared with 61% at 1 month. The amount of time spent in getting things done, preparing for and going on outings, and in caring for the infant was all-consuming despite feelings of greater competency and having more sleep. Except for sleep deprivation, age differences were not significant in difficult mothering tasks.

Ideal Image of Motherhood

Failure to live up to one's ideal image in a role may lead to role strain and depression. To determine something of the women's conception of ideal mothering behaviors and whether there might be a potential gap between their ideal mother image and their own mothering, they were asked to list five characteristics of a good mother.

The women's ideal mother image was a woman with ability to accomplish a wide variety of tasks. Their image of an ideal mother was one who meets/is responsive to infant's needs (64%); teaches (56%); provides love/is unselfish (42%); provides nourishment (40%); keeps clean (34%); provides stimulation/exposure to outside world (31%); maintains appropriate environment/safety (31%); plays with (29%); has patience/calmness (22%); soothes/cuddles (14%); keeps well informed/reads (12%); takes care of self (11%); promotes loving family (9%); respects individuality of infant (8%); promotes infant health (8%); fulfilled/happy as a mother (6%); dresses infant appropriately (6%); disciplines (5%); and fosters her infant's independence (3%).

The teenagers more often listed the following: keeps the infant clean (52%, 27%, and 32%), dresses the infant appropriately (21%, 3%, and 2%), and (with Group 2) is happy/fulfilled with mothering (10%, 9%, and 0%). Groups 2 and 3 more often listed teaching (37%, 62%, and 60%), respects individuality of infant (0%, 9%, and 11%), and takes care of self (2%, 9%, and 18%). There were no significant group differences in other categories.

The teenager's conception of a good mother tended to include concrete mothering tasks more often; fewer considered teaching, and none thought of the individuality of the infant. These differences seemed to be related to their level of maturity and perhaps to their values. Their greater focus on outward appearance—cleanliness and clothing—may reflect the kinds of feedback they received from others.

Self-Image of Motherhood

Women were asked to rate themselves in the mothering role on a scale of 1 to 10, with 10 being considered the ideal mother. The range of scores was from 2 to 11, with only 1% rating themselves as 4 or less. Five percent rated themselves as 5, 3% as 6, 13% as 7, 36% as 8, 24% as 9, and 18% as 10. Two women rated themselves as 11, indicating that their mothering was particularly excellent. There were no significant group differences; the group means ranged from 8.2 to 8.3.

Maternal Role Attainment Behaviors at Four Months

A common belief is that teenagers do not assume responsibility for care of their infants; this was not true in this population. Ninety percent of the women reported that they were the major caretakers of their infants (92%, 87%, and 94%). Three percent reported sharing responsibility with the father of the baby 50–50; 2% named the father as major caretaker; 2% shared with another person other than the father (usually their mother); and 2% said a housekeeper or babysitter was the major caretaker. There were no significant differences by age group.

The measures of maternal behaviors indicated increased competency, feelings of love for the baby, and satisfaction in the role. These findings were congruent with the mothers' high ratings of their self-image in the role and their positive reports about motherhood during the interview.

Feelings of Love   From a possible score of 40, the range of scores for the total sample was 23 to 40, with a mean score of 25.7, standard deviation of 2.62. There were no significant age group differences, but all age groups' scores increased from 1 month: from 35.4 to 35.8 for Group 1, from 35.1 to 35.6 for Group 2, and from 35.3 to 35.6 for Group 3. This finding is consistent with the observations of Robson and Moss (1970) who reported that by the end of the third month most women felt strongly attached to their infants.

Almost one-third (29%) of the variance in feelings of love for the baby was accounted for at 4 months. The demographic variables (educational level, marital status, and race) were forced into the regression model at the first step and accounted for 1% of the variance. In order of their entry into the model, other variables were as follows: infant-related stress, 13.4%; child-rearing attitudes, 4.8%; infant persistence, 3.6%; empathy, 2.7%; mother–infant separation following birth, 1.3%; self-concept, 1.2%, and informational support 1%. Less infant-related stress from changes in their life-style and household continued to be a major predictor of higher feelings of love.

Gratification in the Role The total sample range of scores was from 24 to 70, with a possible range of 14 to 70; the mean score was 56.8, standard deviation 6.72. All group means were higher at 4 months, supporting the greater gratification in the role than at 1 month reported by the women: Group 1, from 56.3 to 59.4; Group 2, from 54.8 to 57.3; Group 3, from 51.0 to 54.4. There were significant group differences in these means; groups 1 and 2 reported significantly higher gratification in the role than did Group 3. This is consistent with the group differences at 1 month and with the findings of both Russell (1974) and Steffensmeier (1980) that more highly educated parents derive less gratification from mothering. However, if these findings were totally consistent with Russell's and Steffensmeier's, Group 2's level of gratification would have been significantly lower than Group 1's because Group 2 women had more education than the teenagers.

An indication of the source of the women's gratification in motherhood was obtained by having them describe what was the most rewarding about motherhood. Their answers centered around what the infant provided for them and positive changes that they observed in themselves. The most rewarding event for one-third (34%) of the women was watching their infants grow and develop. Almost one-third (30%) described the infant's response to and love for them as the most rewarding. Significantly more of the women in groups 2 and 3 reported the infant's response as the most rewarding facet of motherhood (15%, 34%, and 39%). The increasing babbling, smiling, and mobility of the infant evoked much pleasure. One-fifth (19%) described loving the infant, taking care of the infant, or just "the baby" as the most rewarding thing about motherhood. Fifteen percent of the women described reward in the accomplishment and pride in being a mother; comments related to their sense of creativity in having produced the infant and their greater respect for life.

Teenagers more often than older women described having someone who wouldn't leave them, someone to keep them company, something all their own, or someone to play with as the most rewarding thing about motherhood (25%, 8%, and 7%). It is sad that one-fourth of the young women perceived an aloneness such that their infants appeared to be the major persons in their lives.

Seven percent noted that their infants' health was most rewarding. Four percent felt rewarded by the extended family's response to the infant. Only two women denied any rewarding feature of motherhood, one each from Groups 1 and 2.

One-fifth of the variance in gratification was predictable at 4 months: Educational level, marital status, and race accounted for 5%, with educational level being the only variable that was significant; empathy, 3.6%; rigidity, 3.0%; child-rearing attitudes, 3.3%; perception of the birth experience, 1.6%; appraisal support, 1.4%; and maternal mood, 1.6%. Although the women described their infants' behavior as a major source of their rewards in mothering, infant temperament variables did not enter the model. Temperament traits did not measure the infant's affectionate responses to their mothers, however. The mother's personality traits and attitudes were more important in the satisfaction derived.

Observed Maternal Behavior Maternal behavior scores ranged from 22 to 42 from a possible range of 14 to 42; the mean was 37.3, standard deviation 4.37. There was an overall increase in observed competency behaviors at 4 months: Group 1 from 31.6 to 34.8; Group 2 from 33.7 to 37.6, and Group 3 from 34.4 to 38.5. The observed increase in competency behaviors was congruent with the women's self-reports. There were significant group differences; the two older groups, although not differing significantly from each other, were functioning at a higher level of competency than the teenage group.

Just under one-third (31.1%) of the variance in maternal behavior was predictable at 4 months. Predictor variables included the following: educational level, marital status, and race, 13.9%; child-rearing attitudes, 8.0%; self-concept, 4.9%; infant-related stress, 1.5%; infant rhythmicity, 1.1%; maternal health, 0.8%; and maternal adaptability, 0.8%. All three of the forced variables were significant and were the largest predictor of maternal behaviors, with child-rearing attitudes and self-concept being the second and third best predictors. However, an easier infant who was less stressful and more predictable contributed to more competent or adaptive mothering.

Infant Growth and Development The infant's growth and development did not reflect any disadvantage from somewhat less adaptable maternal behaviors. Teenage infants were ahead of the two older groups' infants in the growth factor, although their mothers scored lower in maternal behavior.

Just under one-fifth of the growth factor was predictable (19%). The predictive variables were as follows: educational level, marital status, and race, 4.4%; size of support network, 3.4%; physical support, 3.5%; maternal age, 1.8%; child-rearing attitudes, 2.0%; informational support, 1.2%; maternal intensity, 1.3%; and emotional support, 1.1%. Support was clearly an important factor in the infant's growth and development at 4 months. The teenager's support system probably contributed to her infant's care and made it possible for her to provide the kind of care the infant needed.

Role Conflict and Role Strain

Although there was an overall increase in achievement of maternal role attainment behaviors, one-third of the women voiced their primary concern as role conflict, and 41% of the mothers were employed. Because of the change described in mate relationships, this was another potential area of role conflict.

With increased role conflict, an increase in role strain is expected. Role strain had not been measured at 1 month; however, with a possible range of 1 (none) to 5 (very high), the observed range was from 1 to 5. The means for the age groups, from youngest to oldest, were 2.77, 2.67, and 2.49, respectively. Group differences were not significant. Eleven percent had no role strain (score of 1); 39% had low role strain (score of 2), 33% had moderate role strain (score of 3), 12% had high role strain (score of 4), and 6% had very high role strain (score of 5).

Just over half (51%) the sample of women experienced moderate to very high role strain at 4 months. One-fifth of the women experienced either high or very high role strain (25% of Group 1, 19% of Group 2, and 12% of Group 3). This finding suggests that the older the woman, the better able she is to handle role conflict and/or the greater her resources for dealing with conflict. Her higher level of development as indicated by her greater flexibility and higher level of personality integration also would contribute to her greater ability to deal with role conflict.

Since the interview responses suggested that stress was increased because of employment roles, women were grouped as either employed or nonemployed. There were no significant differences in role strain between these two groups.

Twins and Role Strain Although the group of five mothers with twins was extremely small for comparison with the 259 mothers of single-born infants, there were no significant differences in maternal role strain experienced. Role strain was actually lower and less variable in the small twin group of mothers (average, 2.0; standard deviation, .71, compared with an average of 2.6; standard deviation, 1.0).

However, there was a preoccupation with mothering tasks that had preceded the ability to relate to the twins emotionally by their 34-year-old mother:

> A woman who had twins visited me in the hospital and said, "Don't worry if you don't have feelings of love for them now." I had forgotten that she said it. She called last week, and when she restated it, it was an immense relief. I love them now, but earlier I was so busy coping, I had no time for love.

A 23-year-old mother with twins was Italian and had a lot of help from her family, husband, and godparents. Her husband's mother lived with them and provided a lot of help with the twins. She took outings by herself while her husband took care of the twin girls. She was an extremely well organized person, and the twins were on a predictable schedule. Her attitude was, "What is the big deal about having twins?" When people made comments about "double trouble" or wondered how she managed with two, it made her angry; her reply was "I can handle it."

The 26-year-old mother of twins was having more difficulty; she was from Canada and had no family or friends to help her, and her husband was busy with graduate school. In addition, she reported that she had had a dilatation and curettage just 2 weeks previously to remove placental tissue that was growing into her uterine wall, and she also had an infection at the site of her epidural anesthesia with localized back pain. The twins kept her very busy so that she had no time to apply makeup or fix her hair. Both her son and her daughter had diaper rashes and green stools, which were diagnosed as allergies. The lack of family support and her infants' and her own poor health status were major factors in this mother's having a more difficult time in managing twins.

An 18-year-old mother of twins viewed the earlier months as a very hard time, but things were going much better by 4 months. Her husband was also helpful with the twin girls. She was successfully breast-feeding both infants. A 19-year-old mother of twins felt that her infants gave her life much more meaning and that her relationship with her husband was much improved since their birth. She was the oldest of seven children and noted that she had had a considerable amount of experience caring for children. She was calm and confident in her mothering role and was warm and loving with both infants.

Thus, while a sample of five is too small for making generalizations, only one mother was having difficulty adapting, and her own ill health and isolation from family and friends were major factors in her inability to manage.

IMPACT OF INFANT ON LIFE-STYLE

There were no significant differences by group in ratings of the extent that the infant was influencing or changing their life-style or home environment at 4 months. Almost three-fourths of the women (72%) reported that they had experienced either a good bit or a great deal of change in their life-style.

How Infant Had Changed Life-Style

Women were asked how the infant had changed their life-style. A change in their personal schedule was reported by 85% of the women. Women reported that they had no time, were home more, had new priorities or plans, the baby came first with responsibility and time requirements, and a very few (3%) were depressed or bored.

Both positive and negative changes in the household schedule were reported by the majority (60%). Almost half (46%) noted that the household schedule revolved around the infant. Fifteen percent reported that they were better organized, more on schedule, or had a routine for the first time. One third had difficulty in getting things done or just had to let things go. Two teenagers reported that the infant gave them something to do.

Two-thirds of the women described changes in the mate relationship. Half of these changes were positive; one-third of the women reported that their relationship was closer or more sharing than before. Two-fifths of the sample reported that they had less spontaneous time together, less time to talk or pursue common interests, or their mate was not around much. Five percent reported that they were having mate problems (25%, 25%, and 12%). Five percent of the sample reported that they were either separated or in the process of getting a divorce. Sixteen percent reported more arguments, sexual problems, or their mates' failure to understand their needs.

At 4 months, parenthood was exerting a strain on the majority of the mate relationships but was more problematic for the women less than 30 years. These younger women had had less time to work out conflicts in their relationships prior to the birth of their first child. Forty-two percent of the women reported that they were married the year prior to the birth of their infant.

One-fifth of the women reported that their extended family relationships were closer, but 2% reported that they received more criticism from their family. Two teenagers enjoyed being treated as adults by their family.

One-fifth of the women identified specific family stressors that had been troublesome for them during the past 3 months. Stressors included financial problems, divorce or separation, partner problems including sexual adjustments, mate's incarceration, moving or living conditions, family member out of work or fired, family drinking or drug problem, major illness of mate or a parent, and a single custody battle for the infant. These represent the vicissitudes of life rather than crises specific to motherhood; however, these stressors may have a greater impact when the person is responsible for a very young infant.

Infant-Related Stress The group means reflected that over-all women were bothered less than "somewhat" but more than "not at all." With a possible range from 23 to 115, the total sample range was from 23 to 91, with 23 indicating no bother from infant-related changes and 91 representing much bother. Group differences in infant-related stress were not significant, and the group means had changed little from 1 month: Group 1 from 52.0 to 52.7, Group 2 from 52.5 to 51.4, and Group 3 from 50.6 to 50.3.

Since two-thirds of the women had reported the changed relationships with their mates, a subscale from the Checklist of Bothersome Factors was derived that related specifically to the mate relationship. From a possible range of 7 to 35, the mean scores reflected little bother or stress from mate relationships because of infant-related change: Group 1, 14.3; Group 2, 13.4; and Group 3, 13.0. Older women's scores reflected slightly less stress from relationship change, which was congruent with their reports. This measure did not seem to reflect the amount of discord that was reported, however, only one-fifth reported severe problems. In general, the mothers' verbal reports were indicative of greater mate-related stress than they committed to ratings on paper. Their greater joy in a more responsive infant capable of expressing affection may have offset some of the bother from changes caused by the infant.

COPING STRATEGIES: RESOURCES FOR
MOTHERING AT FOUR MONTHS

To manage or cope with the infant-related changes in their lives, almost half (49%) of the mothers stated that they planned and adjusted their priorities and schedules, maintained flexibility, and shared work when possible. Two-fifths (41%) noted that they just stayed home more; 11 women postponed school or career plans to manage mothering. Sixteen percent reported that the change was slow to allow time for adapting or that they just made the best of a difficult situation. Three percent of the women emphatically said they had not adjusted "period." Four women were seeing a therapist. Two percent stated that they changed themselves to adapt to the situation.

Vacations, sports, or outings without the infant were especially important for one-tenth of the mothers. A vacation was described by one woman as "turning things around." One-tenth reported they either talked to others or friends with children, or went to parents' groups to help them cope.

The only coping strategy in which there were significant group differences was planning and adjusting time. The teenager less often reported taking this responsibility (22%, 57%, and 54%). This probably indicates their lesser sophistication in organization and planning ahead skills and their dependence on other adults they lived with.

Size of Support Network

The size of the social support network that helped with day-to-day mothering situations did not differ significantly by age group. The range was from no one to four persons: 9% listed no one; 37% listed one person; 28% listed two persons; 15% listed 3 persons; and 11% listed 4 persons who helped them. The mate was the most frequent helper listed by two-thirds of the women. Their mothers or mothers-in-law were listed by one-third, and friends were listed by one-third.

The composition of the network had changed somewhat at 4 months. The inclusion of friends had increased from 13% at 1 month to 34% at 4 months. Teenager's mates were more frequently named in the social network, an increase from 30% to 49%, indicating that they may have been moving away from dependence on their mothers. This is an expected developmental process if they became more independent as an individual and were moving toward increased ability for intimate relationships, as opposed to transferring dependence from their mothers to their mates.

As Much Help as Needed

Teenagers significantly more often than older women reported that they had as much help or more than they needed. Their perceptions of what they needed may have been less accurate. However, with increased mate support, the emotional component that mates tend to provide for mothers may have bolstered the teenagers' perceived support.

Type of Support Received

Except for emotional support, there were no significant differences by age group in the type of support received. Although more teenagers reported their mates as a member of their support network, there were still fewer teenagers than older women who reported mates. Mates appear to be a major source of emotional support.

Physical help, largely in caring for the infant and to a lesser extent in providing maternal recreation and diversion, was the most frequently described type of help reported by three-fourths of the women. Over half (56%) reported emotional support in the form of someone to love them and to provide moral and emotional support. The older the woman, the more often she reported emotional support (43%, 56%, and 65%).

One-fourth of all women reported receiving informational help in the form of advice, questions answered, or shared experiences with other women. Very few women (14%) reported appraisal support. Appraisal support included such statements as "reassured me that I was doing a good job of mothering."

ADDITIONAL INFORMATION MOTHERS WOULD GIVE ABOUT FOUR-MONTH-OLDS

Despite the greater adaptation and achievement of competency in mothering, less than half of the women (44%) offered information that would be helpful to other mothers. Their suggestions, however, were quite sensitive to needs.

The most frequent response was one of encouragement for mothers. Mothers need to know that things improve by 4 months and that it is a different experience. Mothers should be told that the baby is entertaining; to relax, play with, and spend a lot of time with the baby.

Others expressed the importance of patience and a sense of humor in dealing with the unexpected. Recognition of the child's moods and wants that are constant and continually changing requires much flexibility. A mother should use her own instinct and set her own priorities because she knows her infant best. However, priorities should include providing for the infant's safety.

Several stressed the importance of mothers getting help with the baby; that although mothering was very hard, it is worth it. Some who lived a great distance from their families noted how difficult it was to be away from their families at this time. Association with other mothers or attending mothering groups was also recommended, as was reading or attending classes.

SELECTED WOMEN'S EXPERIENCES AT FOUR MONTHS

As earlier, women in the vignettes are presented by sequence. Group 1 mothers' names begin with "A," Group 2 with "B," and Group 3 with "C." The first two in each sequence were single or separated at birth, and the last two are married.

Alma

At 4 months, 16-year-old Alma was neatly groomed and casually dressed for the interview. She was confident and poised with the interviewer. She was obviously very proud and felt very capable. Her mother-in-law's house, where they were living, was immaculately clean, well furnished, with many infant age-appropriate toys, quilts, and pillows in a playpen. She rated herself as 10 in mothering.

Alma reported that she was able to rest more and felt good overall. Except for not getting enough outdoor exercise, Alma felt healthy. Alma's husband was present and was obviously proud of his son; he handled him gently, talked to him, and played with him during the interview with Alma. (Alma reported she was single at early post-partum but now referred to her mate as her husband.) She described motherhood:

> My mom said it would be hard, but he's doing well. He lets me sleep at night [Alma complained of lack of sleep at 1 month]. He likes to play, and he giggles a lot.

> My husband helps me when I'm really tired, so it's been easy for me [at 1 month he was praising her for her mothering]. Things have gone smoothly. It's fun to have a little kid around to take care of when there is no one else around but us ... He likes to look in the mirror, have his tummy tickled, be thrown up in the air, play with his toys, swing, and walk in his stroller. I tell him stories, show him around the room and show him things and name the things and show him pictures. I help him hold and reach things.

> I go out less. I plan to start school next month. But I take him with me if I want to go bowling or to a drive-in movie.

> My husband has been more help than anyone else. When I'm tired, he takes care of the baby. He bathes, diapers, and puts him to sleep most of the time at night.

> He [baby] wants to be carried all of the time. He can't be, so I just talk to him and tell him.

> The most difficult thing is not being able to go out. I'd rather just stay home. The easiest thing is taking care of him.

Alison

Eighteen-year-old Alison was casually but very neatly dressed. Her home was immaculately clean and neat. However, she reported that she had been blue a little bit because she was breaking up with her son's father. She reported her health was very good and that mother-hood was wonderful. She rated herself as 9 in mothering:

> I love it. I just like to see the different things that he does every day. He does something new every day, and it excites me [she smiles and seems very pleased].

> Being a mother makes me feel a lot better about myself. It gives me a lot more to do; I'm not just sitting around. It takes my mind off things. It gives me someone to be with all the time.

> His godfather has been the most helpful to me with mothering. Some-

times my mother will help me or let me go out, and she'll take care of it [the baby] ; if not, I stay home and stick it out.

I play with him; he likes to play. He likes patty-cake and feet- and body-play and likes to bounce. He is starting to roll over. He likes to pull up and sit up. He laughs and screams.

Having someone around is the most rewarding, and watching him grow up. The hardest thing is being around him *all* the time. My major concern is his growing up, and hoping that nothing serious happens to him.

Alice

Nineteen-year-old Alice had just arrived from her mother's with her baby when the interviewer arrived. She had missed several appointments. She had been working from 7:00 p.m. to 1:00 a.m. on the swing shift and going to school in the mornings taking an EKG class for the past month. Alice was dressed neatly in a skirt and blouse. Her new apartment was a little cluttered, but she had just recently moved. Alice apologized for having missed appointments. She appeared happy and was very animated. During the interview she played with her baby, often spontaneously interrupting the interview to talk to, smile at, hug, or kiss her baby.

Alice described her health as very good, but mentioned that she hadn't had a period yet, although she didn't suspect pregnancy because she is still nursing. She spoke of motherhood:

I don't believe I'm a mom! It's hard to believe. I see him as something given to me, my responsibility. He looks like me, not my kid per se. But I'd die if I lost him. Hard to have someone dependent on me. Hard to see that one day he'll look up to me.

The sitter said he cried too much. I think she has too many kids—the others are walking. I feel guilty when they aren't quiet and laughing at the sitter's.

I feel more adult. I don't drink, but feel like I'll have to do adult things. In a way, I don't feel I want to grow up yet [laughs] .

I used to be bored. Now he gives me something to do. He is not wasting my time. He changed my value of the dollar. I believe in a budget. Now I want him in nursery school—more stimulation. I love my job, and it forces my husband to stay here with him.

God has been the most helpful to me, and quiet time. I pray a lot. I meditate; it helps.

He [baby] laughs, talks baby talk, holds his bottle, tries to sit up and turn over. He crawls backwards and reaches for things. He looks at himself in windows. I talk to him, tickle and cuddle him. I play with him and show him the mirror, pictures, and let him feel different things. He loves aluminum foil.

When he doesn't need something he wants I take him away, put his mind on other things. I rate myself a ten in mothering. I think all moms should give themselves a ten; you do the best you can. I am giving it my best.

The most rewarding thing is that I helped bring life into the world. I made my husband happy. The hardest thing is his crying—depends on my mood how much it bothers me. Loving him is the easiest thing.

Amy

In contrast to Alison, 18-year-old Amy lacked self-confidence in her mothering ability. When asked to rank herself in the mothering role, she said 5, then asked what 5 was. When the interviewer said, "In the middle," Amy repeated, "Five." She lived with her family, and her husband was not very involved in helping her with her infant. Although she was dressed stylishly for the interview, she was reserved and lacked the animation evident in Alice. When her baby fussed, she took the baby to her mother who was in another room. Although her family seemed to be helping her with child care, Amy also used health professionals in seeking help. She had difficulty in understanding the interview questions; the interviewer had to rephrase and give examples, which indicated Amy's cognitive development was not at the same level as the other teenagers.

Amy's response to motherhood was more positive than it had been following birth, when she saw that it would be all worries, or at 1 month, when she described it as hard and tiring.

It's fun [laughs]. I like babies. I don't know how to take care of babies all that good. I don't feel no different about myself.

He's changed things a good bit. I have to do a lot of things for him. I just do it. I have to. No one else will.

His doctor has been the person that has helped the most the past months. She's nice. She says everytime I need something to call her up.

He can hold his head up high without wiggling. He tries to stand up when I hold him up [laughs]. Holds his bottle. He knows when I'm bathing him. He turns toward people when they walk into the room. I play with him all the time. He always wants me to be there.

attention but not too great. I love her and am enjoying it more than I expected. I don't want any more [children] because I want both a career and baby and don't want to overdo either. I feel overall better being a mother. I'm more conscious of not abusing my baby.

She's changed our life a good bit; we have a family now. I always felt free, I'm still free, but am more careful of impulsive change. I try to keep the house cleaner [laughs].

My relationship with my man is good now—much better. It's really opened up. Elsie is a source of inspiration for both of us. Having a child gives a chance to grow. Elsie sleeps with me and my man.

My man has been the person who has been the most helpful with mothering. My girl friend has helped also. He supports me very lovingly and sees me as doing something as a great benefit and feels good about how I mother. I am so surprised that others will suggest what I should do—too much advice even from strangers.

She is sitting up by herself. She is totally frustrated with trying to crawl. I can see she is impatient—has that personality. She mimics our eating habits. She likes for me to balance her as she goes from sitting to standing. I wear bright colors and patterns, and she loves it. I sing and exercise her legs. I take her to the park in a Snuggly® [cloth body carrier that holds baby against breast]. I usually play one to three hours with her every day.

If she grabs my breast, I might say, "Ouch," and she laughs. It's novel to her. I just say no when she wants something she doesn't need.

The most difficult thing about motherhood is not enough time to myself. I love to read. The easiest thing is that it feels natural, so easy to love her. The most rewarding thing is watching her develop.

Oh, a good mother is patient, playful, cautious, loving, affectionate, attentive, and concerned about nutrition and the family.

My major concern is with myself, family, relationship with my man. I am working on balancing these.

Bea

Twenty-one-year-old Bea was very neatly dressed in a casual skirt and blouse. Her home, although modest and furnished with "make do" furniture, was neat and clean. Her son was very alert, happy, clean, and well-dressed. He spent the entire interview in a stroller near his mother or in her arms. Bea responded very sensitively to her son. She rated herself as 9 in the mothering role.

She rated her health as very good and said that she had felt good—
no problems. When asked what motherhood was like, she responded:

> My life is pretty much the same. I haven't had to adjust that much. I
> have to start earlier to get things done, but otherwise, it's the same. Have
> been at home more since we moved from Arizona. I don't feel differently
> about myself. I feel good about myself, though.

> He's changed our life-style a moderate amount. It takes longer to do
> things. I used to just go. I can't imagine him not being here. I don't plan
> to go back to work while he's little.

> My mom has been the person who has been the most helpful to me.
> She lives in Palo Alto and brings gifts for me and the baby. She comes
> to visit me once a week—it's a lot of moral support.

> He has a positional deformity of the feet. Tomorrow he has to get casts.
> He is sociable and smiles a lot—coos and goes strong and blows bubbles.
> He can almost sit up. He smiles at me and talks a lot. He's just discovered
> his feet. He loves to be kissed and nuzzled and talked to. I sing to him.
> He likes to be exercised and to go for stroller walks. I sing, "One little,
> two little Indians" to him and show him his fingers as I count. I hold
> things for him to reach for. I name things for him—little doggie, body
> parts, and features as I touch them.

> The most difficult thing about motherhood is my weight—my body.
> It's hard on your body to have a baby. I'm adjustable, and I'm so used to
> him I can't imagine not having him.

> Everything is easy about motherhood—maybe playing with him and
> watching him grow and develop is the easiest. Watching the baby grow and
> develop is the most rewarding.

> My primary concern is finances—the loss of my income. Yet both of
> us feel it is best for me to be home.

Bonnie

Bonnie, 28 years old, was nicely dressed in a dress and leotards and
had just returned from the spa. Bonnie yawned a lot and appeared
bored throughout the interview but did mention that she was on
tranquilizers. She expressed frustration at being "fat" (she was
definitely overweight). Although not openly affectionate to her infant, she handled her with ease. She rated herself as 10 (ideal) in
the mothering role and commented, "I'm still not on a schedule,
but I'll still give myself a ten."

Bonnie rated her health as very good and noted that she was seeing a psychiatrist, who told her her problem was the frustration of being a new mother. She didn't think her frustration could be related to childbirth, but the therapist assured her it was natural. She described what motherhood was like:

> I'm second and my baby is first. All my thoughts are occupied for her well-being. A whole lot of additional responsibility. Mostly my likes and dislikes have changed. My priorities have changed. I used to be manipulated by others. I feel like my psychological self is more under my control even though I'm seeing a therapist. I used to think that I should always be on the social scene—like disco every week. Its not important now.

> Motherhood has given me a great sense of pride. I'm very proud of myself. I have something to live for. I feel that being a mother motivates me.

> She has changed our life-style a great deal. I can't focus on myself. I value time more. Everything has changed. She's my first responsibility.

> My mother has been the most helpful to me with mothering—telling me what I should be doing. She taught me how to bathe her.

> The hardest thing about motherhood is feeling that you're doing the right thing. The easiest is just giving her love—loving and hugging. [yawn]. The most rewarding thing is looking up and seeing a beautiful baby that's happy.

> My weight is my major concern right now. I don't want to go see my friends because I got so fat. I used to see them several times a week.

Carrie

Carrie gave the overall impression of still lacking direction in her life at 4 months despite her age (33 years). She was casual in slacks and a shirt, and her home was free of clutter but did not appear overly clean or neat. Her daughter was asleep during the interview.

Carrie rated her health as very good, although she noted she had been very depressed for about a week. She had talked with a lawyer about her husband, from whom she is separated. She indicated that she would like to get back with her husband. She rated herself as 9 in mothering and referred to motherhood as follows:

> It's a lot of fun. I like it. It isn't as hard as I thought. I thought babies cried all the time. It's a shifting of priority.

Motherhood enhances me [giggles]. I feel it is an accomplishment. She has changed my life-style a good bit. But it's making me more responsible. I was only responsible for myself, so now I'd rather buy a toy for her than new clothes all the time for me. I have to be more organized, I have learned to delegate more responsibility and to communicate better with the babysitter.

My friend has been helpful during the past months, but now my husband comes over more. He calls to see if I'm OK and will stop by on his day off. He is helpful with finances. We've had a lot of good talks examining what things in our relationship didn't work out. We're friends now, but I would like to have some romance in my life now.

She makes a lot of sounds, has learned how to scream. She rolls over, and sits up if I hold her fingers. She likes to go places and have people talk to her. She gets a lot of attention. Likes her toys, and likes being in a car seat.

The most difficult thing about motherhood is change in freedom—have to have a babysitter if I want to go out. The amazing thing about babies is that they are with you all the time. The easiest thing about it is the pleasure, when she smiles, and the responsiveness. You get a perspective on yourself, learn patience. The most rewarding thing is the love—interaction of love.

My major concern is my relationship with my husband. We're getting on better terms. A friendship is developing which is nice, but if it doesn't go beyond that I would like some romance in my life.

My advcie to other mothers would be to introduce your baby to a lot of people and situations. Some of the mothers I've been around have been a lot more protective, but she loves getting out and going places.

Cathryn

Cathryn, 36 years old, looked tired; her hair was uncombed, and she was dressed in a sweater and slacks for the interview. The interview took place in the dining alcove of her parents' home. Cathryn is a clothing designer but has not pursued it actively. Although Cathryn appeared open to the interview, she was unable to be clear in her responses on occasion; this may have reflected her European background.

Cathryn was attentive to the baby, who fussed shortly after the interview began, but her mom came and got the baby so that the interview would be uninterrupted. She rated herself as 9 in mothering.

Cathryn rated her health as very good but reported that she got tired. She often forgot to eat and was continuing to breast-feed. Things seemed to be coming more into focus for her, she noted. She began talking about motherhood very seriously but soon was quite animated:

> I usually am chattier but am tired today. I didn't get to sleep until three a.m. Sometimes I still can't believe I'm a mother. At the same time I feel I've known him all my life. I don't have a husband, no other duties or activities to take my concentration, so my relationship with him is intense. I'm with him all the time. The minute I'm without him, I miss him.
>
> Motherhood has made me feel more solid. I'm not so concerned about what others think of me. He has changed my life a great deal. I'm more in contact with certain immediate things. I've always been good at postponing things. The baby puts things into perspective. The baby shows me what I want to do—what I should do now related to his care first, then things I want to do. I am more organized, use time better. It amazes me that I am not resentful of losing freedoms.
>
> My mother has been the most helpful to me during the past months. She does a lot of physical work. Sometimes she feeds me. She's an energetic person. She has good intuition—doesn't remember all that I'd expected but she helps me find my own intuition.
>
> He jumps on his feet, bounces, likes to stand. He is fascinated with his feet. He tries to crawl. He is also teething. Normally in the morning he can spend a long time by himself. He likes for me to make faces or any kind of rhythmical movement. I hold him over my head; he likes to look down on faces. I talk to him, rock him, sing to him. He doesn't understand his stuffed animals. I play with him four or five hours a day, off and on.
>
> When he wants something that he doesn't need, I treat it differently each time. I let him play with it for awhile. Then if it bothers me, I accompany it with words, take it away.
>
> A good mother makes him laugh, keeps him healthy, makes all his moments as worthy of what they are. I'm angry at myself, I'm sleepy in the morning and he's awake a lot, but I am afraid he'll tone down a lot because of how I react.
>
> The most difficult thing about motherhood is being drained. If I go past a certain point, I might not be able to cope. While I'm healthy, it's not hard. Missing one meal can make you faint. Its hard to keep regular meals. The easiest thing is being with him. The most rewarding is the uniqueness of the relationship. It's so self-fulfilling.

My major concern is toilet training. I've heard kids here are trained late—two years. I've been geared to think about it early. It's made to be a positive way—type of emphasis. Make it a practical thing; try to get the child to use the pot. No repression behind it. I have decided I'll do it. Especially him with his sensitive skin—diapers are a bit of a hassle.

I am grateful that I could spend so much time with the baby the first three days. I could cultivate it; it takes time. I am glad I'm breast-feeding. At first I thought what's the big deal, but now I really enjoy it.

Cynthia

Forty-year-old Cynthia was neat and well groomed for the interview, and her house was spotless. Cynthia looked tired and was very tense during the interview, not at all open to expressing her feelings. Her baby, who had been asleep in the bedroom, awakened and cried for 15 min during the interview. Finally, at the interviewer's suggestion, she went to the baby. She brought him to the dining room and held him on her lap, but away from her body, and did not cuddle, talk to, or play with the baby. Her son was thin and appeared immature; he was not standing or sitting up well. He was quiet and passive, not smiling or gazing at the interviewer. He would not maintain eye contact with the interviewer or the mother. Although Cynthia was very efficient, she did not seem to be relaxed or spontaneous in the care of her son. She rated herself as 8 in mothering.

Cynthia rated her health as very good and noted that things were better now, back to normal. She reported, "I go back to work next week. I think I'll be tired. I'm tired thinking about it."

She described motherhood:

> I feel more adjusted than I did at first. I am more confident with the passage of time. The first month I was tired. I wondered how I could cope. Things just sort of fell into place, automatically.
>
> Being a mother is something I always wanted. I feel complete. He has changed our life-style a great deal. I used to have all my time to myself. Now it's hard to find time. Not seeing friends as frequently. I no longer have time to sit with my feet propped up. We don't go out much—never have. Don't go for a walk or anything.
>
> My husband has been the most helpful to me in mothering. His emotional support and helping with the baby in the evening and taking over if I need him to are ways he has helped.

The baby plays with his cradle gym, rattle, and toys. He is alert and stronger than before. He talks, smiles, and giggles. He is doing well. He likes for me to play giggle, laugh, and peekaboo. I occasionally play toys with him. I sometimes leave him by himself to play. I play with him about fifteen minutes out of every four hours.

I don't tell him no if he wants something he doesn't need yet.

The most difficult thing about motherhood is leaving him to go back to work—being away five days a week for ten hours a day. The easiest is the satisfied feeling. He's more responsive now. The most rewarding thing is the responsiveness of the baby.

A good mother provides physical and environmental needs, plays with the baby, keeps him clean and dry, and I can't think [laughs]. My major concern now is returning to work and coping with the baby and housework.

Carmen

Carmen, 31 years old, looked rested and was casually dressed. Her home was neat. The baby's playpen and stroller were in the living room. Carmen was very warm, and although more relaxed than at 1 month, she was still nervous about her baby. She interacted warmly and sensitively with her baby. She and her husband were having disagreements about child rearing, but Carmen deferred to her husband and seemed to accept this. She rated herself as 5 in the mothering role, saying, "I have a lot to learn."

Carmen rated her health as good and reported that she had been fine and free of illness, colds, or flu. She described motherhood as follows:

Getting a lot better. It's easier. It was my first time. I was afraid to take care of him. I really leaned on my sister-in-law. She left when he was two months old. Now it seems that he's all mine—easy to care for. It's hard to say no to relatives—wouldn't do it again, but the help was great.

In the beginning I was confused in thoughts. I was very sentimental. I'd get frightened when he cried. I didn't want anyone to come see the baby. I was afraid something was wrong. I am back to what I used to be like now.

He has changed our life-style a great deal. I used to work. Everything I do is for my baby. My husband adores him. He doesn't want to leave the baby. He has changed a lot. At first he wasn't as concerned or enthusiastic

about the baby. Now he is enthusiastic about the baby, but he is overwhelming about it. He wants me to drop everything if the baby is crying—
even unnecessary. We have less time for ourselves and time out in the evenings. My husband falls asleep at seven p.m.

My husband has been the most helpful to me the past months. He takes
care of the baby as soon as he gets home. If the baby wakes at night, he
often takes care of it. Often feeds the baby in the morning. He feels a little
guilty because he is gone all day.

The baby grabs everything. Everything goes into his mouth. He tries to
turn over, turns his head everywhere, and follows things when it's called
to his attention. He talks, likes to stand. I talk to him, play with the
mobile over his crib, and play peekaboo. He loves it. I play with him for
ten to fifteen minutes off and on for a total of about two hours a day.

When he wants something he doesn't need, I hold his hand and say no.
Sometimes he responds.

Nothing is difficult about motherhood now. The easiest thing is taking
care of him. The most rewarding is to see him smile when he wakes up.

A good mother takes care of the baby, feeds them, shows love to them,
makes sure they are OK all of the time. My major concern is that I tend to
be more emotional now. I think more about things in the future. What
would happen to the baby if we weren't here—if we died.

ANALYSIS AND IMPLICATIONS FOR
NURSING INTERVENTION

Analysis

A common misconception is to assume that teenagers are less likely
than older women to be major caretakers of their infants. In this
sample of 15-to-19-year-olds, teenagers did not differ significantly
from older women in reporting they were major caretakers of their
infants. Thus, generalizations cannot be made; individual family
situations have to be considered. Several general problem areas stood
out at 4 months that are important to consider when counseling
mothers.

Although the women were enjoying their infants more at 4
months, it was striking that only a few referred to their infants by
name. The majority still said "he," "she," or "the baby." There was
no doubt about mothers' competencies overall or their feelings
of confidence in the mothering role; two-thirds of the women had
internalized the maternal role. But the infant had not fully taken

on her or his identity by name. The expectation was that through the transactions with the playful and affectionate infants and mothers' increased feelings of love for their infants, the infants would have been more often referred to by their names. However, the 9-month long habit of referring to "the baby" during pregnancy may be difficult to break.

Households tended to revolve around the infants, with 85% of the women describing changes in their schedules. Half of the women adjusted to this household schedule change by adapting and planning schedules so they could cope. Older women were twice as likely as teenager to report adapting and planning their schedules; more of the older women were employed and had to meet schedules. Planning ahead requires abstract conceptualization of events to come, and adapting to the unexpected requires flexibility. Older women had developmental advantages in such areas, but teenagers are developing in these areas and may be helped to improve their skills.

Older women also may need help in planning ahead. The randomly selected women in the vignettes illustrated that increased chronological age does not necessarily mean an increased level of cognitive and social development. Alma at 16 years had a greater grasp of questions and explanations than Amy at 18. Carrie at 33 years was working hard at sorting out relationships and seeking romance, and she seemed less secure in her identity than did Alma and Alice.

Spotless homes with no sign of infant occupancy or maternal fatigue may signal a lack of stimulating mother–infant interaction. Cynthia, who was very uptight during the interview in a home with no sign of infant occupancy, had a son who did not maintain eye contact and was very placid. Similarly, Betty, who described herself as very tired, and who lacked knowledge about infant stimulation had an infant who was very flat and asocial. Bishop (1976) reported that she considered a relentlessly clean house a negative and critical signal because a mother's energy is limited during the first 6 weeks postpartum. A very clean house after that early period also may indicate that mother–infant interaction is not a top priority.

Changes in household and personal schedules meant less time for mates. Two-thirds of the mothers reported a change in the mate relationship. Although half of the changes were positive, many were negative. Others without negative changes were in conflict about how to balance mother–mate roles.

The importance of self-concept in both observed and self-ratings of maternal behavior was evident. Self-concept was predictive of observed maternal behavior. Amy from Group 1 and Carmen from Group 3 both rated their mothering as 5. Amy had no help from her husband, and Carmen and her husband were experiencing conflict regarding child-rearing attitudes. Both Amy and Carmen felt they "didn't know" or "had a lot to learn." Appraisal of their role performance from their mate or other important person seems to have much influence on mothers' self-perceptions in the role.

The importance of social support in the infant's growth and development from 1 to 4 months was evident. Social support variables predicted just about half of the variance accounted for in this area. Physical help and the size of the network played a larger role at this time in infant growth and development than informational and emotional support. Physical help both frees the mother's time for social interaction with the infant and offers additional interactional opportunities for the infant. The teenagers who reported more overall help than older women also had infants who scored higher in the growth factor.

Career conflicts and issues around going back to work were problematic for several; however, role strain did not differ significantly between those who had returned to work (41%) and those who had not. For some women, returning to work was therapeutic, and that may be why role strain was not increased for employed women:

- I feel better now that I'm back at work, relating to the real world and not a baby's world. [Group 3]
- I really like to go to work, rather than staying home with her. I send her out six days a week, and on the seventh day I have her. [Group 2]

The prospects of returning to work introduced conflict for Cynthia, who viewed this as the most difficult area of motherhood at 4 months. Barbara, who was taking her daughter to work with her, experienced no conflict. Alice, who was attending school and working a swing shift, reported that she "used to be bored," and her son gave her something to do. Alice was enjoying her job, but her husband was taking care of her son during the evenings.

Interventions

Because the major areas for intervention are not specific to any one age group, interventions are addressed by general areas of difficulty.

Time and Household Change Anticipatory guidance about the dramatic change that occurs with the birth of the infant is critical. Women need to be prepared for the household to change to revolving around the infant and for the enormous demands on their time. If women do not know about these critical changes, they feel that it is their disorganization and incompetency that are at the root of their problems in trying to have an orderly household, rather than the additional work imposed by an infant.

Any preparation that fosters a woman's feeling better about herself is vital; otherwise, she is vulnerable to blaming herself when things don't work out as planned. When she has a low opinion of herself, this interferes with her ability to interact with and care for her infant, as indicated by the association between self-concept and maternal behavior. The nurse, on learning that women are feeling overwhelmed and unable to manage, can offer to review a routine day with the mother. In going over daily schedules, the woman can prioritize those activities most important to her and identify those that may be dropped, done less often, or even delegated to someone else.

Change in Mate Relationships The support from the mate, whether physical, appraisal, or emotional, played an important role in the woman's self concept and in her mothering abilities. Caplan's (1959) observation several decades ago still seems to hold true: the husband's role in "charging his wife's battery" appears to provide energy for mothering.

The infant's integration into the family changes the previously exclusive mate relationship. Both parents need counseling about these changes, *before* they occur and *during* the first year of motherhood. Some women may benefit from therapy, as did Bonnie in handling the frustrations of early motherhood. The old saying that "a baby brings the couple closer together" needs to be discussed because the baby may bring out any existing differences in opinions about every activity within a family. With differences, compromise must occur so that each partner feels a sharing in the decision-making process. Children need consistency from adults; therefore, it is important for parents to agree on a style and work together, rather than against each other with the infant caught in the middle.

The household revolving around an infant means that sexual intercourse is less spontaneous and that it is likely to be interrupted by a crying infant. These changes, if thought about and discussed beforehand, are less resented when they actually occur.

Infant Stimulation The infant's early social and motor development is enhanced by parental and other adult involvement with the
infant. Parents, however, respond to infants according to their perceptions of what they think an infant is capable of. Snyder and
associates (1979) found that what a woman expected of her baby
was what she got, that is, the woman who expected an early performance from her baby was more likely to provide early stimulation
for her baby. Infant competencies and development over the first
year should be taught during pregnancy and emphasized during
subsequent contacts with the mother at public health nurse visits
or well-baby visits to the clinic or physician.

Any examination of the infant may be used to illustrate the infant's reflex abilities and ability to track sound and respond to
voices. The pediatric nurse practitioner or pediatric clinical specialist has an excellent opportunity on each well-baby visit to discuss the
current development and what the mother may look for or expect,
as well as how to prepare for it. For example, mothers of 4-month-
olds need to be prepared for the fact that within 4 months their
infants will be very mobile, able to reach and pull and to stick their
fingers or objects in electrical outlets or in their mouths.

In the Snyder et al. (1979) study, women with lower developmental expectations of their infants had fewer years of formal education, lower family income, less social support, less positive feelings
about pregnancy, more perinatal complications, and more self-
reported negative perceptions about their birth experiences. At
birth the women in the study reported here differed significantly
by age group in naming the age at which infants become aware of
surroundings (teenagers less realistic than Groups 2 and 3), age for
teaching the infant (older women significantly earlier than teenagers), and the infant's age for hearing sounds and voices clearly
(Groups 1 and 2 ahead of Group 3 here).

These differences by age group in beliefs about infant competencies point out that a woman may stimulate an infant in one area
but not in another. Differences in maternal care were observed by
Roberts and Rowley (1972), who reported that a mother could be
above average in one area of care on the observed maternal competency scale and be average or even below average in others.

Some mothers may learn more about child development in group
settings than in one-to-one counseling (Chamberlin, Szumowski, &
Zastowny, 1979). However, not all women have access to classes
or are inclined to participate if they have access, so both group and
individual counseling are important. Infants who had experienced

positive contact with their mothers were more advanced developmentally at 18 months (Chamberlin et al., 1979); activities that foster early positive interactions also foster infant stimulation.

Social Support Social support variables were major predictors of infant growth and development at 4 months. Women most often listed their mates and their mothers as individuals who had been most helpful to them in the mothering role. Logically, both the father and the grandmother would benefit from the opportunity for classes to learn about child care and child development. The grandmother might appreciate being updated so that she is more confident in role modeling for her daughter. Among first-time parents, the father knows as little about infant care as the mother; as a major supporter, he would benefit enormously from counseling.

The problem with counseling men is that their schedules often prohibit their attending class sessions, or they do not see class material as worthy of their time. They go to childbirth classes under duress and may remain aloof. Yet as major supporters and battery-chargers, they need to understand the emotional and physical changes the mother is experiencing as well as changes in the infant.

Health care providers also should spend some time discussing how things are with the mother and infant or with the mother alone. The mother needs the opportunity to express any concerns she might have.

Friends are the third greatest source of help for mothers at 4 months. Mothers sought out women with young children. The number of friends involved almost tripled from 1 to 4 months. Mothers' support groups are a place to meet friends; other women reported meeting friends in parks or playgrounds when they take infants on outings.

The number of persons available (size of the social network) and physical help were especially important at 4 months. Amy, who had no one to do things for her, viewed her pediatrician who told her "to call every time she needed anything" as the most helpful person in her network. Giving a woman "permission" to call is very important.

Conflicts in Employment Roles Satisfaction with child care is positively related to satisfaction with employment roles, and work satisfaction is positively related to mother-child interaction (Harrell & Ridley, 1975). Mothers need to begin during pregnancy to inquire about available child care in their community and about individuals who come to the child's home for care. Visits to day-care centers can help allay anxiety if the mother sees that there is adequate staff for the number of children, that the environment is cheerful, clean, and healthy, and that children are happy and well cared for. Other alternatives for child care also should be examined.

Although the cost may be greater for an individual to come to the child's home, the parents must weigh the convenience of not having to get the child out of bed, dress her, and take her out on cold, rainy days, as well as not having the child exposed to colds and other communicable diseases. Consideration of backup care is also critical for times when the infant is ill, the mother's work hours are changed unexpectedly, or some other emergency arises.

Women who adapt well to work were observed to adapt well to childbearing (Jimenez & Newton, 1982). Slesinger (1981) reported the same finding among low-income mothers and concluded that work experience indicated an ability to keep schedules, accept responsibility, accept a commitment to an outside institution, and to communicate with strangers. Nineteen-year-old Alice is a good example of a mother who had adapted well to both roles. Cathryn at 36 years was not employed, remained dependent on her parents, and did not appear nearly so well adapted to motherhood as Alice.

CHAPTER 7

The Eighth Month: New Challenges

At 8 months over two-thirds of the mothers were positive in their responses about motherhood. Their infants were more direct, with specific responses that were easily interpreted. However, the more mobile, interactive infant also required different mothering skills. Mothers who felt competent earlier felt incompetent at 8 months. In addition, over half (55%) of the 250 women continuing in the study were employed. It was not surprising that major concerns were infant care and finances.

This chapter highlights the women's responses to and feelings about motherhood at 8 months post-birth (43 in Group 1, 119 in Group 2, and 88 in Group 3). Following a brief overview of expectations at 8 months, the women's responses are presented. Employed and nonemployed mothers are compared on several variables. Following the selected women's experiences, an analysis of major themes during this period is presented, and implications for nursing interventions conclude the chapter.

OVERVIEW OF EXPECTATIONS AT EIGHT MONTHS FOLLOWING BIRTH

Infants

Sander (1962) described a period from 5 to 9 months during which the infant reaches out to the mother and stimulates her to respond to him. The infant learns to anticipate his mother's response and to reproduce her responses. One of the women in her twenties illustrated this ability well. "It starts at about 6 months; they're trying to test you. If you get upset about coughing, he'll cough. He tries to fool me. If he thinks it'll work, he'll try it."

The infant's increased ability to direct her mother's attention provides the mother with more opportunities to respond to the infant's social behaviors, so that during the second half-year of life mother–infant interactions become quite different in their content and structure (Green et al., 1980). Although there is consistency among mother–infant interactions over time, changes in infant developmental behaviors seem to assure continued maternal involvement through play, affectional, and stimulating responses.

Infant–mother social interaction also plays an important role in the infant's development. The more sociable the infant, the more stimulation he elicits from his mother. Eight-month-old infants' mental development scores were predicted by their social responses to interviewers and to their mothers (Lamb, Garn, & Keating, 1981). This relationship did not differ by social class, race, or infant gender.

Mothers

Over the past 30 years the number of women in the work force has grown by 173%, from 16.7 million in 1947 to 45.6 million in 1980 (Associated Press, 1983). Over half of the mothers in the United States are employed, and over one-third have children under 6 years. The movement of mothers into work roles has not resulted in any change in the usual wife or mother role responsibilities. The working mother continues to assume major responsibility for the household and child rearing (Harris, 1979; Shainess, 1980; Yogev, 1981).

The potential for role conflict that leads to role strain is increased when there is a proliferation of roles. This is even more likely when social support for the mother role is not increased (Zambrana, Hurst, & Hite, 1979). Majewski (1983) did not find differences in role conflict between employed and unemployed mothers, however. Mothers who viewed their work role as a career had more conflict than those who viewed the work role as a job. This indicates that employment may be less of a strain when commitment to that role is less. Greater role conflict was associated with greater difficulty in the transition to the maternal role.

Eight months following birth was identified as a time when parents experienced a general decrease in their sense of well-being

(Miller & Sollie, 1980). Mothers also reported higher marital stress at 8 months.

OVERALL FEELINGS: PHYSICAL AND EMOTIONAL

Physical Feelings, Problems

Overall, the women's health status at 8 months had improved since 4 months. Physically, mothers were in better shape to cope with the more mobile infant. The majority of the women (87%) rated their health as either good or very good at 8 months, with only 13% rating their health as fair. More teenagers rated their health as fair (19%, 14%, and 8%).[1]

Some of the women's comments indicated that the return to feeling normal or their usual selves did not occur until around 8 months:

- She's completely weaned now, and there's a big change. I didn't like it at first. Now I feel like I've got my body back to myself. I've lost some weight. I'm feeling more in control of me.
- I'm just now beginning to get my vigor back—feeling like my old self again. I'm surprised how much it took out of me.

Health Problems More than one-third had no health problem (38%); 40% reported one health problem; 16%, two health problems; 5%, three health problems; and 2%, four health problems. The older the woman, the greater the likelihood that she reported *no* health problem (24%, 36%, and 45%).

The most frequently reported health problem was upper respiratory infections (colds, flu, bronchitis, sinus, throat infections), reported by 38% of the women. Other more frequently reported problems included either over- or underweight (8%); reproductive tract infections (6%); a chronic illness such as arthritis, diabetes, multiple sclerosis, or asthma (6%); and orthopedic problems such as disc problems or backache (6%).

Less frequently reported problems included gastro-intestinal problems (3%); menstrual irregularities (3%); headaches (3%); men-

---

[1] Series of three figures in parentheses indicates percentages for the three groups from the youngest to the oldest, respectively.

strual extraction or dilation and curettage (2%); abortion (2%); hospitalization (2%); anemia (1%); injury (1%); and urinary tract infection (1%). Two women sustained fractures as a result of their mate's physical violence.

Six percent of the women were pregnant at 8 months postpartum (5%, 8%, and 2%). Fewer than half of the women (43%) had seen a physician since the fourth month postpartum. Over one-fourth (27%) went for treatment of a health problem, and the remainder of the physician visits were for regular checkups only.

Health Status Although teenagers were at an advantage the first month in their health status, their score was significantly lower on the maternal health status factor than the two older groups at 8 months. Teenagers tended to have more ear, nose, and throat infections, anemia, menstrual irregularities, and urinary tract infections. The menstrual irregularities and anemia are not surprising because menstrual patterns sometimes take a few years to become established, and iron demands are high during the teen years. The tendency toward higher infections may be related to their care of themselves.

Emotional Feelings

The majority of the women (68%) reported more positive emotional feelings; they reported they had been "fine," "good," "better," or "things were easier." A few reported that they were feeling great or very good. However, almost one-third did not feel so well. Fatigue continued to be a problem for one-fifth, and 12% described a state of emotional disequilibrium. Differences were not significant by age group.

MAJOR CONCERNS AT EIGHT MONTHS POSTPARTUM

Concerns about Infant's Growth and Development

There were fewer concerns expressed about the infant's growth and development than at 4 months. In order of the frequency reported, concerns were as follows: gross motor development/not crawling, 8%; inadequate social development, 6%; no teeth, 5%; not growing, too thin, too short, 5%; too tall, fat, or big, 4%; inadequate speech, 3%; feet turned/hip dislocation, 3%; aggressive behavior, 2%; eye problems, 2%; and one each reporting undescended testis, hernia, tongue-tied, and head too large. There were no significant group differences in these concerns.

Primary Concerns Reported

Many of the women said they had no primary or major concerns at 8 months. Other women listed more than one primary concern. However, mothers would sometimes say they had no major concern, then in their advice to other mothers they voiced a major concern.

One-fifth of the women reported that the infant and his care was their primary concern at 8 months. With the infant more mobile and more socially interactive, women began to be concerned about moving to a larger or better apartment or to a suitable house in a good neighborhood.

Over one-third had concerns around role conflict. Finances were a major concern for almost one-fifth so that employment was necessary. Career and mother–career role conflict continued to be problematic. Mother–mate roles also continued to be problematic, although fewer women focused on mate relationships. Getting back into school or attending school was a primary concern for some whose schooling had been interrupted by the infant's birth.

Fewer mothers were worried about the future, but those who did wondered whether they'd be able to provide for themselves and their child. Those who were pregnant were concerned about the second pregnancy and the coming baby. A few in Group 3 were concerned about politics and the world situation.

Except for concern about the future, there were no significant group differences. Teenagers appeared more worried about future security (16%, 3%, and 2%). Their financial situations in the present and lack of education or preparation for careers indicated that this was a realistic worry.

WORK TOWARD MATERNAL ROLE ATTAINMENT

Overall Feelings about Motherhood

Almost half (47%) responded with positive feelings about motherhood when asked what it was like for them now: "rewarding, wonderful, great, enjoyable, fun, better, easier." The infant's responsiveness to them was central to their remarks. Almost one-fifth (17%) commented that it was "both good and bad," or "work and enjoyment."

Roughly one-third of the women continued to have difficulty adapting to the maternal role; they described motherhood as either "more difficult, hard, frustrating, tiring" or as a direct conflict with their career roles. A few responded rather flatly with noncommittal responses such as "OK," "I'm used to it," or "It's the same." Age groups did not differ significantly in their reported feelings about motherhood.

Feelings about Self as a Result of Motherhood

The majority of the women (61%) reported positive changes in themselves as a result of being a mother. Women saw themselves as more responsible, unselfish, or other-person oriented. Others described feeling more mature, older, more confident or creative. A few saw motherhood as contributing to their feeling more feminine, complete, or fulfilled. Illustrations of positive changes were evidenced by comments:

- Before I had a baby I thought of myself as a young girl, not experienced with life. I feel matured. I had to grow up. It is such a responsibility. I see myself more clearly, and I was doing a lot of soul searching. I have been through an experience that lifted me to another level.
- I was told I had a bone disease and couldn't bear weight. So I decided to try, and I proved that I was a woman. I could put up with those nine months; now I want to prove it again.
- I feel more like I can think of myself as an adult and also act that role more around my parents, whereas before I'd get sucked into the child role with them.
- For a long time I was under treatment for infertility—felt like I had no role or career. . . . She's put some definition into my life—has given me a wonderful purpose.

One-fourth of the women maintained that their feelings about themselves had not changed as a result of motherhood (13%, 25%, and 27%). Significantly fewer teenagers felt that motherhood had not changed their feelings about themselves; the adult role of mother could be expected to have a greater impact on an individual just entering adulthood.

Almost one-fifth of the mothers felt more negatively about themselves since becoming mothers. Negative changes centered around their lives being more restrictive, and their feeling depressed or being fat.

- I'm just not ready for it yet. It's very rough. I've gone back to work.
- Motherhood has confused me more than anything. I used to feel who I was.
- I feel the same, but it's different—confusing to put into perspective.
- Sometimes I feel like a feeding, diaper-changing machine.
- I understand child abusers now. It can drive you up a wall. All I can do is leave him in his room and walk out of the house and let him scream.
- Out of all the professions I've had, this is the biggest challenge.
- I don't have patience. Sometimes I don't like her. I yelled at her sometimes; my family didn't like it. [Mother took her infant to her family in Taiwan to raise for the first few years while she is so busy working.]
- I feel like I'm getting old. I'm twenty-two years old, and I forgot how old I was. I thought only old people did that. It just slipped by; we all forgot it was my birthday.

Motherhood and the Mother–Daughter Relationship

The process of reconciliation between pregnant daughter and her mother that researchers have observed during pregnancy (Ballou, 1978; Bibring et al., 1961; Lederman, 1984) continued following the birth of the child and well into the first year of motherhood. Some of the mothers who observed a change in themselves compared themselves with or related to their own mothers. Several comments made by women from groups 2 and 3 reflect change in self-identity as a result of reviewing their mothers' mothering:

- Sensations of my mother come through to me. She died when I was two. I feel her. I feel so akin to my mother now; I can see the bond.

- There is a conflict between my mother and myself. Mother is very dominant and efficient. . . . I question my capabilities. Can I handle this?
- I find myself looking at my mother and seeing what kind of a mother she is. I don't want to be like her.
- I find I am a lot more like my mom than I thought. She has even admitted there were times she couldn't take it [motherhood].
- I see my mother as an excellent example. I feel some inferiority. I was scared. [This Group 3 mother named her mother who is in Japan as the person most helpful to her in the day-to-day mothering.]

These women are awed at their mother's performance overall, except for the one who rejected her mother as a role model. This is an example of introjection–projection–rejection in the process of maternal role attainment described by Rubin (1967a). The mother who admitted there were times she "couldn't take it" was sharing a confidence that seemed to give her daughter permission to find mothering difficult at times. Lederman (1984) reported that women whose mothers reminisced with them took on the mothering role during pregnancy more easily.

Easiest Mothering Tasks

The majority (60%) saw mother–infant interactions, which they described as being with the baby, playing with the baby, loving or seeing the baby, as the easiest thing about motherhood. Caretaking tasks such as feeding were easiest for one fifth of the women.

Women focused on pleasure derived from infant interactions far more frequently than at 4 months (42%, contrasted with 26%). This finding reflected the infant's increased ability to initiate interaction as well as to return love and affection. A few women (8%) continued to argue that nothing was easy about caring for an 8-month-old.

Most Difficult Mothering Tasks

The most difficult tasks in mothering or the major challenges for women at 8 months were the same as those that had been reported at 4 months with one addition: the infant's behavior, such as getting into things, persistence, and anxiety toward strangers was reported as difficult. The infant's changing behavior was mentioned as most difficult by 14% of the women. The changing behavior was related to both their perceived role incompetencies and role responsibilities.

More women reported role incompetencies as most difficult at 8 months (14%, compared with 9%). Women were concerned about whether they were teaching or doing the right thing for their more capable infants and felt both guilty and vulnerable. The infant's crying, clinging behaviors resulting from anxiety toward strangers evoked guilt when mothers left infants with babysitters, yet they had no other choice because their employment was necessary for family finances.

More mothers reported their responsibility in the role as the most challenging at 8 months (an increase from 8% at 4 months to 18% at 8 months). The constancy of total responsibility for the infant's well-being seemed greater for some as the infant's needs for mobility and exploration increased.

Far fewer women cited the challenge of the time required in the mothering role—19%, contrasted with 58% at 4 months. More of Group 3 reported being pressed for time than did the younger groups (14%, 15%, and 27%). This finding indicates that the infant's schedule was blending more into the household schedule. One example of this blending of schedules was that many infants were reported to be eating three meals a day at 8 months.

Sleep deprivation had changed little overall from 4 months (from 8% to 9%). A few reported that their infants who had been sleeping through the night earlier were waking at 8 months. Women attributed this night waking to teething.

Ideal Image

Women's perceptions of the ideal mother were derived from having the women list five characteristics of an ideal mother. In the order of their frequency, responses included the following: provides an appropriate environment, 81%; is loving, giving, enjoys motherhood, 71%; teaches the infant, 61%; plays with the baby, 48%; comforts, nurtures the baby, 48%; provides developmental stimulation, 47%; feeds the baby, 35%; keeps the baby clean, 21%; disciplines, instills moral values, 15%; involves mate, responsible for family, 11%; stays healthy, 10%; and sees baby as individual, 9%.

Teenagers more often listed "keeps the baby clean" (47%, 20%, and 11%). The older the woman, the more likely she was to list "plays with the infant" (26%, 45%, and 64%) or "comforts and nurtures the infant" (23%, 48%, and 61%). The 20-to-29-year-old mothers more often noted personality characteristics of the ideal mother as loving, giving, and enjoying motherhood (60%, 82%, and 67%). Group 2 women may be more influenced by the stereotypical image of motherhood portrayed in the media.

Maintaining an appropriate environment became very important at 8 months (81%, compared with 31% at 4 months). Safety was a big concern as women put safety latches on kitchen cabinets, gates across stairways, covers over electrical plugs, and moved harmful objects out of the crawling, cruising infant's reach. The category "loving, giving, enjoys motherhood" was named much more often at 8 months (71%, contrasted with 6% at 4 months). The importance of the discipline responsibility increased from 5% at 4 months to 15% at 8 months. Thus, changes in infant development required somewhat different emphasis on what was considered ideal mothering behavior.

The smaller the gap between what women considered as ideal mothering and what they perceived as their own performance, the more positively women could feel about motherhood.

Self-Image

As a whole, the women held positive views about their mothering; 80% rated themselves as 8 or higher. The women's ratings of themselves in the mothering role from 1 to 10, with 10 considered ideal, ranged from 3 to 11. Only 1% rated themselves as 3 or 4; 4% as 5; 3% as 6; 11% as 7; 31% as 8; 30% as 9; 19% as 10; and one woman rated herself as 11. Age groups did not differ significantly in their ratings. There was a very minimal increase in self-image means from 4 months: Group 1, 8.33 from 8.20; Group 2, 8.29 from 8.23; and Group 3, 8.42 from 8.30. The mothers' self-image in mothering changed little with the additional 4 months' experience.

Maternal Role Attainment Behaviors

The quantitative measures of maternal role attainment behaviors reflected the women's reported feelings of incompetency and responsibility that were described as more difficult at this time. Although the mothers' self-image had changed little, the reader will recall from Chapter 2 that their self-concept had decreased significantly at this time. Rather than a linear increase occurring, as might be expected with increased experience in the role, there was a decrease in maternal role behaviors at 8 months, with the exception of the infants' growth and development.

There were no significant group differences in whether the mother was the major caretaker of the infant; 83% of the mothers reported they were the major caretakers (83%, 87%, and 78%). Ten percent reeported they shared caretaking 50-50 with either the mate or another person (who was usually her mother). Six percent reported that they spent less than 12 hr per day as responsible for their infants, and three women (one from Group 1 and two from Group 2) reported they shared caretaking 50-50 with either the mate or another providing the total care for these infants. One infant was in a communal nursery at 8 months, but her mother visited her and took her turn working in the nursery.

Feelings of Love   There were no age group differences in feelings of love for the baby. The mean scores were as follows: Group 1, 35.0; Group 2, 35.1; and Group 3, 35.1. The overall sample mean of 35.1 was significantly less than the mean at 4 months (35.7). Group 1's mean had dropped from 35.8 at 4 months, Group 2's from 35.6, and Group 3's from 35.6.

Only 15.4% of the women's feelings of love for the baby was predictable from the studied variables at 8 months. Variables that predicted these feelings were as follows: race, marital status, and educational level, 0.2%; personality disorder, 8.1%; infant-related marital stress, 3.1%; sadistic child-rearing attitudes, 2.4%; and role strain, 1.6%. The woman with a healthier personality, less infant-related marital stress, more positive child-rearing attitudes, and less role strain scored greater feelings of love for her infant.

Gratification   At 8 months the young women in Group 1 scored significantly higher in gratification in the mothering role (mean, 58.0) than Group 3 (55.2); however, Group 2's mean did not differ significantly from either of the other two (57.1).

The overall sample mean was 56.4; standard deviation, 7.77. Although this was a decrease, it was not significantly different from the mean at 4 months (56.8).

The infant or the infant's responses was the most rewarding thing about motherhood at 8 months for most of the women (87%). Women described their rewards as the infant's growth and development (36%); the infant's responses (25%); the infant (being with, having, closeness) (21%); fulfillment, self-awareness (7%); infant's health and traits (5%); and reinforcement from others (4%).

Role strain and physical support were the major predictors of gratification in mothering at 8 months, indicating that women experiencing high role strain and having little physical help were less able to enjoy or derive rewards from their infants' responses. Almost one-fourth (23.7%) of the variance in gratification was predicted by race, marital status, and educational level (3.2%); role strain (7.3%); physical support (5.9%); marital stress (3.4%); size of network (2.2%); and empathy (1.7%).

Observed Maternal Behavior As had occurred at 4 months, Groups 2 (37.2) and 3 (38.3) means were significantly higher than Group 1's (33.8). All had decreased slightly since 4 months (Group 1, 34.8; Group 2, 37.6; Group 3, 38.5). The overall scores ranged from 18 to 42 (mean, 37.0; standard deviation, 4.63), which was a nonsignificant decrease since 4 months (37.5; SD, 4.24).

Role strain was also the major predictor of observer-rated maternal behavior, with educational level, marital status, and ethnicity as the second greatest predictor. At 8 months maternal behavior was 45.7% predictable from the measured variables. Predictive variables were the following: race, marital status, and educational level, 14.2%; role strain, 19.1%; low-boiling-point attitude, 4.4%; disciplinarian attitude, 2.8%; maternal adaptability, 2.1%; emotional support, 1.1%; infant in hospital during the first month, 1.1%, and size of network, 0.9%.

Self-Reported Ways of Handling Irritating Behavior The most positive score for handling irritating child behavior is 0, and least positive is 20. The range at 8 months was from 0 to 13 (mean, 7.2; SD, 1.90). The older the age group, the more positively the mother handled irritating child behaviors (8.0, 7.5, and 6.8).

Race, educational level, and disciplinarian attitudes were the greatest predictors of the way a mother would handle irritating child behaviors. Being Caucasian with a higher level of education and with less strict disciplinarian attitudes was associated with more positive self-reported ways of handling irritating child behaviors. Just under one-fourth (23.3%) of the ways of handling irritating behaviors was predictable. Predicting variables included race, marital status, educational level (12.1%); disciplinarian attitude (9.8%); infant health status (1.4%).

Infant Growth and Development There were no significant group differences in the factor measuring infant growth and development. Group 1 infants had gained more weight than had infants in the other two groups and weighed significantly more at 8 months (9,032 g, 8,591 g, and 8,840 g). There were no significant group differences in social or motor development.

Little of the variance was predictable in the growth factor (13.4%). Predictive variables included the following: race, marital status, and educational level, 0.5%; low-boiling-point attitude, 6.9%; maternal mood quality, 3.7%; and role strain, 2.4%. Growth and development is probably related to genetic variables more so than to variables measured here. It is noteworthy that social support variables did not predict growth and development as they had at 4 months. Attitudes continued to play a role at 8 months, but maternal mood, marital stress, and role strain played a role that they had not played earlier.

IMPACT OF INFANT ON LIFE-STYLE

The age groups did not differ significantly in the extent that the infant influenced their life-styles. Two percent said, "none"; 8%, "very little"; 17%, "a moderate amount"; 26%, "a good bit"; and 48%, "a great deal."

Mothers' descriptions of how their life-style and home environment had changed included similar responses to those at 4 months. Practically all women reported some change. Decreased mobility and an inability to go whenever they pleased resulted in more homebound time for 98% of the women. Along with the decreased mobility was a lack of spontaneity that had previously enriched their lives. A Group 2 woman noted, "I'm always within a few steps of her; she's very demanding of my attention and is very insecure if I leave the room."

The older the woman, the more likely she was to describe the infant as changing her priorities (10%, 42%, and 56%); 42% reported changed priorities, compared with 29% at 4 months. Almost one-third (29%) reported changed relationships with their mates, only half as many as had mentioned this fact at 4 months. Women described their relationship with their mates as either different (9%), closer (11%), more conflicted (4%), or having negative effects on their sex life (6%). This finding seems at first to be in conflict with Miller and Sollie (1980), who reported increased marital stress at 8 months; however, they were reporting the increase from 4 to 6 weeks postpartum. Whereas the concern about changed mate relationships had been highest at 4 months postpartum, the concerns at 8 months were higher than at 1 month, which agrees with Miller and Sollie's observations. The increase at 8 months over 1 month seems to be related to the negative impact on their sexual life and more vague changes that could not be articulated.

Over one-fifth of the women described changed relationships with their friends; Group 2 women less often mentioned this (24%, 16%, and 31%). There was a tendency for women gradually to drop friends who had no children and seek friends who had children. Because more women have their first child between the ages of 20 and 29 years, the women in Group 2 had more peers with babies, and consequently their friend relationships did not change as much as did the teenager's or the older woman's. The infant presented an opportunity for meeting people, however. A teenager's comment reflected this: "I meet more people now. I'll be out and people will say how cute he is and we start talking."

Other ways in which 13% reported that their life-style had changed included both greater responsibility and personal stability (21%, 17%, and 2%). The teenagers perceived the assumption of responsibility for an infant had forced them to be more stable and reliable individuals; in this sense, motherhood fostered their development.

Fifteen percent of the women reported they were closer to their families; 12% mentioned changes in their home environment that included childproofing, infant equipment, or a cleaner house; 7% reported their lives were more enriched, fun, or happier; 6% reported greater financial strain; and 5% were concerned about having their plans for school interrupted. None of the teenagers expressed conflict about school.

Two-thirds of the women reported from one to three stressors that had occurred since 4 months; 38% reported one stressor, 15% reported two stressors, and 8% reported three stressors. This was a decided increase from 4 months, when only 15% reported stressors. Problematic situations included their own illness, possible pregnancy or pregnancy scare, infant's illness or injury, work factors, mate (jailed, battered her, increased conflicts, or separated from), housing problems or living conditions, death of a parent or grandparent, increased conflicts with friends, neighbors, or relatives. There were no significant differences in stressors by age group.

Infant-Related Stress

There were no significant group differences in infant-related stress at 8 months. The group means indicated that the more active 8-month-old infant caused more stress than the 4-month-old, however. Group 1's mean increased from 52.7 to 54.5; Group 2's mean increased from 51.4 to 53.0; and Group 3's mean increased from 52.7 to 54.5. Although group mean increases were not significant, the overall sample mean increase was: 52.5 (SD, 12.05) from 51.1 (SD, 12.10).

There were no group differences on the mate-related stress subscale means. The overall sample range was from 7 to 27 (mean, 13.7; SD, 4.51). The group means varied little: Group 1 from 14.3 to 14.1 at 8 months; Group 2 from 13.4 to 14.0; and Group 3 from 13.0 to 13.3. Fewer talked about stress from changes in the mate relationship at 8 months, but that may have reflected the increase in other general stressors in their lives during this period, which may have been worse than the minimal change in infant-related marital stress.

Since financial problems were reported by some, one item related to financial problems was analyzed separately. The teenagers' score was significantly higher for financial stress than those of groups 2 and 3 (3.4, 2.9, and 2.6, with 3 indicating somewhat of a bother and 5, very much of a bother).

Role Conflict and Role Strain

Women talked about their feelings of ambivalence and conflict around career–mother and wife–mother roles very openly at 8 months. Further, 55% were employed, and only 10% of the women reported sharing caretaking responsibilities 50–50 with either the mate or another person.

Almost half of the women (48%) experienced from moderate to very high role strain. Nine percent of the women did not reflect any role strain, 43% experienced low role strain, 32% experienced moderate role strain, 9% experienced high role strain, and 7% experienced very high role strain.

However, despite the increased reports of ambivalence regarding other roles, role strain had not increased at 8 months. There was little change from the role strain means at 4 months: Group 1 from

2.77 to 2.76; Group 2 from 2.67 to 2.51; and Group 3 from 2.49 to 2.66. There were no significant group differences in observed role strain.

Maternal Individuation Although the mothers' responses were largely positive, there was a sense of maternal impatience at having been unable to move on with personal plans. The consuming nature of being a mother made it difficult for the women to see themselves apart from the infant. One woman in her twenties expressed her frustration: "I'm me, a person who happens to be a mother. It comes naturally. I do lots of things. She's just with me while I do them. I'm no longer 'a working woman' or a 'sexy person.' " A woman over 30 years stated, "I'm thinking more about things I want to do than I did before, and I'm not as willing to wait."

Some of the mothers' descriptions of the impact of their infants indicated an inability to separate the infant from the maternal self. Much has been written about the infant's individuation; however, such comments as "I don't think of myself apart from the baby" indicated that women had not achieved the polarization process described by Rubin (1977), in which the symbiosis that began during pregnancy is severed with the establishment of distinct body boundaries for mother and infant. Although a physical break occurs at birth, an emotional symbiosis continues (Deutsch, 1945).

The polarization process described by Rubin (1977) is analogous to maternal individuation observed in this sample. Rubin defined polarization as the "physical and conceptual separating-out process of the incorporated infant of pregnancy into a separate, external and constant entity postpartally" (p. 70). She described polarization as beginning during late pregnancy and continuing through the 4- to 6-week postpartum period. A "bursting out" was described at the third to fourth week, when the mother ventures into adult society and reidentifies the infant as a "you" and restores her "I." The "I" was not completely restored at 8 months postpartum for many women.

Mothers were asked when their infants first seemed like real persons; their responses may suggest something about where the mother was in individuation from her infant at 8 months following birth. Their responses ranged from birth or immediately (32%), 1 to 3 months (21%), and 4 to 6 months (36%), to 7 to 8 months (8%). There were no significant differences in group responses. One teenager stated that her baby was like a person "when he started talking and making noises and could wear clothes." Group 2 women gave illustrations such as the following:

- At two months, when she began to really look at me.
- At six months, when he was beginning to be more physical, sitting up, turning over.
- When she sat up and noticed differences and had preferences.
- At five months, when the lady at the day-care center referred to her as Elizabeth. This reminded me that she was a separate, unique little person, and I realized that she had her own little life and saw and did things that I wasn't a participant of.

Group 3 responses included:

- When he started laughing, at three months.
- Always—even before birth.
- I had an amniocentesis and sonogram and saw him paddling water and knew he had his own motivations, but at eight months he became a *real* person.

Their comments indicate that mothers are observing the infant's evolving self as described by Stechler and Kaplan (1980) in Chapter 4, and as the infant develops awareness of self, mothers were also seeing their infant's uniqueness as an individual person. However, over half (54%) of the mothers reported that their infant had become a real person to them by 3 months; Robson and Moss (1970) reported that most of the mothers in their study had felt this at 9 weeks.

Mothers also were asked when their infants first recognized them. Over two-thirds (69%) said their infants recognized them during the first 4 days following birth. Another fifth (18%) noted that their infants first recognized them during the first month; 6% stated that their infants first recognized them at 2 to 4 months. Mothers' feelings when their infants first recognized them ranged from 9% who were vague or unsure to the great majority who really felt good and were excited about their infants' recognition. Two percent expressed a feeling of being frightened by the infant's recognizing them as the mother because of their responsibility to a helpless human being.

During the process of maternal individuation, 87% of the women perceived that their infants recognized them as their mothers very early. But it wasn't until 3 months that over half (54%) of the women viewed their infants as separate, unique persons. Some women from groups 2 and 3 were continuing to struggle for the retrieval of their "I" as individuals who had other important adult roles apart from mother:

- I'm totally different; my metabolism is different, my body is different.
- There are times when I feel trapped and frightened about the future.
- I'm trying to figure out how I fit in all of this; I don't think of myself apart from the infant.

Teenagers did not appear to allow themselves to become enmeshed with their infants to this extent. The question is raised whether only a person who is comfortable with an established adult identity (the major developmental task of adolescence) is able either to permit, recognize, or verbalize the disequilibrium of the self system to incorporate a child.

COPING STRATEGIES: RESOURCES FOR MOTHERING AT EIGHT MONTHS

Coping Strategies

Women were asked specifically how they managed difficult times with their infants. Half described self-initiated caretaking action that met the infant's needs either by soothing, distracting, or changing the infant's activity. One-third reported that they gave the infant to either their mate or another person to care for. One-fifth directed self-action inward by regrouping after they had gotten the infant quiet; they regrouped by either napping, praying, or meditating. One-sixth of the women reported that they cried, bitched, yelled, or became otherwise angry and upset. One-sixth just put the infant to bed, walked out, and let the infant cry it out. One-tenth reported that they went for a walk or an outing, and one-tenth talked to someone—a friend, mate or a physician.

Five percent of the women reported that they had *no* difficult times. One or two women reported each of the following: smoking pot, drinking, biting nails, turning the stereo on loud, voicing frustrations to the infant, and taking frustrations out on the husband.

There were no significant group differences in coping strategies, except for the category of meeting the infant's needs by soothing;

the older the woman, the more often she reported this (8%, 22%, and 30%). This indicates that with increased maturity an individual is able to recognize infant frustration that needs soothing as distinct from, and having priority over, self-frustration.

Size of Support Network

The number of persons in the women's social support network who helped with day-to-day mothering situations did not differ significantly by age group. Only 4% reported that they had no one to help them with mothering. Most mentioned either one person (31%) or two persons (27%). Nineteen percent listed three persons, and 19% listed four or more persons.

The pattern of the mate being reported more frequently by groups 2 and 3, and the mother being reported more frequently by Group 1 continued at 8 months. Mates were listed by almost three-fourths (71%) of the women (51%, 74%, and 75%). Over one-third (38%) reported the mother/mother-in-law as being helpful (51%, 39%, and 30%). Friends continued to increase in the support network at 8 months (reported by 47%, contrasted with 34% at 4 months). The older the age group, the more often friends were reported in the social network (35%, 43%, and 56%).

Teenagers listed their mates as often as their mother/mother-in-law in their social networks at 8 months. They also listed friends more frequently than at 4 months. The equal importance of mates and increased importance of friends to teenagers may indicate a shift toward independence from their mothers and increased social skills in establishing friendships.

The teenager more often reported having more help than she needed (16%, 7%, and 6%). Groups 2 and 3 indicated more often that they had as much help as needed (52%, 72%, and 65%). One could conjecture that around 10% of the teenagers may have viewed their mother's or an adult's help as intrusive rather than as helpful; other comments did not indicate that they actually had more help than was needed.

Type of Support Reported

Most of the women (92%) reported physical support such as help with child care, errands, housework, cooking, or financial help and gifts. Only 7% described reassurance in their role performance, and almost one-fourth (23%) reported receiving advice or information that was helpful. There were no group differences in these types of support.

Almost half (48%) reported receiving emotional support that included having someone understand their feelings and someone to listen to them. The older the woman, the more often she reported receiving emotional support (34%, 46%, and 60%). Fewer teenagers reported emotional support at 8 months than earlier at 4 months (43%); although there was a reported increase in friends, they apparently did not provide emotional support.

Help Other Than People

Over half of the women (56%) reported that books and magazines were helpful to them in their mothering. The older the woman, the more likely she was to report books or magazines as helpful (39%, 58%, and 65%).

Seven percent of the women reported that parenting classes were very helpful. Other help came from the following: television or radio, 8%; previous experience with children, 3%; getting away or out, school, or work, 3%; religion, 2%; infant equipment such as walker, playpen, or disposable diapers, 2%; toys, 1%; money, 1%; and participation in this project, 1%.

EMPLOYED VERSUS NONEMPLOYED MOTHERS

The interviews raised many questions about employment for mothers because 55% were employed and 48% experienced moderate to high role strain. The literature indicated that working mothers did not receive additional help with mother or wife roles, and Majewski (1983) did not observe differences in role conflict between employed and nonemployed mothers; however, questions were raised about differences in perceived help and infant schedules. As was noted above, only 10% of the women reported having shared caretaking of the infant 50-50 with a mate or someone else, and another 6% said that someone cared for the infant 12 hr or more a day.

The average age of the infants when the mothers as a whole went to work was 15.2 weeks. The older the age group, the younger the average age of the infants in weeks when their mothers were employed (20.4, 14.7, and 13.8). Jimenez and Newton (1982) reported that women who had higher interest in their work tended to wait longer before starting a family, work longer during pregnancy, and planned to return to work sooner postpartum.

All women were grouped as either employed (n = 128) or nonemployed (n = 114). There were no significant differences by employment status in the number of stressors reported, maternal health status, perceived help in mothering, reported regularity of infants' schedules, role strain, ratings of self in the mothering role, or in maternal attitudes. There were no significant differences in the maternal role attainment variables for feelings of love for the baby, gratification in the mothering role, observed maternal behaviors, and self-reported ways of handling irritating child behaviors.

There were significant differences in the infant growth and development factor between employed and nonemployed mothers, however, with infants of employed mothers scoring lower. This raises questions about whether infants' day-care situations provide the quality of stimulation and nurturing that mothers do. One teenager had a retired couple caring for her infant who kept her infant in the crib all day while she worked. Another teenager had her infant in a situation in which there were 15 toddlers for 1 adult. Some parents could not afford day care, so they worked at night when husbands were home and cared for their infants and slept during the day. Older women in Group 3 were more likely to have either live-in help or persons who came to their homes to care for their infants.

Although there were no significant differences by employment status for any of the variables in the teenage group, it is of interest that their infants' growth and development factor differed by a greater margin than for the total group or any group individually. Because of the smaller sample size in Group 1, this greater difference did not reach a level of significance (Chassan, 1979). Employed teenagers scored higher in observed maternal behaviors (mean, 34.84) than nonemployed teenagers (mean, 33.12). The teenager who sought employment may have been a more mature individual who performed all roles well. This finding and interpretation are in agreement with Slesinger (1981) who found that among a sample of low-socioeconomic-status (SES) mothers aged 15 to 45 years, employed mothers scored higher in mothercraft than nonemployed mothers.

Within Group 2 significant differences were found in role strain (employed mean, 2.71; N = 65, nonemployed mean, 2.24, N = 49), observed maternal behaviors (employed mean, 36.49, nonemployed mean, 38.24), and infant growth and development factor (employed mean, – 0.38, nonemployed mean, 0.26).

Within Group 3 no significant differences were found in any of the variables except for feelings of love for the infant. Employed mothers (n = 46) had more positive feelings of love for the infant (35.63) than nonemployed mothers (N = 40; 34.42). It is noteworthy that although differences were not significant, employed Group 3 women also scored higher on gratification in the maternal role (55.62, compared with 54.72). Nonemployed Group 3 mothers' infants also scored lower on the growth and development factor (-0.07, compared with 0.11).

The failure to find significant differences in role strain by employment and nonemployment is congruent with Majewski (1983), who did not find differences in role conflict, with the exception of Group 2. The difference between employed and nonemployed women was only 0.47 in Group 2 and 0.44 in Group 1, and nonemployed women had higher role strain in Group 3 (0.35 difference). Group 2 was larger, so a smaller difference could reach a level of significance. However, Group 2 listed their mothers in their support group less often than teenagers and were financially less able to hire live-in help than women in Group 3. Group 2 also listed the ideal mother as one who was loving and giving and enjoyed motherhood significantly more often than the other groups. The difference in physical help along with different images of what was ideal mothering behavior could account for differences in role strain.

The group differences in the infant growth and development by employment status also raises the issue about whether factors such as readiness for the pregnancy, gratification in the employment role, or SES may affect infant growth and development more than employment status per se. Further research is warranted to look at these relationships. The reader will recall that there were no group differences for infant growth and development, role strain, or feelings of love for the baby. Teenagers scored significantly lower on observed maternal behavior, but employed teenagers scored higher than nonemployed teenagers, whereas employed women from Group 3 scored higher on feelings of love for the baby. The older group of women had opportunity to develop a career prior to childbearing and may have enjoyed their more accomplished employment roles more. This interpretation agrees with Harrell and Ridley (1975), who found satisfaction in one area of life was related to satisfaction in other areas and that adaptation to employment roles was related to high adaptation to the childbearing role.

Group 2 women were moving into the mothering role without the benefit of having achieved in a career role to the extent that most of

Group 3 had, and the employment role may have been less attractive, more difficult, and less clearly defined for them. As discussed above, other factors such as their image of an ideal mother, along with support received, may have also been influential.

ADVICE MOTHERS WOULD GIVE TO OTHER MOTHERS OF EIGHT-MONTH-OLDS

Sixty percent of the women did not offer information for other mothers from their experiences. This was a last interview question, and fatigue may have been a factor in their lack of response to this item. However, of those who offered advice, the most frequent response was that flexibility in dealing with the infant should be stressed. Others mentioned that playing with or enjoying the infant were important. The rapid infant changes should be stressed because these changes necessitated closer supervision.

Getting help from others was considered important advice along with the admonition that a mother needs breaks from the routine and diversions for herself. Socializing with other mothers was frequently mentioned as one way of getting needed help. A few women stressed that readiness for an infant was critical.

SELECTED WOMEN'S EXPERIENCES

As a reminder, all women in Group 1 have names beginning with an "A," those in Group 2 begin with a "B," and those in Group 3 begin with a "C." The first two women in each of the three groups reported they were unmarried at the initial interview, and the last two reported they were married.

Alma

Sixteen-year-old Alma and her husband were still living with his mother. Alma appeared rested and was neat and well groomed. The baby's residence was evidenced by toys everywhere; the playpen was in the living room. Alma's husband was present for the interview and played with the baby throughout. He took the baby to the mirror, later to a window, talked to him sensitively, and pointed out things.

Alma was not employed, nor was she attending school. She planned to take the high school equivalency test the following week and had been studying at home for it.

Alma reported that she had felt good for the past 4 months except for a cold and sore throat a month ago that lasted 2½ weeks. She rated her health as good, stating that she needed more exercise. Alma talked about motherhood:

> I thought it would be hard; it feels easier. Nothing bothers me about it. It feels good to be a mother. I have more responsibility, and have to work things out on my own. But that feels good.

> My life has changed a moderate amount. I am closer to my family than before. I have more responsibility than I used to have. It makes me feel good to have him around.

> My husband has helped me the most the past four months. He gives the baby a bath, puts him to bed, watches him while I do chores, plays with him and feeds him—does everything. He does a great deal in taking care of the infant.

> The baby likes to play peek-a-boo, to have me chase him, and play with balls. He used to like to be tossed around, but now it scares him. He likes to be tickled and sung to. He says "Da-Da," "BaBa," and "Hi." He opens and closes his hands, crawls, pulls to standing, moves a lot, picks up really fast, talks a lot, picks up tiny things, plays peek-a-boo, and imitates.

> I teach him something is unsafe by saying, "No, that's bad," and pat his fingers. He looks at us; I distract him. He became a real person at five months when he started learning everything. I first felt love for him when he was born. He first recognized me at two to three months; it felt good [laughs].

> Everything is the same; nothing is difficult. Baby care isn't hard. The easiest thing about mothering is feeding him. I'd rate myself as 'ten" in mothering. The most rewarding is taking care of my family.

> My future plans are to let him grow to be whatever he wants; I want him to have karate lessons when he is five and go to public school.

> My greatest concern at this time is our future. What kind of jobs can we get? Getting off welfare.

> I'd tell other mothers that it's easy. People say to me, "you're a baby yourself, something might happen." I know what is right for the baby. We take good care of him, like we took him camping. We know what to do.

Alison

Alison, aged 18, was casually dressed, had makeup on, and her hair was carefully done up at the time of the interview. Her mother's home was neat. Alison had a nervous laugh throughout the interview and did not seem to be completely open. Her pregnant cousin was present during the interview, and some of her responses may have been for the cousin's benefit. Alison directed some of her answers in her cousin's direction. Alison's infant was happy and smiling; Alison was warm and affectionate toward the infant and obviously very proud.

Alison stated that her relationship with the father of the baby was now over. (They were in the process of breaking up at 4 months.) She described how she felt:

> I've felt OK the past four months. I'm trying to lose this "jelly" in my middle. I've had a couple of colds. He [baby] caught one from me. I'd rate my health as very good.

> I like motherhood [laughs]. It teaches me a lot. More patience [laugh]. I like to sit back and enjoy watching him grow up and seeing him do new things. I don't mind not having as much time to myself. I'm happy with myself; I wasn't too happy with myself before. I have someone to take care of—responsibility.

> The baby has changed my life-style a great deal. I feel closer to my family now [laughed and appeared more nervous]. I stay home a lot more now. I used to go out a lot more.

> My mother has helped me the most the past few months. She helped by giving me free time for myself and advice about what to do. In the beginning it interfered, but now I appreciate it more. I read a lot of baby books—an old one of my mom's. I like the old-fashioned way. Our relationship [with mother] has improved a lot.

> He [the baby] is doing a lot of new things. He stands up by himself, and says "Ma-ma," plays with toys, crawls, gets into stuff, likes to walk, and is learning what "no" means. He likes for me to tickle him and walk with him, play peek-a-boo and patty-cake, brush his hair. He goes crazy. He likes for me to play with his toys, and bounce him up and down. I teach him something is unsafe by saying no and removing him and slapping his hands.

> He became a real person to me at six months. I first felt love for him when he was first born; it just grows stronger as he grows up. He recog-

nized me immediately. He stared right at me right away. It made me feel happy [loving type of laugh].

The most difficult thing about motherhood is all the time I have to put into it. The easiest is taking care of him. I'd rate myself "eight" on mothering. The most rewarding thing is knowing you have decisions to make for another person.

My future plans for him are school [laugh]. I haven't looked very far yet. My primary concern is about his growing up—that nothing will go wrong.

Alice

Alice, aged 19, looked rested but somewhat disorganized. She was dressed neatly in a skirt and blouse. She was enthusiastic about mothering and seemed happy. She asked the interviewer questions about options for career and school. She was spontaneous with her baby and had age-appropriate toys, but she slapped him frequently during the interview for normal curiosity-type behavior.

Alice reported that she had gotten depressed about her job (has been working 7:00 p.m. to 1:00 a.m. since 4 months) and that she'd like another job but only if it is a daytime job.

Alice had not been ill the past 4 months and rated her health as very good. However, she reported that she had a bad scare:

> I forgot my period wouldn't be regular. It was delayed two and a half to three months, and I thought I was pregnant. We got into an argument. My husband doesn't want more kids. I used to be against abortion, but I couldn't afford another. I cried. Finally two days later, I started. I was so relieved.

> Motherhood is nice. I really like it. Fun! I don't see him as someone who depends on me. I see me helping him to learn. I want him to learn to depend on himself. I won't be here forever. I really know my baby, and he knows me. Motherhood hasn't changed how I feel about myself. When I leave the house, I'm me. I don't forget about him when I'm home—I'm a mom.

> He has changed our life-style a great deal. We usually have to stay home. We [baby and self] really depend on each other now. It's fun to watch his curiosity. I understand he's not just tearing things up. My mom and I are closer. She's calling me more. Friends are a little more distant—don't go out as much; it's hard to arrange it. My priorities have changed. I can accept change; I know it won't be constant. I'm not going to school anymore.

My husband has been the most helpful to me. When he gets home at 4:00 p.m., I'm wound up. The baby needs a new energy level. He helps some with the baby so I can cook; he distracts him. He's more worried about his health.

The baby walks along furniture, still scoots—can't get up on his knees. He tries to stand alone. Says "Ma-ma," "be" or "ba," claps with patty-cake, waves bye-bye, plays peek-a-boo, likes to tear things up, likes noise, and loves kisses. The toilet and shower fascinate him. He likes for me to play patty-cake, peek-a-boo, horse, puppet (we talk), and with his squeezy toys. He likes for me to hold his hands and walk him, and to toss him into the air, and to bounce and tickle him.

I teach him something is unsafe by saying "no" real firm and talking to him. I put plugs in the outlets and moved dangerous solutions to the back of the cupboard. I slap his hands when he gets into places [she slapped his hands frequently during the interview].

The baby became a real person to me right about now—eight months. He knows what he wants; he's more mobile and he gets to what he wants. I first felt love for him the day after birth. I was disappointed, I wanted a girl—felt the world was against me. He first recognized me when he was a few weeks old; I was really happy.

The most difficult thing about motherhood now is that I'm afraid I won't motivate him enough. I know that motivation and stimulation are important. The easiest thing is loving him. I rate myself a "seven"; I wish I could motivate him more [rated self a 10 at 4 months]. The most rewarding thing about motherhood is him—he's a gift—a reflection of my mothering. He reflects what I feed in.

My future plans are for him to go to a private school—a French bilingual school. I'll pay two arms and four legs to pay for it. I don't have any major concerns now.

Amy

Amy, aged 18, still had on her night clothes at 3:00 p.m. when the interviewer arrived. Her room was immaculate, but the house was quite cluttered (they were living with her mother). The baby shares her room. The maternal grandmother cared for the baby during the interview.

Amy reported that she had had no problems since 4 months, and she rated her health as good. She responded to what it was like as a mother:

I feel good. I feel proud. It's getting better. I don't have to carry him so much. He crawls and plays by himself. I feel more responsibility—but I'm going through with it.

He has influenced our life-style a great deal. My husband and I are getting along good with my folks. We don't hardly ever go out now. I went back to school when he was two weeks old, so see friends at school. But I miss going out.

My mom has been the most helpful to me the past months. She always helps. She likes it—just her and me usually take care of him. We share about fifty–fifty except when my mother is on vacation. I just don't go to school if I can't find someone to take care of him. Three times a week I go to school. There is no nursery there. I wish my husband would take care of him more. He lives with his parents in Alameda, and he sees the baby two times a week.

The baby wants to walk, climbs, stands up by himself. He's so cute [laugh]. He eats a lot. Says, "Ma-ma," "Pa-pa," and calls my mom "Mama" too. He uses his hands a lot. He likes for me to talk to him. I didn't believe in that; now I talk to him. He likes for me to chase him, play peek-a-boo. We hardly ever go out.

I don't teach him things are unsafe yet—he's too young. He was a real person when he was born. I first felt feelings of love for him when he was about three months. [She described him as "skinny and hopeless" at birth.] He first recognized me when he was five months old. I felt good about it; I liked that.

The most difficult thing about motherhood is just spending time—being with him all the time, and I'm hardly ever around. He might not know me when he grows up. The easiest thing is playing with him—his smiles. I rate myself "five" in mothering. I don't know too much. I'm not good. I'm just putting up with it. Maybe I'm not giving him enough. Sometimes I don't have time. I'm not here enough. I've been cancelling his appointments a lot—they keep calling me. [She rated herself as 5 at 4 months also.] The most rewarding thing about motherhood is seeing him growing.

My future plans for him is to have a house, and when the three of us start living together. My major concern is what our future will be.

Betty

Betty, aged 22, appeared rested and was casually dressed at the time of the interview. She still lives with her mother and is unemployed. Her health had not been problematic, and she rated it as very good. She was enthusiastic when asked what it was like for her as mother now:

> I feel good. I want more kids. I love it. It's neat now that he's able to return feelings toward me. This is what I've always wanted. He's been a wonderful kid. No problems. I'm stunned, he's so good. Motherhood has changed my life for the better.

> He has changed our life-style a great deal for the better. I'm responsible, not able to do as much. It hasn't changed as much as I'd expected. He's always accepted where ever I take him—eighty percent of the time he goes with us.

> His father has been the most helpful to me the past months. He takes care of him and comforts me if something is wrong.

> The baby stands up and walks in his walker. He walked with support at six and a half months. He crawls, climbs stairs, babbles, puts everything into his mouth, drops things, and holds his bottle. He likes to have his toes chewed, to be nibbled, blown, and kissed all over. He likes for me to crawl on the floor and play chase.

> I teach him something is unsafe by saying "no" and removing him. He's not into much yet. Starting at seven months he first became a real person to me. He's changing. My love for him is stronger as he gets older. He'll show affection now. He first recognized me at four months. Now he jumps up and laughs and reaches for me. It made me feel really good. He's part of me. I've always wondered how they got attached.

> The most difficult thing about motherhood is the worry. He's no burden physically. I'd rate myself as "nine" in mothering. The easiest thing is taking care of him. He's the most rewarding thing about motherhood. He shows his love for me—returns affection and love now.

> My future plans for him are little boy things—baseball, girl friends, school, to be an architect. My primary concerns at this time are to be happy, and I always wonder about our health.

Barbara

Barbara's kitchen where the interview was held was very cluttered, but this was clearly not a priority. Barbara, aged 26, was very self-confident and comfortable with herself and obviously enjoyed her daughter. The daughter was all smiles and responded warmly to her mother. Barbara breast-fed her, talked to her, and caressed her. She gave her a fresh peach later, which the infant dropped on the floor several times. Barbara patiently retrieved the peach, washed it, and gave it to her daughter again. She was baking a special bread for the daughter also.

Barbara rated her health as very good. She commented that she was a little overweight and had more yeast infection—having trouble shaking it. Her response to what it was like as a mother was enthusiastic:

> It's wonderful; I'm having the greatest time. I'm a career woman with a flexible schedule. I take Elsie to work with me. I'm very happy she is a girl. It is very rewarding—precious time. Really bittersweet. I totally enjoy it—frustrations—how I'll get housework done. Nothing is insurmountable. I've always been confident; motherhood has made me more confident. When I was first home from the hospital, I was scared—she seemed fragile; now I'm confident.
>
> She has changed our life-style a great deal. Socially—we almost never go out. I have social time with people I work with. I can't run out impulsively. I usually take Elsie with me. It feels very good.
>
> My mate has been incredible the past few months. Elsie is a remarkable child, not difficult. I talk to other mothers and read a lot as often as I can. My mate is very supportive. I can say anything I want. He listens whether it is his belief system or not. He loves her a lot.
>
> She wants to walk; is starting to take steps. She holds on. She plays hard. She has a great personality, a good sense of humor. She loves for me to sing to her, show her a book, mimic, get down on the floor, and put voices behind toys.
>
> I teach her something is unsafe by saying, "Hot, no, no." I really expound, and I don't let her touch it.
>
> She was a real person to me when I saw her at birth. I loved her right away, when I first touched her. She recognized me in the delivery room. She grasped my finger, and stopped crying, and nursed me. I felt exquisite —fulfilled.
>
> The most difficult thing about motherhood now is the intense vulnerability that motherhood brings. I always felt that I could handle things really well. When I became a mother, I felt someone poked a hole in my confidence. I worry about how other people will treat her. I worry a lot. I wish to give her the best skills like I got, and what if she doesn't get them. The naturalness of motherhood has been the easiest. It is very easy to love this baby—to spend time with her and care for her needs. Motherhood has been better than my expectations. Sensations of my mother come through to me. She died when I was two. I feel it. I feel so akin to

my mother now. I can see the bond [breast-feeding her infant]. I rate my-self as a "ten." The most rewarding thing about motherhood is her re-sponse.

My future plans are I would like an alternative or primary home in the country. Or at least a better neighborhood than where we are now. My pri-mary concerns at this time are the neighborhood, finances—looking to-ward a more stable income, and my appearance—losing weight.

Bea

Twenty-one-year-old Bea was casually dressed, very informal, re-laxed, and happy during the interview. The interview took place on her front steps in the sunshine, watching the baby play. The infant played happily with assorted toys. Bea frequently showed him a new toy and how to play with it. She showed him the cat and helped him pet it, showed him flowers and let him smell them.

Bea reported that she had felt fine since 4 months. She rated her health as very good. She described motherhood:

I'm managing fine. It feels good, very happy; I've not noticed a lot of change. It's been natural, a gradual change in my life. I knew it would be a big responsibility. Now I know it is more than I thought it would be [laughs]. I was meant to be a mom. It has not affected how I feel about myself.

He has caused very little change in our life-style. It takes longer to get ready to go anywhere. Financially—less money—fewer places to go. Nothing bad has happened. We're closer. We do the same things—it just takes longer.

My husband has been the most helpful to me. He helps with James. Feeds him, puts him to bed, pitches in and really helps. I haven't needed much. He's a good baby.

He's doing really good—healthy. He's scooting—moves a lot, feeds himself finger foods, into things. He likes to touch things. I'm trying to teach him "no." He mimics and initiates games. He repeats sounds—*ball, dad, mom, kitty*. He likes for me to read books to him. He turns pages, plays patty-cake, likes for me to sing, likes lap games, to walk, and to go to the park to swing.

To teach him something is unsafe I say "no" and smack his fingers. I started at seven months when he started crawling. I'm childproofing, slowly but surely.

He has always been a real person to me—at birth. I loved him at birth [smiles, hugs baby]. At three and a half months he recognized me as his mom; special, he has a strong attachment to me. It really feels good.

The most difficult thing about motherhood is getting up in the morning when I would like to sleep, going out and needing four arms to do it. I get tired sometimes. The easiest thing is playing and having fun with him. I have a lot of fun. I rate myself a "nine" in mothering. The most rewarding thing is watching him grow and seeing his development, and seeing that he's happy and well adjusted.

I don't have many future plans for him. We're trying to find property to buy and fix up to make a good home for him. We're making a future for him. My primary concern is finding a place to live. We'll move in a couple of months.

Bonnie

Bonnie, aged 28, was dressed in her robe, and her hair was in rollers when the interviewer arrived at 3:00 p.m. Her home was clean, the kitchen and dining room table were cluttered. She seemed open with the interviewer but yawned a lot (as she had at 4 months) and inquired whether amphetamines and barbiturates were addicting. Bonnie seemed self-focused; she noted that she didn't need friendships.

Bonnie's home was childproofed, but toys were not age-appropriate. There were no noisy, bright-colored, or moving toys—only dolls and stuffed animals.

Bonnie reported tha· she was a whole lot better the past 4 months, that she was now adjusted to motherhood. She mentioned that she had seen a psychiatrist earlier to help her adjust to motherhood. Working seemed to help; she teaches English to foreign students for 3 hr 4 days a week. Bonnie is also taking a 3-hr class once a week and is on a citizen's advisory board committee.

She had gotten pregnant; it was a terrible experience, and she felt she couldn't handle another baby, so she had an abortion. Her grandfather died a week ago. Although she rated her health as very good, she noted her weight is not good. For this she is going to a health spa and is on a 500-calorie diet; the physician gave her amphetamines and barbiturates for her diet.

Bonnie was reflective about what it was like for her being a mother:

I enjoy being a mom. I'm able to relate to the word *mother* now, especially since the baby can say "Ma-ma." I'm not sure if it's mother-hood, but I sure do like myself. I never liked myself before. People relate to you like you don't like yourself [friends]. They change their behavior when they realize how you like yourself.

She's changed our life-style a great deal. She is first. I'm no longer in-volved in myself totally. I have gradually accepted it in stages. I am at the final stage of acceptance, a supportive women's group and therapy helped with that.

My husband has been the most helpful the past four months. He is very encouraging, very helpful. Actually, he's a "good mother." Men are now better; he observed at birth—it helps them to be better. [Yawns, takes out pill box and takes a pill.]

She loves commercials; loves TV. Likes watching people; she has a long attention span, is bright, receptive. She says, "mama," "dada," "bottle," "thank you." She knows when we are going out. She can identi-fy people. She likes for me to play patty-cake—grab things. Likes for me to chase her around; she is very independent. We talk and play.

She likes to pick pebbles out of the plant. I take her hand and slap lightly. At first she laughed. After I hurt her, she understands now.

She first became a real person to me just recently, around six months. The first day I brought her home from the hospital I thought I loved her, but recently I felt a lot more. I didn't know it was normal to have doubts. She recognized me at birth. The nursery nurses mentioned it. It was fright-ening. [Could or would not explain this comment any further as to why it was frightening.]

The most difficult thing about mothering now is all the time demands. There are things you have to eliminate. It's good—also helps get your life together. The easiest thing is that I don't have to go through childbirth again soon. I rate myself as "ten" in mothering. The most rewarding thing about motherhood is that it's a blessing to have a child. I feel honored that this is my responsibility.

I want her to be an artist. It's up to her. I want her to develop creative-ly, to be spiritual. That's very special.

Carrie

Carrie, aged 33, looked rested and was dressed in matching slacks and blouse. The interview took place in a home where she babysits. She has had this job for 2 months. Carrie was happy and had begun dating. She seemed to be handling the separation from her husband well. She was animated in her responses to her daughter and encouraged her daughter's exploratory behaviors.

Carrie reported that she was lucky that she had excellent health. However, her skin has been blotchy since pregnancy; she had hoped it would go away. She responded enthusiastically as to what motherhood was like now:

> Pretty nice. A good situation. I am babysitting, so with her it is easy. I don't have to work, but I get here at eight and stay till six p.m. The babies entertain themselves. Its nice to get close to the baby and see her personality develop. I feel more like an adult [33 years]. I'm more compassionate as a person; I can relate better to others who have difficulties. I feel important. I now use belts in the car, don't get high with friends. I take better care of my health.

> She has changed my life-style a great deal. Before, my priorities were to buy nice clothes and travel. Still, they are nice and I am still social. I am very busy with her, so that is not important. She fits in easily. Some friends are closer, and some aren't. A lot of friends have found out that my husband and I separated during pregnancy. He is now helping me financially. He has come around a bit on his own. He plays with her. She looks like him. He thought if you have a child it would alter your life. I have been dating. Have taken baby on dates; men are receptive I've found [pleased].

> The woman I share a house with has been the most helpful to me with mothering. I could count on her in an emergency. She reinforces what I'm doing. She has good advice, has had good experience. She spontaneously helps if I'm busy—cooking, et cetera.

> The baby crawls on all fours. She cruises holding onto furniture, crawls up the stairs, holds her own bottle, imitates sound, and loves mirrors. She likes physical play such as swinging. She likes for me to play with dominoes with her, to ride her in the baby seat on my bike, to dance with her, to look in the mirror with her. She chases the cat. If she grabs at the cat, I pull her away and slap her hand, and say "no" very firmly.

> She has always been a real person to me. When I nursed her in intensive care, I noticed it right away. The nurses were even keyed into her personality. I loved her right when she was born. They said to kiss her. When I was in recovery, I missed her—a longing to be with her. She was jaundiced. She knew my voice, so exciting. She recognized me the first day, when I saw her in ICN. She recognized my voice. I felt great [smiled, pleased].

> The most difficult thing about motherhood is it takes money. Always a parent, it never ends, every minute has to be organized. The easiest thing

is they give you love back. I rate myself as "nine" in mothering. I'm really ready for the experience—not frustrated at all. I am glad I didn't wait for the "right time." The most rewarding thing is the closeness, the intense feeling. It's like falling in love with a man, an incredible closeness, the strong bond. Nice to experience.

My future plans for her are to view her as a buddy, take her roller skating, put her in my backpack. I'll take her on the vacation back home at Christmas.

Cathryn

Cathryn, aged 36, was still overweight and was dressed in jeans and a sweater. She was still living with her parents. Her parents' home was very clean. Cathryn looked a little tired. Her mother chatted with the interviewer a few minutes, then left the room. Cathryn was unaware of aspects of babyproofing her home.

Cathryn was watchful of her infant during the interview but did not seem happy when interacting with the baby; she rarely smiled at him. Her attitude was one of coping. She seemed depressed. She said she had felt good until the last couple of months; since then she has been in a "haze." Cathryn has been trying to find a place to live in the East Bay—a place that would let her have a baby. She went on:

I feel fogged. I feel drained even though I don't do much except take care of him. I feel drained. It may be my uncertain situation. I feel like a guest here and want to rest, find a place. I can't do what I want. I'd rate my health as fair. The tiredness; want to rest and I can't find a place. I sleep a lot. It's not a good sleep. He's up a lot at night.

I feel like motherhood should be exciting, but I feel drained [sad, pensive]. He's amazing, changes every day; called me "Ma-ma" the other day. I feel more secure about myself now compared to early months, a feeling of living together. I am into daily life things that used to interest me and have new things too. I'm thinking of school. He needs activity, other kids.

He's changed my life a moderate amount. First of all, my work. I don't get to it. In evenings I'm just too tired. My social life—see friends a bit, but less. Also the last two months, I went to bed late, now I can't. I go to sleep early; yesterday it was seven p.m. Usually nine thirty to ten p.m. The work I miss. The social life I miss, and I do miss seeing movies. I do miss going out in general. I really miss not feeling strong at night. I think that'll change when I get my own place, own routine, have my own time.

My mother has been the most helpful with mothering; a friend has helped for moral support. My mother is very positive about everything. She helps me physically with diapers, babysitting on occasion, and is very encouraging.

He crawls now, pulls himself to standing, makes sounds—sound like words; when he's tired, makes a gurgle. He says "Ma-ma," "baba" [grand-mother in Russian], "Pa-pa," "amom" [food in Russian]. He is interested in everything. He likes for me to play hide-and-seek with him, and to play a lot of things on the floor—rolling around, touching, bouncing, toys— anything that's around. I don't bombard, have one thing at a time. He likes intricate shapes, a thing that rolls, rattles, et cetera.

I teach him something is unsafe by talking to him, then take it away, such as plants. He has always seemed like a real person to me. I felt love for him when he was born. He recognized me from the beginning. I had the feeling, it's my turn. Other mothers knew this, and now I know what it is like.

The most difficult thing about motherhood is being tired. The easiest is how fast they grow up. I might miss something. His independence. I rate myself "eight" to "nine," normally "ten," but I don't feel good. The most rewarding thing about motherhood is I'm happy. I want to find a play group for him. My primary concern at this time is to do my settling down.

Cynthia

Cynthia, aged 40, still had on her nurse's uniform (interview at 7:00 p.m.). She was very restrained and noncommunicative, as she had been at 4 months. Her answers were all brief, nondiscriminating, such as "fine." She was attractive, well-groomed, and did not look fatigued after having worked all day.

Her home was comfortably furnished, orderly, and clean. Her husband took Joshua to the den, and the interview took place at the dining room table.

Cynthia noted that she had been in very good health since 4 months. She described what motherhood was like:

Very rewarding. I work Monday through Friday. I feel good about myself. I went back to work when he was four months old.

Joshua has influenced our life-style a moderate amount. We do many of the same things we did before except we include him.

My husband and my sister, who has children, have been the most helpful to me with mothering. My husband helps get Joshua ready in the mornings. He helps dress him and helps with the feedings. He also does some of the shopping and cooking. We take Joshua to a licensed day-care center in the mornings.

He is crawling with his abdomen off the floor. He pulls himself up to his knees and looks around—he doesn't stand yet. He can't pull himself up to stand yet. He likes for me to swing him, play peek-a-boo, and laugh with him.

I teach him something is unsafe, such as hot, by saying, "hot" and putting his hand near to feel the heat.

He first seemed like a real person around five months. He was more responsive then. I felt love for him from the beginning. He first recognized me at about three months. It was a great feeling.

The most difficult thing about motherhood is finding enough time for everything. The easiest is just being with the baby. I'd rank myself as an "eight" to "nine" in mothering. The most rewarding thing about motherhood is when he comes to me—that's very rewarding.

My future plans for him include nursery school in a couple of years. My primary concerns at this time are my husband and baby—to have time for them.

Carmen

Carmen, aged 31, was dressed casually in slacks. She looked a little tired and as if she had gained weight since 4 months. She was interviewed in her living room, which was clean but filled with a variety of infant's equipment—highchair, swing, playpen. Carmen was very open but at times did not seem to be listening to the interviewer's questions. She is bilingual, speaking Spanish and English.

Carmen vented her feelings five or six times during the interview about the discrepancy between her and her husband's methods of disciplining. She is trying to teach the baby "no," and her husband comes home and says, "Everything here is the baby's, and he can have anything he wants." Carmen was clearly upset by this, and pointed to a palm plant that had been almost destroyed by the baby. Her husband also doesn't want them to use babysitters.

Carmen was affectionate with her son during the interview. After feeding him in her lap, she held him several minutes and kissed him several times.

Carmen reported that she had felt pretty good since 4 months but that she was tired. She also had had the flu a couple of weeks ago. She rated her health as good. She described what motherhood is like for her very seriously:

> It's pretty good. Pretty interesting. It's hard to keep up with him now that he's growing up. It's a challenge keeping up with him. [Pointed to glass-top table]. Had to move it; he gets into everything. I tried to teach him "no," but it's too hard. I feel the same about myself as I always have. When he does something new or different, I like it.
>
> He has changed our life-style a great deal. I'm still not working outside the home—my husband won't let me. Everything I used to do—do it only when the baby lets me; I wait until he sleeps. Most of my friends have kids. I only go out with Carlos [the baby]. It's difficult.
>
> I know I'm happy, but it's an adjustment. I used to think I'd not have more fights as others have after babies, but it happens. My husband comes home and tells me what to do with the baby. He wants me to feed him all the time. After I've been with him all day, I know what he needs and cries for. My husband won't let me go back to work yet, so now I'm going to go back to school. My niece will care for him [stated very defiantly].
>
> The baby stands by himself for awhile. [Very pleased and animated when talking about the baby.] He won't crawl—he rolls over only. I need to teach him to crawl. He talks—"Da-da," "Ma-ma"—meaningful. He yells a lot. When he's happy, he smiles, moves his head. He loves to look at himself in the mirror. He likes TV a lot more now than he used to. Likes commercials. He likes for me to talk to him. I hide and he finds me. He loves my glasses. I put him on the rug to teach him how to crawl. He laughs and rolls to me.
>
> My sister-in-law has been the most helpful to me. She lives in Los Angeles. She calls a lot. She was here one month. It was great; she took care of him [same sister-in-law who had been a great help at 1 month but had given a lot of advice and helped almost too much]. She helped so much entertaining the baby. She is so good. When Carlos was fussy, she said, "Why don't you offer a bottle?" I would never have thought of it. Also, she said to try cereal before bed so he'd absorb it better. I was giving it in the morning. She suggested mixing vegetables with applesauce—practical suggestions.
>
> I teach him something is unsafe by saying, "Don't do it," and I pull him away from it. If I say "no" and pat his hand, he gets mad and hits at me.
>
> He became a real person to me at six months, when he started to use

the walker. I felt love for him when he was first born, but I felt another surge around three to four months. He first recognized me at four months. Even now I can see the difference; he cries when I leave the room. It feels great.

The most difficult thing about motherhood is to keep up with him. I'm tired. I want to be alone sometimes. He doesn't understand. The easiest thing—now it feels like I know how to do—as if I have been doing it all my life. Not like the first few months; I was crazy then. I was always worried that I'd do something wrong. I'd rate myself as "seven" in the mothering role. The most rewarding thing about motherhood is to know I'm giving him the right food.

My plans for him—to take him to the park, play with him. To show him trees; he loves it. I take him; we watch people play tennis. I don't have any major concerns. I would tell other mothers that it's a challenge. My main concern is that I'm not sure if I'm doing everything right. [Talked about five minutes about her uncertainty.]

ANALYSIS AND IMPLICATIONS FOR NURSING INTERVENTION

Several themes emerged from the 8-month data that crossed all age groups. Yet some subtle differences by maternal age were also observed.

Major Themes

Responsibility as Organizer and Time Demander Pervasive throughout the interviews was the feeling of *responsibility* that the women felt. This responsibility was linked with change in identity that reflected to the women a maturation indicative of adulthood. Although the responsibility demanded time, it was an organizer. They reprioritized and reassessed goals and plans. Alison at 18 years saw the "responsibility of making decisions for another person" as the most rewarding thing about motherhood. To a teenager, this kind of responsibility or admission to adulthood may also be equated with a degree of power or control—something they may not have enjoyed as a child. For the majority, responsibility and time that the responsibility demanded were prominent among mothers' major concerns and problems that were the most difficult for them.

Infant Development The *infant's behavior,* the source of the greatest rewards in the mothering role, also brought the greatest challenge to the women. The mobile, manipulative, and demanding infants created a challenge in providing for their safety, in beginning to discipline them, teaching them what was safe in the environment, and in providing the kind of stimulation that they craved. The perceived role of an ideal mother changed accordingly. There was a 261% increase in women listing "maintains an appropriate environment," an 85% increase in listing "loving, enjoys motherhood," a 69% increase in "changes priorities," and a 33% increase in "disciplines."

The degree of bother scale mean score indicating the extent of infant-related stress showed a significant increase over the 4-month mean score.

Social Support The *social support network* of persons who helped them with day-to-day situations had changed at 8 months. More friends were included in the support network than had been included at 4 months. Teenagers were shifting from their mothers to friends, which may have indicated work toward achieving their own developmental task of independence. Friends at 8 months were more likely to be persons with children. Bonnie did not seek out friends for socializing, but she commented about friends without children relating to her as if she didn't like herself but changing their behavior when they found out that she did. Bonnie also was having difficulty adapting to the mothering role.

The *kind of social support* mothers received at 8 months varied. Almost all mothers reported physical help with the infant, household tasks, or financial help. Very few reported reinforcement in their mothering role (7%); thus, most women did not receive appraisal support for their role. One fourth reported informational support, and one half reported emotional support. The teenager's reported emotional support had decreased at 8 months, with emotional support tending to increase with age. The social skills to elicit emotional support were probably better developed among the older women.

Employment and Mother Roles *Employment role* had increased at 8 months, with over half of the mothers now employed. This increased the potential for role strain; however, except in Group 2, role strain did not increase significantly with employment roles. It is noteworthy that almost half of all the mothers (48%) were experiencing moderate to very high role strain. Although 55% of the women were employed, only 10% reported sharing responsibility for child care 50–50 with another person.

Employment seemed to mean different things to different women. For example, Bonnie at 28 years viewed going back to work and to school as contributing to her adaptation to the mothering role, whereas many women reported conflict around their employment status.

The total sample's lower scores in infant growth and development and the groups 1 and 2 employed women's infant's lower scores raise questions for further study. Group 3 women, in which the opposite was found, more often had live-in help or babysitters who came to their homes. Women from groups 1 and 2 who were less well off financially, often had to work evening hours when mates could watch infants, or relied on persons who were keeping infants under less than desirable conditions. For example, babysitters included a retired couple who were keeping several children in their home and a mother who was keeping eight toddlers. In these kinds of situations, infants would receive less adult stimulation and perhaps less conscientious attention to food intake.

Primary concerns of women at 8 months reflected their added employment roles. *Care of their infants, finances, career and maternal-career role conflict,* and *relationships with their mates* were all dominant. Marital stress, role strain, and maternal attitudes about child rearing were consistent predictors of the maternal role attainment behaviors. Financial problems necessitated the mothers' seeking employment, led to career and maternal role conflict, and decreased their time to spend with their mates.

Health Status Another theme that emerged regarded the mothers' *health.* There has been a tendency to assume that after the puerperium (first 6 weeks following birth), physiologically things have returned to normal. Over one fourth of the mothers were treated for health problems between 4 and 8 months following birth. One eighth of the mothers rated their health as fair. Some of the women reported during the interview that their vigor and usual sense of physical well-being were just now returning. The comment "Having a baby takes a lot out of you" was made by a few. Enough attention has not been paid to the mother's health following the puerperium. Miller and Sollie (1980) observed a decrease in overall well-being at 8 months; the teenagers tended to experience this decrease more so than the older women.

Cultural Context The mothers' comments present the problem encountered by a *minority culture within the majority culture.* Carmen dramatized this by the conflict that she was experiencing with her husband (both are Hispanic). Carmen was very depressed, and her husband refused to let her go back to work. She was rebelling by going back to school. Her need for outside stimulation and the probable influence of the acceptance of an employed wife by the dominant culture may be influencing Carmen but not her husband. Barbara, on the other hand, in a biracial relationship (she is white and he is black) was having no problems. She reported that her mate was most helpful: "He listens, even if it's not his philosophy." Barbara's concern about how her daughter will be accepted by others in the future, however, probably relates to the infant's biracial status.

A woman from Group 3 noted that the area in which their lives changed the most was in their relationship and how they related to their baby. "Once you have a baby many things come up that have to be confronted; your value differences come up."

Maternal Individuation: Time to Regain Oneself A final theme was dissatisfaction with the status quo and an emerging *impatience* to move on with one's life as it had been before motherhood. Events such as school or a career had been postponed, and some women felt it was time to get on with their plans for their personal lives apart from motherhood. Some felt that during their merged identity with the infant they had deteriorated mentally.

Age Differences

Teenagers The myth that teenagers are not primary caretakers of their infants did not hold true with this sample of Bay Area teenagers. The teenager was no less likely to be primary caretaker than the older woman. However, the absence of any teenager less than 15 years old in this sample, and the fact that two-thirds of the sample were 18 or 19 years old, must be kept in mind. Age and maturity make a difference here.

The tendency for teenager parents to live with their families is probably related more to their unmarried status than to age. For example, Betty and Cathryn, older single mothers, also lived with their families.

The teenagers were more concerned about the future. Alma was concerned about the future and their ability to "get off welfare." Amy, who lived with her mother while her husband lived with his parents several miles away, was concerned about their future as a family and whether they would be able to get a house of their own. Amy, who was initially negative toward motherhood, was still not committed to it at 8 months: "I'm just putting up with mothering" and "I'm going through with it." She sounded as if she felt trapped, and seeing her husband only twice a week did not help her feelings.

Teenage mothers also had poorer health at 8 months. Health problems related to anemia, urinary tract infections, and menstrual problems. Alice had been depressed that she might have been pregnant; she did not want an abortion, and her husband wanted her to have one, so her menstrual period brought much relief.

Teenage mothers, while assimilating more friends into their social networks, received less emotional support than older women. Although friends are able to help in many ways, teenagers also need alternative sources of persons available for emotional support.

Twenty- to 29-Year-Old Mothers This group of women was more enthusiastic in its responses to motherhood than other groups. They responded with the "naturalness of motherhood," or how they "were meant to be moms." The reader will note that all of the Group 2 men in the vignettes above were very involved. Even Bonnie, who had difficulty adjusting to motherhood, felt it was a "blessing" that she was "honored" to have. Her husband's involvement with their infant, along with therapy, was probably playing a role in her adjustment.

Group 2 women experienced greater role strain, however. Careers were less meaningful to these mothers who felt so natural in the role. Without the commitment to an employment role, the conflict and, consequently, the role strain was greater.

Group 2 women were less likely than the other groups to change friends in their social network. Because more women have first infants during their twenties than at any other age and the overall tendency was to move toward becoming closer to friends with infants, this group experienced fewer negative cues from the larger societal environment. They were not "out of step" with the majority. Role transitions that are either "early" or "late" for the social times in which events typically occur are more stressful (Hogan, 1980; Neugarten et al., 1965).

Mothers 30 Years and Older This group of women dramatizes the importance of the situational context or environment in studying mothering behavior. Cathryn's depression and fatigue, the extent to which she missed work, friends, and going out all seemed to relate in part to her living situation. She was tired of living with her parents and not "having a life of her own." The difference in the depression between Amy and Cathryn is that Cathryn more directly attributed her problems to living with her parents, rather than motherhood per se.

The illustrative cases above suggest that Group 3 men may be somewhat less involved with child care and helping out with the infant than younger men. However, when women were asked whether mates were helping out as much as they should, there were no age group differences in responses. One case in which a couple had been married 12 years illustrated different expectations from a long-time marital relationship: "He doesn't understand why I can't go play five sets of tennis with him, or why I don't feel like going to the theater. He just isn't as involved as I am with the baby and feels that it is time for my involvement to decrease." (This type of prompting from the mate may also facilitate the maternal individuation process.)

On the other hand, these mates of older women apparently were more skillful in providing emotional support. Women from Group 3 more often reported emotional support than younger women, and their mates were most often named as their major support person.

One important difference emerged about this older group of women. Nonemployed mothers scored lower on their feelings of love for their infants than did employed mothers. Employed mothers also tended to derive greater gratification from the maternal role, and their infants tended to score higher on growth and development. There was a significant positive relationship between feelings of love for the infant and gratification in the role. Career roles had been part of this group of women's identities for a much longer period of time; thus, giving up an employment role meant giving up a part of one's identity. Cathryn and Carmen both illustrate the depression of not accomplishing in previously successful career roles. A Japanese mother from Group 3 described going back to work as being most helpful: "I am a teaching aide. I feel needed and useful. I am not so preoccupied with my own child. I'm more objective when I see other children. It was hard on me being home. I feel I gained myself back again in a way. I have my perspective."

Interventions

Interventions will be directed to the major themes first and followed by age-specific suggestions.

Responsibility as Organizer and Time Demander Since responsibility played dual roles in both contributing to the individual's maturation and detracting from time for creative endeavors for the majority of women, there needs to be communication of and preparation for the responsibility that occurs with motherhood. Responsibility might even be used synonomously with both motherhood and adulthood. Becoming an adult means that an individual is a responsible person; becoming a mother means that an individual is responsible for a dependent child until that child reaches adulthood. Perhaps parenthood is not viewed this way during pregnancy or earlier, when fantasies of "what will it be like as a mother" are rampant.

The demands of the responsibility of motherhood are less consuming when shared and when one has help. Single mothers will benefit from close alliances with a person who can be supportive, share responsibility, and offer reinforcement that their decisions and actions are those to promote the infant's health.

Infant Development With career roles, there is usually a linear progression in achievement. This is not true with motherhood. With each developmental phase, a new repertoire of mothering skills is warranted. Women were not prepared for the change in skills required in caring for a dependent, immobile infant to those required in caring for an infant who was mobile, more demanding, and manipulative. Most women used magazines and books for additional information. However, teenagers less often utilized these resources, more often turned to their mothers or other older, more experienced family member.

Parents' classes in infant development can alert parents to upcoming changes so that they do not feel incompetent in dealing with new behaviors. Childproofing the environment is an area of vital importance to parents. The importance for gates around floor heaters and across stairways, cabinet safety locks, electrical outlet covers, and removing breakables and other attractive hazards can be stressed at well-child checkups. These safety precautions could be illustrated on posters in well-child clinics, compiled in booklets, or presented on video filmstrips for women to peruse while waiting for appointments.

Social Support The importance of support groups, friends with infants, and available resources such as day-care centers is critical for the new mother. If there are no licensed, quality day-care centers in the community, a committee should be gotten together to approach the city planning committee with arguments for why such a center is needed.

Pregnant women tend to be less social during the last trimester, but at that time, if the health care provider stresses the importance of developing friends who share common interests (largely children), they may begin to think about this. Many women become friends with other pregnant women whom they meet in the office while waiting for appointments. This common history provides women with a mutual bond and provides a confidante. However, it is important for the repertoire of friends also to include persons with infants somewhat older than her own infant. These friends can offer invaluable advice and can reinforce their newly acquired mothering behaviors.

Comments from nurses provide much support, often when they are not intended as support. Carrie felt good about the uniqueness of her daughter, and nursery nurses had mentioned her personality. Bonnie reported that her infant recognized her from birth, and even nurses had commented on this. Nurses must be aware that even the most casual comment may be taken quite seriously by a new, insecure mother, and as such, should be helpful and reinforcing as much as possible.

Employment During pregnancy some women may know that they will need to or may wish to return to work following their infants' birth. Since research has indicated less role conflict when women have "jobs" that are not important long-range, women who are going back to work for the single purpose of supplementing the income might be advised that a position with fewer demands may exact less stress. Career women may be more conflicted because of their long-range commitment to establishing a career as part of their future identity and security.

However, the importance of good, reliable day care and the availability of care for sick infants is central to a mother's peace of mind in maintaining employment. Many larger companies are being pressured into providing day-care centers within their buildings for employees. A sitter who comes to the home is more expensive but less of a hassle than having to get up 30 to 45 min earlier to dress an infant, pack his supplies for a day, and take him off to a strange environment. During toddlerhood, play with other children becomes more important; however, during the first year, the luxury of not having to take the child out compensates for slightly higher fees. In addition, exposure to multiple colds and illnesses is avoided.

Backup care is always important. Individuals will sometimes agree to care for an infant for a few days when they would not take on the responsibility full-time.

Women have less conflict with career roles when their husbands are supportive of them. This does not mean that husbands automatically assume half of the responsibility for child care, but the verbal support as opposed to arguments is very meaningful.

If individuals care for the infant, it is important that the mother educate the individual about infant growth and development, and the importance of talking to, stimulating, and showing the infant things must be stressed. Cuddling and play time are very important to the infant, who is learning the art of socializing very rapidly.

Help with household tasks is important if the women is to have any time for herself and for her mate. Are there high school students who can clean house, do the laundry, or run errands? How many of these activities is the mate willing to take over?

In some situations, the father may be at a place in his career in which it is preferable for him to stay home as the major caretaker. This assures that the child receives care from a parent, and for some this outweighs the inconvenience of a year's leave of absence from work. However, a father also may be expected to experience role conflict in assuming the major caretaker role.

Health Status It takes some women longer to recuperate from childbirth than others. The responsibility demands on time take away from time to enjoy leisurely meals. Many times mothers forget to eat until they become hypoglycemic, then they may snack on handy nonnutritive foods. Anemia, infection, and fatigue all zap a mother's energy amd leave her depressed and feeling inadequate.

The pediatrician or pediatric nurse practitioner should routinely inquire about the mother's health. Many women never go back to a physician after the initial postpartum checkup and may need medical attention. Persistent fatigue may indicate anemia, infection, depression, or all three.

Cultural Context Sensitivity to the minority mother who is struggling with motherhood in a majority culture is critical. The minority mother is often torn between following the advice of her own mother and that of her physician. She may be even more vulnerable to the media. Her self-confidence reflects this lack of fit in either culture and her questioning of the values of each culture.

The cultural context also dictates many child-care practices. The health professional must inquire about special practices if she is unfamiliar with a particular culture. With such knowledge any treatment or regimen can be adapted to be more congruent with the mother's cultural practices.

Maternal Individuation: Time to Regain Oneself With the infant's beginning mobility and separating out from his mother, the woman also seemed to feel it was time to regain "something of her pre-mother self" at 8 months. If school had been postponed, or if a career had been put aside, women began to be impatient to take up previous activities.

Even for nonemployed women, activities outside the home provide stimulation and private time to enjoy something for themselves. Whether it is a shopping trip or a trip to the museum, outings replenish energy and motivation for mothering.

Teenagers The teenagers' increased concern about their futures is understandable. Enlistment of social workers, high school counselors, and career counselors who can provide opportunity for rap sessions with young women is very important during the second half of the first year of motherhood. Social workers know the financial resources available and are sensitive to many community resources that could be helpful. High school counselors can help young women make decisions about the preparatory courses they need to take to complete high school. Career counselors can help the young woman decide whether she wishes to take a business, cosmetology, or technician course. Future social mobility is very directly related to education. If the appropriate recognition is not made of prerequisites, and necessary preparation, much time may be lost by the teenage mother, who is already a year behind her peers at best.

Follow-up on the teenager's health is critical. Iron needs are greater at this time than any other period of her life if she is still growing. Has she received counseling regarding good nutrition?

Has she received counseling about how to avoid infections from sexually transmitted disease? Does she know that she should void before and after intercourse to help prevent urinary tract infection? Her anxiety during pregnancy may have been too high for her to have heard counseling in these areas at an earlier time.

The teenager needs to be in contact with an adult whom she sees as supportive. Many persons available to the teenager for support are those who may also be a source of conflict (Barerra, 1981; Crawford, 1985). Helping the teenager identify a person that she is comfortable in disclosing her feelings to and who is willing to serve in this capacity will help her move toward obtaining emotional support resources.

Mothers in Their Twenties These women appeared to relish their motherhood roles. Their advantage of fitting the "cultural norm" of bearing a first child in their twenties may be far greater than is realized. As mentioned earlier, Neugarten et al. (1965) referred to life events being more stressful when they were unexpected or out of step with societal expectations. Group 2 women had not become firmly entrenched in career identities, they were more mature than the younger teenage mothers, and their expressed enjoyment at 8 months surpassed the other two age groups.

As a consequence, when financial circumstances required their return to employment status, many experienced conflict about doing so. This group of mothers really needs to go through a decision-making process. This process must include career options at this time as opposed to long-range goals; other ways of earning money that do not require separation from their child; and facets of daily activity that may be relinquished when additional roles are assumed. The process of finding day care, as discussed above, is very important, as is the discussion on social support.

Mothers 30 Years and Older This group of women who were more competent in both observed and self-reported maternal behaviors derived less gratification in the mothering role. The differences between employed and nonemployed mothers indicated that employment may have contributed to their satisfaction with the mothering role. This greater satisfaction was related to feeling more love for their infants. Women who rated themselves higher in work-derived satisfaction also felt their employment had a positive influence on both their and their child's life (Squires, 1985). Whether or not mothers were employed had no effect on 5-year-old children's math, language, motor and social skills, but a stimulating home environment was the significant factor (Squires, 1985).

These older mothers need reinforcement for their mothering behaviors so that they can feel successful in this role. They demand more of themselves, as indicated by their attendance at antepartum classes. Knowing that they can find satisfaction in work roles without handicapping their children may help alleviate some feelings of guilt. They are accustomed to success and achievement, so the information that providing a stimulating home environment that includes reading to their child can provide them with something positive to work toward. Pickens (1982) reported that most career women had resolved their loss of confidence in career and mothering roles by 4 months. The ambivalence and dissatisfaction observed among the older women in this study indicated that many had not resolved these feelings at 8 months.

CHAPTER 8

One Year: Integration of the Maternal Role

By the end of the first year most of the mothers were more relaxed in the mothering role, and had integrated the maternal, wife, and other roles into their self system so that they were enjoying the new family unit. Their infants were walking or cruising as they moved into toddlerhood and required greater maternal creativity in providing a safe but stimulating home environment for them. Demands of the women's multiple roles of wife, mother, and career woman were evident, but some now felt more confident and comfortable in handling these roles, which were at times conflicting. Almost two thirds of the women were employed (62%).

Although the majority of the women described motherhood as easier and more enjoyable at 1 year, the challenges of this first year of motherhood and what was entailed in bearing and rearing the child had been unanticipated by the women. There had been no social preparation, and there had been little social assistance for most of the women as they had struggled through the first year. The mothers had experienced vast reorientation in relation to their mates, their mothers, and themselves. They viewed motherhood as growth producing and as admission to adulthood, regardless of maternal age; however, patterns of growth differed.

This chapter presents the women's responses at the 1-year interview and contrasts them with earlier responses at 8 months. A total of 242 women continued in the study at 1 year; 40 were in Group 1, 114 in Group 2, and 88 in Group 3. The final vignettes of the 12 women present challenges that single women parenting alone experienced as well as challenges that women with mates experienced. Following an analysis of these data, nursing interventions for the transition to motherhood, and in particular for the transition to parenting a toddler, are suggested.

EXPECTATIONS AT ONE YEAR

Similarly to the four first-time mothers over 30 studied by Hees-Stauthamer (1985), the women in this study, although feeling more competent and at greater ease in the maternal role, were also astonished that it would take an entire year to reestablish a sense of their lives apart from their children. Others also reported the women's identity being merged with their children; a woman reported that when she went out socially, it took awhile to lose the motherhood role (Grossman et al., 1980).

At 1 year, less anxiety and less depression were observed than at any other period during pregnancy or following birth (Grossman et al., 1980). A lower socioeconomic status (SES) was associated with higher anxiety and depression, as well as more medical problems experienced during pregnancy. The mother's health and well-being at 1 year was positively related to the father's marital satisfaction and anxiety level at 2 months postpartum. The greater the stress that was experienced by mothers, the lower their self-image (Grossman et al., 1980).

OVERALL FEELINGS: PHYSICAL AND EMOTIONAL

Physical Problems

Almost three-fourths of the women (71%) reported a physical health problem since 8 months: 48% reported a single problem, 17% reported two problems; 5% reported three problems; and 1% reported four problems. There were no age differences in the physical health problems reported. The incidence of those with *no* health problems did not vary from 8 months (38% at 8 months, compared with 39% at 1 year).

Upper respiratory infections and flu were reported by 43% of the women. Other health problems included the following: nausea/gastritis, 8%; orthopedic/back problems, 5%; chronic disease, 5%; rashes/allergies, 5%; cysts—ovarian/pilonidal, 4%; vaginal infections,

3%; abortion, 2%; headaches, 2%; weight loss/run down, 2%; dys-plasia/cancer, 2%; urinary tract infections, 2%; menstrual problems, 2%. Three women had a cholecystectomy, three had fractures of either hand, foot, or knee, and two had anemia. There were no age differences in health problems reported. The husband of a wo-man from Group 2 fractured her hand twice. They separated, she went back to him, and they separated again; she was in the process of obtaining a divorce at the time of the interview. This woman was abused as a child by her mother who hit her over the head with a coat hanger and with her knuckles.

Eight percent of the women were pregnant at 1 year; 3% of Group 1, 8% of Group 2, and 10% of Group 3. Two teenagers and one wo-man in Group 2 had delivered second babies. One teenager and four women in Group 2 had had abortions. In this study, teenagers were no more likely to have a second child or a second pregnancy in the first year following birth than were the older women. The health status factor did not show any significant differences by age group at 1 year.

Emotional Feelings

The women's feelings during the 4-month period since 8 months were rank-ordered from depressed/sick, up and down, tired, better, OK/fine/good, to great. Nine percent of the women had been de-pressed, 1% up and down, 17% tired, 15% better, 51% OK/fine/good, and 7% great. Thus, well over half had felt from good to great; however, a large portion of women (42%) had felt *less* than good. The teenage group responded significantly more positively, with Group 2 responding the lowest overall. One woman in Group 2 was depressed to the extent that she had considered suicide (see com-ments below from Group 2). Two women in Group 2 and four wo-men in Group 3 were seeing psychiatrists or other therapists for emotional problems. One woman in Group 3 reported that she was an alcoholic. The Shereshefsky and Yarrow (1973) study of 78 wo-men reported seven women who had psychiatric problems following childbirth; that rate is higher (9%) than was self-reported in this study (2%). One woman from Group 3 who was lost to the study after the first test period was hospitalized during the first month for depression and other problems that she had had prior to child-birth.

In summary, the time required in regaining mastery of their physical and psychosocial lives was a shock to the mothers. Comments by women in Group 3 dramatized this point:

- I thought as soon as the baby was born our sex life would get together. I'm still not completely back together. My pelvic muscles aren't as strong. I don't feel good about my body. He [mate] feels parts of my body are not his anymore. I leak milk all over the bed.
- I felt the whole past year was disruptive. . . . I still don't see myself as "Mother." I'm performing the role. I don't identify myself as "Mother." My mother is a mother. I think the total dependence of infancy was hard for me. I'm enjoying her responsiveness and her independence.
- I don't have a picture of myself at this stage. I'm not thinking of myself as a mom in a way because I'm not involved in any social life now—am living a sheltered life.
- The feeling that I don't have one hundred percent of my mind to focus because part of me is always with Bobby [infant]. You can't tell someone this. You need to experience it. I can't focus professionally, I can't compulsively put one hundred percent into medicine, go to the library, and so forth.
- It took me longer than it should have to recover from the cesarean. For four or five months I was sick with colds, bronchitis, lack of sleep.
- Until eight to nine months it was a problem. I was *never* well rested.
- The adjustment of being parents together after being married thirteen years, and losing your independence and privacy is difficult. You have to accept you'll be bored. Mothering wasn't too much fun at two months; it was a shock.
- The body image is a problem that is ongoing all year. I don't feel as good about my body as before. Physical fatigue has been pervasive—chronically tired. I've not ever felt rested as I did before birth. It colors everything.

Younger women in Group 2 also related the unanticipated demands of the first year of motherhood on their total being:

- I don't like having nothing else to talk about but baby care.
- Mothering is really easy but I don't always feel motherly . . . . The disruption in my life has been difficult—the change of

going back to work. We don't have a babysitter; I work nights. We don't have time to be together. We don't have an end in sight. It can't go on like this.

- At one point my feelings about myself changed. I felt incompetent. I had a terrible complex about the difficult birth, and I had a lot of guilt for being so stubborn. I didn't want a cesarean or medications. My confidence is coming back. I think once I get him weaned I will feel like a whole person again. It's time. . . . Childbirth was a horrible experience; I hated it all.
- I was so down Friday night, I considered suicide; I called my doctor, and he counseled me. I took a high-pressure job [pharmacist]. Super-high pressure. I burned myself out. My mother-in-law made me feel terribly inadequate as a mother. . . . I'm not sure I want another one. I wonder if I was meant to be a mother.
- I'm still feeling the struggle. Am I a woman or am I a mother? I can't decide whether it is worth fixing myself up. Will anybody notice?
- I finally feel that my body is my own. I'm not physically attached to someone else. I haven't been able to do things for myself in eighteen months. Everything stopped for me [age 26 years].
- A third person is expensive . . . . We just haven't had money to do things for ourselves. We've needed a vacation. We've pushed ourselves these past four months.

The younger women (under 20) in Group 1 also keenly felt the emotional disruption in their lives:

- I feel lonely. I feel bad sometimes, not being with her father. I'm doing everything.
- It's been hard adjusting my time, being with her and not excluding myself from the rest of the world. From three to six months was the hardest.
- Finances are hard—I was bored, angry, and jealous when my husband went out.
- I ain't doing nothing but take care of him. I used to go out and party. I don't like it that much. My aunt says I should get up earlier to feed him.
- It's hard. He's a lot of work—a lot of sacrifice. Everything I do

with him in mind. ... Sometimes I wish it wasn't like that; I wish I could think about me.

These remarks all indicate the unanticipated consuming nature of motherhood, which had an emotional impact on the women, and the difficulty that arose in sorting self from the mothering role. The diffuseness of boundary between self and infant was problematic to many of the women during the first year of motherhood. The women's struggle to regain their former physical and social selves suggests that maternal individuation discussed in Chapter 7 is a process following birth that may parallel the separation–individuation process of the infant–toddler.

MAJOR CONCERNS AT ONE YEAR

Concerns about the Infants' Growth and Development

Just over one-third (36%) of the women were concerned about their infants' growth and development. Over one-fourth (26%) had one concern, and 10% had two concerns. In the order of their frequency concerns included the following: not talking, 6%; shorter than other infants, 5%; impact of illness on mental development, 5%; lack of social interaction with others, 5%; no/low weight gain, 3%; bowed legs/feet turned, 3%; teeth/thumbsucking, 3%; temper, 2%; hyperactive, 1%; underweight/appetite loss, 1%; no hair, 1%; stools weird/painful, 1%; and fat, 1%. There were no significant age group differences in these concerns.

Primary Concerns Reported

The major concerns that the women reported at 1 year were more extensive than at 8 months. More women were concerned about the infant's care and/or health at 1 year (one-third, compared with one-fifth). Finances continued to be problematic for 22%. Moving or looking for a bigger house was a major concern for 16%. Twelve percent were having conflict over their careers or returning to work; Groups 1 and 2 reported conflict over careers significantly less often (7%, 7%, and 21%).[1]

---

[1] Series of three figures in parentheses indicates percentages for the three groups from the youngest to the oldest, respectively.

Other less frequently reported concerns included the following: balancing family relationships, 7%; relationship with mate/marriage, 5%; school/getting back, 5%; single motherhood, 4%; own health/weight/fatigue, 4%; world situation, 4%; sex life, 2%; time for managing two children, 2%; husband's job/school, 2%; husband's health, 1%; whether to have another child, 1%; weaning, 1%; remodeling home, 1%; juggling time, 1%; ending relationship with father of baby, 1%; and comfort in role and identity, 1%. One mother was concerned about potty training.

The difficulties of single motherhood were verbalized more readily at 1 year by Group 3 women:

- It bothers me when people react negatively to me being a single mom. I meet women who want to get together with babies, and when they find out I'm single, they don't. It's hard.
- It's no fun to take her with me to friends' houses. I have to watch her; you can't drink. . . . My negative emotions focus on the strained relationship with her father. Sometimes I think I'd be better off without him. Babies do strain relationships.

These more mature women were shunned despite the greater societal acceptance of single parenthood, and they found that a baby strained relationships.

WORK TOWARD MATERNAL ROLE ATTAINMENT

At 1 year, 83% of the women reported that they were primary caretakers of their infants; that is, they were responsible for their infants 12 hr or more per day (78%, 84%, and 85%). Ten percent reported they shared caretaking 50–50 with another person (20%, 8%, and 9%). Five percent reported that they were responsible for infant care one-fourth to one-half the time (3%, 5%, and 6%). Three women, all from Group 2, reported others were responsible for their infant full-time.

Overall Feelings about Motherhood

Over half (57%) of the women described motherhood as easier or enjoyable at 1 year. One-fifth spoke of both the enjoyment and the difficulties encountered. The remainder (23%) found the demands of their multiple roles of wife, mother, and career woman frustrating and described mothering as more difficult. These general feelings about motherhood did not differ significantly by age group.

Feelings about Self as a Result of Motherhood

Women reported a range of feelings from self-questioning and a loss of self-esteem (8%) to a fuller meaning in life or greater fulfillment (10%). In between, 24% reported they felt the same about themselves; 34% reported greater confidence in themselves or increased independence; 20% reported they were more responsible individuals, and 4% reported they were up and down. Groups 2 and 3 were more likely to report greater confidence in themselves as an effect of motherhood (18%, 39%, and 34%), but Group 1 was more likely to report they were now more responsible individuals (50%, 15%, and 14%). Comments reflecting this range of teenagers' feelings include the following:

- I like it. It makes me feel good that he is growing and he is a person.
- She gets into my things; sometimes I feel invaded.
- Teaching her is so exciting; before it was just caretaking, and there were times when I felt it wasn't good to have her in my life.
- This period has been the hardest; he's more mobile and I'm trying to potty-train him and get him off the bottle.
- I can't wait until the baby is older and can help me.

Women in Group 2 expressed their feelings:

- I love it when I'm hugging her and she is patting and loving me back.
- My self image was best when I was pregnant. I lost a little when she was born.
- My mother has Cynthia. I could have her if I wanted. I had her for a weekend; it was hard. I can't handle it by myself. I put a hole in the wall with her here—slammed the door against the wall. I've given her one bath; I haven't changed her diaper three times in the last three months. I can't stand BM diapers. Early in pregnancy I wanted them to adopt her. I resented her

in my stomach. When in labor, I didn't care. Her heartbeat went down. All I wanted was her to be out. I didn't care if she died or lived.

- I think I lost a little self-esteem—being home, not working, not seeing people. I've had to pull myself out of that at times.
- Before I was single. Now I am a homemaker, so I play a different role. But you are the same person just the same.
- I feel left out; I have no part in my husband's life.

Group 3 women's descriptions of a changed self as a result of motherhood included the following:

- I feel a lot different. There is a redefining of yourself.
- Before I had him I was in the mid-thirties crisis. The problems I was having stopped when I decided to have a baby. I am more satisfied now.
- I was bored with my work; what did I want to do, was that all there is?
- I feel fulfilled. I think that every woman should have a child if she is physically able to. Then you appreciate your own mother. . . . I had a hell of a time during delivery and then afterward— was in the hospital nine days, had pre-eclampsia, four units of blood. . . .
- The symbiosis is most difficult; it is hard for me to disconnect easily. I had to give up a lot of independence for one; not sure I want another child.
- I feel less physically connected and have my body back since I stopped breast-feeding.
- I feel more myself. I own myself; I'm more separate from him. I've been able to give up that big bubble of motherhood and let go of my expectations.

Although the mothers expressed positive and rewarding feelings from motherhood, there was a felt need not to be excluded from adult activities with mates, or from the world, and to "own" themselves. Cynthia's mother in Group 2 had not achieved a maternal identity; fortunately, her own mother could care for Cynthia. Her repugnance at dirty diapers and difficulty with handling emotions are signals of her emotional inability to mother Cynthia at this time (Bishop, 1976).

Easiest Mothering Tasks of a One-Year-Old

The infant's social interactions at 1 year were perceived as the easiest mothering task for the majority of the women (58%, compared with 42% at 8 months). These enjoyable interactions with the infant included playing or being with and loving the infant. Twelve percent reported that the independence of the infant was the easiest; 9% reported feeding or other care activities; 7% reported an easy temperament; and 4% reported when the infant was asleep was easiest. Seven percent maintained that nothing about mothering was easy, and 4% stated that everything was easy.

Most Difficult Mothering Tasks of a One-Year-Old

The infant's increased activity level and greater demands were the most difficult challenge reported by 37% of the women at 1 year; this was an increase from 14% at 8 months. The two younger groups tended to report the infant's activity level as most difficult more often than Group 3 (45%, 41%, and 27%).

Almost one-fourth (22%) reported role incompetencies as most difficult at 1 year. Incompetencies largely centered around disciplining the 1-year-old, allowing her the level of independence that was needed, and in general knowing her needs. This was an increase from 8 months, when 14% reported role incompetencies as most difficult. Age groups varied little.

With increased longevity in the maternal role, women learned to manage the responsibilities more efficiently. Only 13% of the women reported the time demands of the role as most difficult at one year compared to 19% at eight months. Only 10% reported role responsibility challenges, a 50% decrease from eight months. A 50% decrease in sleep deprivation was also reported, with 5% continuing to find this problematic at one year. The older the woman the greater was the likelihood of reporting the time required for the role as most difficult (3%, 10%, 22%). Group 2 was somewhat less likely to report the role responsibility demands as most difficult (10%, 6%, 14%). Group 3 reported sleep deprivation slightly more often (5%, 4%, 8%).

Five percent reported the conflict of the mothering role with either school or career roles as most difficult. This was a low percentage considering that 62% of the women were employed at one year.

The Most Difficult Thing About Mothering the Entire Year

When women evaluated the most difficult thing about mothering from the perspective of the entire year, the infant's illness (18%) and sleep deprivation/fatigue (18%) were the most frequently named. The older the woman the more often she mentioned sleep deprivation/fatigue (8%, 15%, 25%).

The first month at home was reported as the most difficult thing by 10% of the women (3%, 12%, 9%). An additional 9% extended this time and reported that the first two to four months were the most difficult (0%, 8%, 15%). The teenagers' fewer reports of difficulty during this critical time of the mother learning the infant's needs and reading the infant's cues indicate that teenagers may have relied on other adults for help. As noted in Chapter 4, infants are also learning to control their state during the first month of life, which may be facilitated by sensitive input from a nurturing person.

Making adjustments in family relationships, largely with the mate, were reported as the most difficult by 13% of the women (15%, 15%, 8%). Group 3's less difficulty here may indicate their higher level of development in achieving the adult task of intimacy (Erikson, 1959), or possible longer time in relationships so that adjustments were easier (data were not collected about the length of the marriage). Seven percent of the women reported finding time was the most difficult (3%, 4%, and 13%). Five percent found the isolation from the outside world that they had experienced as the most difficult (0%, 4%, and 8%).

Financial problems were the most difficult for 3% of the women, and 3% described childbirth as the most difficult thing about the first year of motherhood.

The impact of the childbirth experience is long-lasting. Kutzner (1984) reported that some women described the experience so vividly 3 to 4 years following birth that it was as if the experience had occurred the day before. The childbirth experience was described vividly and graphically by some of the mothers at the one year interview:

- It took sixty hours from start to stop. [Group 2]
- I had a twenty-hour labor and a cesarean section. . . . What I didn't like was all the people who kept coming in. I got tired; I must have had six medical students ask the same question. I finally refused to talk to the last one. I didn't like the catheter being put in. I was naked and strapped to bed [operating

table], and all the doctors were standing around. I had no privacy. [Group 2]
- I had a thirty-hour labor followed by a cesarean section. It was pretty rough. I was disappointed and totally unprepared. I was a little angry at not being forewarned and prepared for that. I don't see how that happened. I had too small a pelvis. I want a complete evaluation before the next birth. [Group 2]
- I don't want to go through labor and delivery again. The memory is too vivid. It was too painful—thirty-six hours, and two hours pushing. [Group 2]
- Suggestions need to be practical. I never went through such unbearable pain. I was told it would be like menstrual cramps. They lay a trip on you that it's not that bad [Lamaze class]. I was totally unprepared for what happened before, during, and after birth, and came home exhausted. I was so helpless and so was my baby. [Group 3]
- I bled and went into shock. I needed nine liters of fluids. [Group 3]

Comments by these women indicate that they had not had opportunity to discuss their childbirth experiences and to resolve their deep feelings of anger and disappointment at the events that occured. The pain of labor and delivery is a subjective experience and is perceived differently by each woman. For example, one woman in Group 2 described a similar very painful labor and delivery as the most rewarding thing about her first year of motherhood: "I feel power in being able to reproduce. It put me in touch with sort of basic values, and I take a stand a lot more—don't back down. I faced an extreme situation [labor] and survived it. Labor was very hard. It was like facing death—the pain was that bad."

The Most Unexpected Happening of Motherhood the First Year

Women were asked what event or occurrence they had least expected during the first year of motherhood. Only 12% denied that any unexpected event had occurred (18%, 12%, and 9%). A range of 35 unexpected events was given; however, the most frequently reported unexpected event was the infant's rapid development and learning (14% overall). The teenagers were more engrossed by the rapid growth and development of the infant during the first year (24%, 15%, and 9%).

Eleven percent of the women were surprised by the extent of the involvement and the engrossment of motherhood (3%, 11%, and 16%). Seven percent were not expecting their infants' illness and/or hospitalization.

Other less frequently reported surprises of the first year included the following: time commitment/responsibility, 6%; easier or better than had anticipated, 5%; the extent of self-change, 4%; that they could be a good mother, 3%; lack of self-confidence, 3%; another pregnancy, 3%; the unreal birth (both in being too long or too short), 3%; difficulty in taking care of infant, 3%; the extensiveness of the transition to motherhood, 3%; fatigue/lack of sleep, 2%; breast-feeding, weaning, 2%; infant injury, 2%; success with mate, 2%; not working, 2%; mate problems, 1%; self-sacrifice, 1%; twins, 1%; decrease in sex life, 1%; baby's love, 1%; difficulty in working, 1%; support from outsiders, 1%; birth easy, 1%; and one each found the financial impact, her own illness, and death of a family member as the most unexpected event of the year.

Self-Image as a Mother at One Year

The mothers overall viewed themselves rather positively in the role. Ninety-two percent rated themselves as 7 or higher.

Their self-ratings in the mothering role, with 10 considered as ideal, ranged from 2 to 10. One (a Group 2 women whose infant was in Taiwan) rated herself as a 2, 3% rated themselves as 5, 4% as 6, 10% as 7, 37% as 8, 22% as 9, and 23% as 10. There were no significant age group differences in their self-ratings. Averages were as follows: Group 1, 8.48; Group 2, 8.30; and Group 3, 8.40. Except for the teenage group there was very little change from the 8-month ratings (8.33, 8.29, and 8.42).

Maternal Role Attainment Behaviors

There was little change in the measured maternal role behaviors at 1 year from 8 months. This was congruent with the women's subjective feelings about motherhood; 8 months was the beginning of a period of increased challenge that continued at 1 year.

Feelings of Love There were no significant age differences in the women's feelings about their infants at 1 year, as was observed at the previous test periods. The overall sample average score was 35.0, with a range of from 27 to 40. This was similar to the average score at 8 months, 35.1.

Only 20% of the variance in feelings of love for the infant was accounted for at 1 year by the variables tested. Predictive variables were as follows: marital status, educational level, and race (forced variables because groups differed on these important variables), 0.0%; self-concept, 11%; empathy, 4%; infant-related stress, 2.7%; and stress from negative life events, 2.4%. The woman's basic feeling about herself as a person was the major predictor of how she felt about her infant.

Gratification For the first time since 1 month postpartum, Group 1 failed to have a higher average score in gratification in the mothering role than Group 2. Group 2 (mean, 58.0) scored significantly higher than Group 3 (mean, 55.1), and Group 1's score did not differ significantly from either of the other two (mean, 56.1). The older group of women were consistent in their reporting of less gratification in the mothering role over the year. The more active infant provided less gratification for teenagers than the infant who smiled quietly from the crib.

Only 12% of the variance in gratification in the mothering role was predictable at 1 year. Predictive variables included the following: marital status, educational level, and race, 0.5%; stress from positive life events, 5%; comfort in meeting infant's needs attitude, 4.1%; and empathy, 2.6%. This finding raises questions about what the major contributors to a woman's gratification in mothering are at 1 year.

Observed Maternal Behavior Just as at the earlier test periods, groups 2 and 3 scored more adaptable on observer-rated maternal behaviors than did Group 1 at 1 year. The average scores were as follows: Group 1, 32.8; Group 2, 36.6; and Group 3, 37.8. The overall sample average was 36.4 (standard deviation, 5.00), which was a slight decrease from 37.0 (standard deviation, 4.63) at 8 months.

Observed maternal behavior was 44% predictable by variables tested at 1 year. The predictive variables included the following: marital status, educational level, and race, 16.0%; maternal attitude reciprocity factor, 13.5%; maternal health status, 8.5%; personality disorder, 4.6%; and the size of the support network, 1.3%. Of the forced variables only race and educational level were significant, indicating that being Caucasian and having a higher level of education were associated with more adaptive maternal behaviors as the major predictor, with maternal attitudes of reciprocity with the infant the second greatest predictor.

Self-Reported Ways of Handling Irritating Child Behaviors The older the age group, the more positively they reported they handled irritating child behaviors (Group 1 mean, 8.6; Group 2 mean, 7.6; Group 3 mean, 6.6). The range of scores for the total sample was 4 to 12 (with 0 the most positive score). The older women in Group 3 consistently reported handling irritating child behaviors more positively than one or both of the younger groups since 1 month postpartum. The overall sample mean was 8.6; SD, 2.06.

One-third of the variance in reported ways of handling irritating child behavior was predictable at 1 year. The predictive variables included the following: marital status, educational level, and race, 19.3%; appropriate control of child's impulses attitude factor, 8%; size of support network, 2.7%; self-concept, 2%; closeness to infant attitude factor, 1.6%. All of the forced variables were significant, indicating that being single, non-Caucasian and having less education were major predictors of less favorable ways of handling irritating child behaviors. Maternal attitudes of control were a second major predictor indicating that attitudes are operationalized into self-reported action.

Infant Growth and Development There were no significant group differences on either the growth and development factor, weight gain, length grown, head circumference, or motor development. Group 2 infants scored higher on social development than infants of groups 1 and 3, however. Although there were no significant differences in weight gain, the teenagers' infants who weighed significantly less at birth weighed significantly more at 1 year (10.2 kg) than Group 2 infants (9.8 kg). Group 3 infants did not differ significantly from either (9.9 kg). Because Group 2 women also reported higher gratification in the mothering role, the question is raised whether their infants' higher level of social development was related to this.

Only 15% of infant growth and development was predictable at 1 year. The predictive variables included the following: marital status, educational level, and race, 4.5%; reciprocity attitude factor, 5.6%; maternal activity level (temperament), 2.3%; and negative life

events experienced during the year, 2.3%. The greatest predictor
was the mother's attitude of reciprocity with the infant; this indicates that women who encouraged and promoted reciprocal interactions with their infants had infants who scored higher in growth
and development at 1 year.

Maternal Role Attainment Index   All of the above maternal role
variables loaded significantly as one factor at 1 year when subjected
to a principal components analysis. Except for the observer-rated
maternal behaviors, more of the variance was accounted for by the
maternal role index factor than by any of the other dependent
variables alone.

Almost 38% of the variance was predictable by the following variables: race, educational level, and marital status, 8.6%; self-concept,
16.9%; reciprocity attitude factor, 7.4%; negative life events stress,
1.7%; infant-related stress, 1.8%; and appropriate control of child's
impulses factor, 1.5%. Race was the only forced variable that was
significant when entered into the regression model. Clearly, when the
maternal role attainment variables were considered as one factor,
the mother's *self-concept* was the major predictor, with race the
second greatest predictor, and maternal attitudes the third greatest
predictor.

Integration of the Role

The assumption that all women would internalize the maternal role
within the period of 1 year did not hold. They named the period
when they first felt like a mother, automatically responding to the
term "mother," and were comfortable with their decisions, which
ranged from 3% who stated, "From pregnancy," to 4% who stated,
"Not yet—I'm still working on it" (5%, 1%, and 8%). One-third of
the women indicated that they had integrated the mothering role
during the first 2 weeks following birth (15%, 35%, and 41%). Almost half (49%) had integrated the role by 2 months (38%, 52%,
and 50%). By 4 months almost two-thirds (64%) had integrated the
mothering role (65%, 66%, and 61%). By 9 months 85% had integrated the role (78%, 90%, and 82%). The time of maternal role
integration did not differ significantly by age group.

A first thought is that other factors, such as life goals and the environmental context, may be more critical than developmental
variables to a woman's integration of the maternal identity. The

three women who were not fulfilling the mothering role at all were from Group 2. However, it is quite possible that of the two-fifths (39%) of Group 1 who were lost to the study, many relinquished the mothering role. This was certainly the case of one who was lost at 4 months; her parents had her infant and did not even know where their daughter was.

Major Role Models for Mothering

The majority of the women (52%) named their mother as their major role model during their first year of motherhood. One-fourth named another woman (aunt, sister, sister-in-law, girl friend), and 23% stated they had not had a role model. Six of the women mentioned their fathers along with another woman or their mother. This finding is not in agreement with Rubin (1967a), who reported that although mothers were major prototypes for mothering initially, they were soon replaced by peers who were less threatening.

Comparison of Self with Own Mother in Child Care When comparing themselves with their mothers in the care of their children, 53% said they were more liberal; 33%, the same; 10%, more conservative; and 4% maintained they did not know. Responses did not differ significantly by age group. Almost half (49%) felt their judgment was the same as their mothers, 39% said their judgment was better, 6% said it was poorer, and 5% did not know.

Almost half (48%) reported the same use of physical discipline with their children, 15% said they used more physical discipline, 34% reported they used less, and 2% did not know. Significantly more teenagers (35%) reported they used more physical punishment than their own mothers, compared with Group 2 (13%) and Group 3 (9%). The two older groups (52% and 53%) more often reported the same amount of physical discipline, compared with 28% of the teenagers.

Despite the similarity in judgment and use of physical discipline, women tended to think they were fairer (45%) or more lenient (37%) than their mothers had been; 15% said they were stricter, and 3% did not know. Age groups did not differ significantly.

Overall, except for the tendency toward being more liberal, fairer, and more lenient, the percentages of women who rated themselves as the same as their mothers in the areas of child care were similar to the percentage who listed their mothers as major role models.

These findings support the conclusion that women tend to mother as they were mothered, while maintaining attitudes that they are more liberal or fairer than their mothers.

IMPACT OF INFANT ON LIFE-STYLE

The majority (55%) of the women continued to report that the impact of their infant on their life-style had resulted in a great deal of change for them; 1% rated no change, 8% rated very little change, and 15% rated a moderate amount. This did not differ by maternal age group.

The changes that had occurred as a result of the infant were both positive and negative. Fewer women (40%) mentioned their decreased mobility and inability to go out than at 8 months (98%), indicating that the walking infant was easier to take on outings. Increased responsibility continued as the greatest infant-related change for 50%. Change in routines that also reflected a change in priority, such as eating, cleaning, shopping, and sleeping, were listed by 40%; 18% felt they were more serious or had new perspectives on life. Twelve percent described the childproofing of their homes and collection of infant equipment as major changes.

Although one-fourth of the women described negative effects on the mate relationship, 12% reported that marriage had resulted as a consequence of the baby's birth. Negative effects included strained relationships, increased arguments, severed relationships, less time together, less privacy, and less depth in their interactions with their mates.

One-fourth of the women described a change in their social life in which they had fewer friends or saw friends less often; 15% described a positive change in which they met more people through the infant or were closer to friends with infants. Eighteen percent described closer relationships to their families, whereas 1% reported more strained relationships with family members.

Eleven percent described a more enriched life since the infant's birth. Five percent of the women reported that they had become more religious.

Nine percent of the women described a change in their life plans such as plans for school or work. This was the only area in which significant age differences were observed (3%, 6%, and 16%).

Infant-Related Stress

Groups did not differ significantly in their rated extent of bother from infant-related change. The overall sample mean (52.3; SD, 12.58) was close to the 8-month mean (52.5; SD, 12.05), with scores ranging from 24 (no bother) to 88 (greater bother).

There were no significant group differences in the degree of bother in mate relationships subscale. The one item measuring financial stress indicated greater financial stress for Groups 1 (mean, 3.3) and 2 (mean, 3.0) than for Group 3 (mean, 2.6).

Role Conflict and Role Strain

The overall percentage of women experiencing high or very high role strain increased at 1 year (21%, compared with 16% at 8 months and 18% at 4 months). This increase may reflect the increase in employed mothers from 55% at 8 months to 62% at 1 year. Thirteen percent of the overall sample did not exhibit any role strain, 31% experienced low role strain, and one third experienced moderate strain.

There were no significant group differences in role strain at 1 year (2.90, 2.66, and 2.80). Role strain scores had increased from 8 months for all age groups (2.76, 2.51, and 2.66).

COPING STRATEGIES: RESOURCES FOR MOTHERING AT ONE YEAR

Coping Strategies

Women listed one or more coping strategies they used to manage difficult times with their infants. Three percent of the women stated that they did not have any difficult times with their infants. Almost two-thirds (64%) stated that they either soothed or distracted the infant by a change in environment or an outing. One-fourth stated that they gave the infant to their mates or another adult.

Other coping strategies involved more personal attention or behavior. One-fourth reported that they either used patience, regrouped, or prayed. One-tenth said they talked to their mate or another adult for help. Others reported less controlled or avoidance responses: crying/yelling/screaming, 8%; ignore infant/let cry, 7%; resting/going to bed, 4%; bite/slap infant when infant bites/slaps, 4%; and wine/beer/joint, 2%.

The method of coping did not differ by age group, except that the younger the age group, the more often they reported "ignore infant/ let cry" (25%, 5%, and 2%), and "bite/slap infant when infant bites/ slaps" (13%, 3%, and 2%).

Size of Support Network at One Year

As was the case at all test periods since 1 month, there were no group differences in the number of persons listed by the women who helped with day-to-day situations. Only 3% of the women reported that they had no one to help them. Just over one-fourth (26%) listed one person; 27% listed two persons; 29% listed three persons; and 14% listed four persons.

The mate was the person most frequently mentioned as helping with day-to-day situations; 73% listed their mates (48%, 76%, and 81%). The mother or mother-in-law was listed by 43%, the second most frequently named helping person (63%, 48%, and 27%). Friends were listed by 39%; the older the woman, the more often she listed friends (23%, 39%, and 47%). There was an increase in the percentage of women reporting mothers or mothers-in-law in the support network from 8 months (38%), and a decrease reporting friends (47%); the percentage reporting help from mates remained consistent (71%).

Type of Support Reported

There were no group differences in the reported physical, emotional, or appraisal support received at 1 year. Over three-fourths (78%) of the women reported receiving physical help with either child-care, household tasks, or financial help. Almost half (48%) reported having received emotional support (39%, 48%, and 51%), and 8% reported appraisal support or reassurance regarding their mothering behaviors. Twice as many teenagers (40%) as older women (20% and 21%) reported receiving informational support. Consistently, the larger number of mothers in the teenagers' support network occurred with more reported informational support. It is of interest that there was a negative relationship between informational and emotional support in the teenage group. This suggests that there may be some conflict in the teenager's support system and that their mothers may be perceived as providing largely informational support. Barerra (1980) noted that the teenager's source of support was often her greatest source of conflict.

ADVICE TO PARENTS OF ONE-YEAR-OLDS

When asked what suggestions they would have for a new mother the first year, almost one-third (31%) would tell a new mother to relax, trust herself, and not to worry. Twenty-two percent would stress taking each day as it comes, being flexible, and that it was fun. One-fifth would stress that rest is important and to be sure to take time for themselves. Sixteen percent stressed the importance of enlisting support from others or going to mothers' groups. Thirteen percent stressed making time to spend with the baby and loving the baby, and 13% stressed the importance of patience.

Other advice included the following: It's hard work the first 4 months, 8%; prepare for by reading/attending classes, 6%; avoid physical punishment, 5%; be sure you want a baby, 4%; stay home/ make no radical change in life, 4%; involve mate from the beginning, 3%; it is good to work, 2%; don't spoil, set limits, 2%; buy practical things for the baby early, 2%; pay attention to mate, 2%; and have an objective party to discuss problems with, 2%.

Teenagers' advice less often focused on enlisting support (0%, 16%, and 24%) but more often included being sure a baby was wanted (14%, 3%, and 2%), avoiding physical punishment (22%, 3%, and 1%), and having patience (19%, 17%, and 4%) than the older women's.

SELECTED WOMEN'S EXPERIENCES

Alma, Alison, Alice, and Amy are teenagers; Betty, Barbara, Bea, and Bonnie are in the 20- to 29-year-old group; and Carrie, Cathryn, Cynthia, and Carmen are in the 30-and-older group. The first two in each group—Alma, Alison, Betty, Barbara, Carrie, and Cathryn— reported they were unmarried when their infants were born. These contrasts were deliberately made because much of the literature supporting differences in teenage parenting does not consider marital status of the woman.

Alma

Sixteen-year-old Alma looked great at her interview at 1 year. This young Filipino woman was slim and very content. She had matured considerably over the year; she was open and friendly with the interviewer. She was very warm and loving in her interactions with her son. Her husband continued to help her very willingly, and it was evident that their relationship was very cooperative. Both Alma and her husband receive a lot of family support. Bob, her husband, has been attending auto mechanics school, and they have been on welfare. Bob was expecting to be called for a job soon. Alma was thinking about going to work in a month or two; she said her mother could get her a job as a telephone operator.

When asked if she had done things differently as a mother as a result of participating in this study, Alma said, "It feels good to talk about it."

Alma said that she had had no problems with her health since 8 months, and she rated her health as very good. She reported that she had been really busy, always having to keep an eye on her son. (There was no gate on the stairs.) When asked who had been her major role model during the year, she responded, "No one really." When asked what it was like for her as a mother, she said:

> I feel good. I'm more responsible. I feel more like a mother now that he's older. When I'm out with my mother, people think he is her baby. It makes mom feel younger. I know that people think I'm too young. If I see friends they think I'm babysitting—people I haven't seen for a long time. I am taking more responsibilities. I think more seriously; I used to act childish, but now I am mature. I first felt like a mother when he was two months old.

> He has brought a great deal of change about in our life-style. I stay home and watch him every day. I try to pay attention to both my husband and my baby at the same time. We both try to keep him company and to keep him busy. We go to the park and feed the ducks instead of going to parties or shopping a lot.

> My husband has been the most helpful to me the past few months. My mother-in-law has given advice. When I get tired and need to rest, my husband takes care of him—feeds, changes, plays, and takes him out with

him. I've had more help than I wanted. He [infant] always wants to be carried. So many people here, they always spoil him, won't let him cry.

He is walking now, says a few words. He can shake hands, do "muscle man," throw kisses, point to things he wants. He understands a lot of things. He likes for me to play ring-around-the-rosey, hide-and-seek, and to chase him. I play with him an hour or so three times a day. We're teaching him with books and story tapes, to name things, to watch TV, and about his past. We're also teaching him how to count and to put different shapes into holes. My husband taught him how to climb off the couch. He eats with a spoon and drinks from a cup, and he eats finger foods.

I tell him no by showing him and saying "no" and moving him and giving him a toy. I rank myself as "ten" in mothering. The most difficult thing about mothering now is that he walks; I have to watch him all the time. The easiest thing is teaching him, feeding and playing with him. The most difficult thing over the whole year was being up at night and those first days at home. Taking care of him was the easiest thing all year. How fast they learn things was the most unexpected thing.

I plan to have him take swimming lessons and go to gymboree. I think he'll complete at least one to two years of college [in response to "How far do you think your child will go in school?"]. I want five children— after I'm twenty; Bob wants a lot of children.

My advice to other parents would include using little tricks about feeding, like play "airplane." If he doesn't like a bath, play first, then wash him.

Our biggest concern is how we're going to live on our own—having our own place, and Bob finding a job.

Alison

Alison is an obese, white 18-year-old who was still in her robe and slippers for a 5:30 p.m. interview at her parents' neat and well-furnished home. Alison's niece who had a 2-week-old baby was present throughout the interview and was very attentive to the interviewer's questions and Alison's replies. Alison's mother and sisters were also in and out a lot. Probably because of the lack of privacy, she was less open and did not make eye contact during this interview, although she talked a lot. She had only superficial insight into her situation and had made no move toward her independence or taking full responsibility for her child. Alison's mother is fully in charge and appeared quite tolerant of the situation. She said that her mother had been her major role model during the year.

Alison's son was happy and playful and appeared well cared for. Everyone passing through interacted with him. Alison was proud and loving toward him but was not overly concerned with him; she did not monitor his movements, and the grandmother redirected or distracted him when necessary.

Alison described her future plans for her son as taking him to Disneyland; she noted that she hadn't been since she was 6. When asked how far she thought he would go in school, she replied that she hoped he would go beyond college—"I kind of want him to be a lawyer."

Alison noted that participating in the study over the year had had no effect on her or her mothering.

Alison reported that she had been fine, having had one cold in the last 4 months. She was still coughing but rated her health as very good. When asked what it was like for her being a mother now, she commented:

> It's something exciting. It's nice watching a little boy—having responsibility for someone else. He's into everything now. I feel more responsibility than I did at four months. I'm still getting help from my family, more curbing how he grows up—not letting him do anything wrong or nothing. Being a mother has taken away a lot of things—not seeing friends as much, not on my own as much, not going out as much. Makes me feel good mentally more than physically. I have someone to grow up with myself. Watching him grow makes me feel more important. I feel fatter. I'm just starting to lose it—gained fifty-two pounds when I was pregnant and never lost it. Once I get exercising and once I lose this weight, I'll go back to work. I have been home with the baby all year. I first felt like a mother at one year. I first realized how important it was the way you raise them and how they grow up.

> He has influenced my life a great deal. He [infant] has helped me in making decisions. I look more to his future than I look to mine. He's brought me closer to my parents. I realize what it's like being a parent—how hard it is and why they were so strict and stuff.

> My mother and father have been the most help to me the past few months. Mom gives advice—what is best to do for him—and takes care of him a lot. My father plays with him, gives him a lot of attention, and changes him once in a while. My mom takes care of him about sixty percent of the time.

> He walks, plays with toys, stands in front of the TV and plays with the knobs. He splashes in the tub, gags himself with his fingers, bangs his head on the floor when he's mad, plays in the sunshine, and likes music. He loves to eat. He holds his cup once in a while and dumps it out. He doesn't

feed himself yet. He likes for me to push him around in his kiddy-car and to play with his shape sorter. I tour the house every morning and name things to him. I do this about four hours a day.

When he doesn't need something he wants, I say "no" and he throws a fit. I ignore it. If he gets into things, I slap his hand and put him in his playpen and let him cry awhile. I'd rate myself as "ten" in mothering. I'd like four children in a couple of years; I don't think I can handle seven like my mother.

The most difficult thing now is watching what he gets into. The easiest thing is playing with him. The hardest thing over the year was when he started crawling—getting into more things—and watching out for him. The easiest thing the whole year was when he was first born. I didn't have to worry about him as much as I do now. My mom did more then. The most surprising thing this year was the time I have to dedicate to him.

Giving birth to him is the most rewarding thing to me as a person. Just knowing he came from me—that I brought someone else into the world.

It's hard to say what advice I'd give to others—watch out for them; keep a close eye on them.

My major concern now is making sure he does OK. I went through a lot of trouble when I was going through school. I don't want him to go through that. I'm watching out for that—drugs and stuff. I want to raise him to be honest and open with me—establish that relationship early.

Alice

Alice, who is a 19-year-old, married black woman, had just returned from school for the interview at 3:15 p.m. Her dress had ice cream spilled on it, and she was tired. Her apartment was cluttered; toys were on the floor. But she is still working evenings 30 hr a week in addition to attending school.

She enrolled in college a month ago and is taking 15 units.

Alice was warm and loving with her infant. It was evident that she enjoyed mothering. She provided a lot of appropriate stimulation for her son. Alice noted that she wanted two more children. Her future plans for her son included taking him to a child-care center next year, then in 3 years his beginning preschool. When asked how far she thought he would go in school, she said beyond college—a Ph.D. "As bad as I want a Ph.D., I won't get it. My mom has her masters's. She gives to him. She didn't have time for me because she was in school."

Alice felt that participating in the study made her more aware of her son, that she concentrated more, and that the questions caused her to look into some things, such as how much time she spent with her son.

Alice reported her health as fine since 8 months and rated it as good. She had been to the doctor to get birth control pills and had a regular checkup. When asked what being a mother was like for her, she became very animated:

> I love it. It's kinda special. Not everyone is a mom. He's a holy terror, but I love him. He owns the whole house now. It has changed how I feel a little. Things that were important aren't anymore—a change of priorities. I first felt like a mother when he was around three to four months old.

> He's changed things around here a great deal. Now that he walks, you've got to be more mobile. He wants to do more; you can't set him down and do your work. I can go more places. People don't mind watching him now. He's not a hassle—one bottle and diaper will tide us over. It's gradual. It's not hard, but you make things happen, but it's not a shock. When they start to crawl, then you put plug covers on. It's amazing how they communicate without talking.

> Charles [husband], my cousin, and my mom have been the most helpful to me the past few months. Charles watches him at night when I work. I can't teach him because I do chores and am busy with that. My cousin and my mom watch him so I can get out. She teaches him—taught him to walk. Charles and I take care of him 50-50.

> He walks alone, tries to talk, makes noises and babbles. He hands things to you, plays with the train, pulls and rolls his toys. He is into wheels, he watches them. His fine motor skills aren't developed—he doesn't put shapes into the right hole. He dials the phone, puts things in containers, gets into my books and tears them apart, reads books and turns pages. He bangs on things, makes noise, loves looking out the car window when he can feel the air coming in through the window. He likes for me to make noises, tickle him, play with his phone. I spend about an hour a day altogether playing with him. Weekends, I spend about two to three hours a day.

> When he wants something he doesn't need, I give him something else. Charles hits him; I don't.

> I rate myself as 10 in mothering. I want two more children.

> The most difficult thing about mothering now is getting him to understand—the discipline. The easiest thing is being able to understand him.

> The hardest thing over the year was at three months. It was hard to get someone to watch him and take time with him. You've been in the

house for so long—that's when it gets to you. I really wanted a girl—he did become a blessing. I can do things with him; I'd have to do a lot of ruffles to keep up with a girl. The easiest thing was accepting him.

The most unexpected thing this past year was I didn't get into school last semester. We'd planned the budget so I wouldn't have to work. I was supposed to quit, had planned to use financial aid. I didn't get into school, financial aid stopped, so I had to work.

The advice I'd give a new mother would be that it's hard work, but it can be done. You can love a child and have time for yourself. Can keep a balance. There's a period where they need more of your time. If you're poor, accept it. If you have to go to work, don't knock yourself out because you have to leave.

The most rewarding thing is that he really loves me. I don't want a dependent child, but I do like that he needs me.

Amy

Amy, an 18-year-old, married Filipino woman, had just returned from school when the interview began. Amy had been back in school for about a month. She and her son share a room in her family's apartment. Her husband lives with his parents across the Bay. The apartment was messy, and Amy asked the interviewer if she minded if she cleaned during the interview. Amy interacted with Jimmy (her son) throughout by putting toys on the floor and offering him food or the bottle.

Amy appeared more relaxed than she had at earlier interviews. She also seemed pleased with her son's "growing" and that he "is a person." Amy had difficulty understanding some of the words, such as "conservative," in the questions, and several questions were reworded for her.

Amy said she'd like a total of three children—but not yet. Her future plans for her son included going to Catholic school. She thought that her child would complete high school.

Amy reported that participating in the study had not had any effect on how she had done things. She noted that she felt the same as before, that nothing had changed, and she rated her health as good.

Amy noted that her mother had been her role model for mothering. In response to what it was like for her as a mother she said:

I like it. Jimmy is growing. It makes me feel good that he is growing and is a person. Being a mother hasn't affected how I feel about myself.

He has changed things around here a moderate amount. I go along with
it. Can't do anything; don't have any time for myself.

My mom has been the most helpful to me the past months. She does
everything that I do that needs to be done. My husband won't change the
diaper. He quit work about six months after Jimmy was born and still
hasn't worked.

Jimmy can clap his hands, open his hands, throw the ball, crawl. He
can stand up—pull on my leg. He yells now—that's all. He likes for me to
play with him. Sometimes I don't have time to watch him play, and then
my little brother watches him and plays with him. I play with him about
thirty minutes a day—I'm never here, at school all day.

When he wants something he doesn't need, I just say "no." I rate myself as "five" in mothering. I first felt like a mother when he was about
four moths old.

The most difficult thing about mothering is they touch everything. I
feel like spanking them. Nothing is easy about it. Looking back over the
year, the most difficult thing is that it's difficult—being a mother is difficult. The most unexpected thing was how tiresome it is.

My advice to a new mother would be "Don't have another one"
[laughs].

My major worry now is his health. He's had a fever lately. [Drainage
from eye present.]

Betty

Betty, a 22-year-old, single Anglo-white woman, looked great although she was tired after just returning from work. She was open,
talkative, and friendly. The infant's father was present. He watched
his son and cooked dinner during the interview.

Betty and her mate had just moved to a new house, which was
empty. Her son explored freely and was very happy. Her son's chest
had recent burns that are healing well, and scarring appeared as if it
would be minimal. However, the kitchen was not childproofed,
i.e., no latches on cabinets, tablecloth on table for infant to pull
down. He had pulled coffee down on himself at the sitter's and was
hospitalized for 2 days for observation of the burns.

Betty said that she would like a couple more children; her mate
interjected "nine or so." Her future plans for her son included
school; she said she had been thinking a lot about that. She thought
he'd complete college, and laughingly said, "He'd better be an archi-
tect."

Betty felt that participating in the study had affected her mothering. The questions had stimulated her thinking.

Although Betty rated her health as very good, she remarked that she had started working when her child was 9 months old and that she was very tired. When asked what it was like for her now as a mother she said:

> Now I'm getting to the point of starting to worry. It's frightening to think of the things that can happen. Schools, accidents . . . I'm a mother. As he gets older, I'm more aware of responsibility. I feel more of what I want out of life. I know for sure I want more. Have kids, raise kids, be a mom.
>
> He has changed our life a good bit. He comes first. I think of him before I think of anything else. I've never been a person that goes out a lot. It gives us more to talk about. We have this main thing between us to share. We've always been close.
>
> My mate and my mother have been the most help to me the past months. If I'm having a bad day, he'll take over. I can depend on that. Mom, she's there when I need her—advice or to babysit. My mate and I share parenting fifty-fifty.
>
> He says "bye-bye," "Ma-ma," "Da-da," dances, walks. He's into everything. He takes things out and puts them in. He cooperates in dressing. He understands a lot. He likes for me to chase him, play peek-a-boo. He hides now. Plays patty-cake. I talk to him and kiss him a lot. On work days I spend about one and a half hours, during weekends about three to five hours playing with him. When he wants something he doesn't need I say "no" and restrain him, and ignore his protest. I slap his hands when he gets into things. I rate myself as "nine" in mothering. [Mate said 10.]
>
> I first felt like a mother when he started walking around at eleven months. He came to me when he needed me.
>
> The most difficult thing about mothering now is when he's in a blue mood and hard to handle and just can't be pleased. Everything is so natural.
>
> The thing that stands out as the most difficult over the year was when he was just brought home, and breast-feeding—nursing at twenty. I was nervous getting used to him, until two and a half months. The easiest thing, looking back, was around six months. I could let him be by himself—easy to deal with. The most unexpected was the financial impact.
>
> My advice to a new mother would be to show that you're available. Try to see what the need is—don't just stuff a bottle in their mouth. They communicate their needs.
>
> The most rewarding thing for me is knowing that he's happy and a part of me.

I'm always worried. Things I read in the paper, what kinds of friends he'll have, whether he'll be a good boy, if I can teach him things to hold him when he is away from us.

Barbara

Barbara, a 26-year-old Anglo-white, was living with the father of her daughter, Elsie. She was slightly overweight, barefoot, and dressed very casually in a loose blouse and jeans. Her apartment was cluttered and not very clean. Many age-appropriate toys were around, and Elsie was dressed in a pretty red dress.

It was obvious that Barbara enjoyed her role as mother very much. She appeared calm and easygoing. She spontaneously demonstrated much affection to Elsie and was very natural in interacting with her. She breast-fed her a couple of times during the 65-min interview.

Barbara's future plans for Elsie included traveling around with her and showing her things through experience. A trip to Hawaii to visit her grandfather had been planned. She hopes that Elsie will complete college; she will probably go further, but Barbara won't force her. "One hopes that her child doesn't get married at fourteen, but she has to make the choice. I would like for her to go to an alternative school. I don't have a lot of trust in public schools."

Barbara noted that she didn't plan to have other children. A possibility would be to adopt when she is less poor, or maybe have another in 5 or 7 years.

Barbara reported that participation in the study had given her a chance to talk and to share her feelings. Her health had been fine since 8 months, and she had had no problems; she rated it as very good.

When asked what it was like for her as a mother, she said:

I love being a mother—no problems at all. Being a mother has made me more aware of who I am. I have more confidence in myself. Mothering is real compatible—a natural thing.

Elsie has changed my life-style a great deal—in every way. To be a mother is to alter life-style. Day by day nothing horrible has happened. Everything is manageable. I'm still working half-time; have been since one month.

My mate has been the most helpful to me. He is helpful by being there to listen and just physically being there. He could do more; he's terrifically together with her physically, but there's so much more—cooking, housework, et cetera. He doesn't have a steady job. We both free-lance.

Elsie has been walking since ten months. She's formulating a lot of words. She is very involved with the telephone; into imitation. She follows me around the house and helps me clean. She draws, loves music, and loves kids at once. She likes for me to look at picture books with her, sing songs, dance, play with animals or toys, eat with her, sleep with her. We're real close—real companions. I do things with her almost all day. I'm with her all the time. I take her to work with me.

When she wants something she doesn't need, I usually put it away from her reach and give her something she can have. I explain and am very firm.

I first felt like a mother as soon as I brought her home from the hospital. As soon as I held her in the hospital. Feels real good. I rate myself as "ten" in mothering. Hard to say who was my role model. I don't have a mother myself. Maybe my father or a combination of women friends.

The most difficult thing about mothering is time usage, time scheduling. I like to read a lot. It's hard to do that even when she takes a nap. The most difficult thing over the year was when Elsie had a urinary tract infection. I had to take her to the hospital for different medications. She hated it and spit it out; it was real hard. Everything else was easy. She has been the absolute joy as a child.

The most unexpected thing is that I hadn't realized that I would have such an opinionated view. I think that we learn caring from our parents parenting us. I understand how abusive parents have been abused themselves. I only knew my mother two years. As I cared for my own child I realized how my own mother actually influenced the way I cared for Elsie. She was a very good mother. I know that I've been parented well. I have had time to sit with Dad to talk about Mom.

My advice to a new mother would be to get a good support system if your mate can't support you. You need to have at least one strong support system—several is better. To help out in the house or drive you around, or just talking. Especially a single mother. That is the most important thing around you. The unknown—having a support system behind the unknown.

The most rewarding thing about motherhood is to watch my child respond to life around her and seeing that she is well fed and happy.

My primary concern at this time is to move out of this neighborhood. I've experienced too many children left on their own at an early age—it's too depressing. I'm amazed at how haphazard parents raise their children. I don't. Children have a large capacity—children will guide parents if we take the time.

Bea

Bea, a 21-year-old, married Anglo-white woman, did not appear distressed with the demands of motherhood at 1 year. She was friendly and receptive to the interviewer. She was dressed casually in slacks, and her home had been made safe for her son. Her maternal pride was evident when she held him and interacted with him warmly and affectionately. Bea misses her friends at work, but overall she appeared serene.

Her future plans for her son include offering him as many things, such as music and other activities, as she can afford. She felt that because her mother was divorced when she was young she didn't have many of these opportunities. She said she had no idea how far her child might go in school, but she hoped he completed high school.

Bea laughed nervously as she replied that she didn't plan to have other children. She noted that participation in the study had had no effect on her behavior.

Bea rated her health as very good and noted that she had felt fine—that only the first months were hard. When asked what it was like for her as a mother now, she stated:

> It's fun. It's a lot of work. I miss work—socializing with people at work. I get bored; I don't have a car. It gets monotonous, but I wouldn't do it differently. It's good for my son's development. That's why I had him—to enjoy him. Motherhood hasn't really affected how I feel about myself. I still feel the same. It wasn't any big adjustment. Just the first few months—being tired.
>
> He changed our life-style very little. If you want to go out, have to find a babysitter. I put him first—no big problem.
>
> My husband has been the most helpful to me over the past months. He helps around the house, does dishes, cooks once in a while, or watches James when I go out.
>
> James walks, talks, plays—that's about it. He likes for me to read books to him, play with his toys, go for walks, go to the park with him. I do these things about ten hours a day. Most of the day is play.
>
> When he wants something he doesn't need, I say "no" firmly. When James has a temper tantrum, my husband is really stern. I think it's a natural thing. I ignore it, but my husband won't.
>
> I've always felt like a mother, even when I was pregnant. I don't think I had a role model. I'd rate myself as "nine" in mothering.

The most difficult thing about motherhood the past year is being patient. Sometimes I have to bite my lip. Play is the easiest thing. The most difficult thing over the entire year was the first month. The easiest overall thing was watching him grow—the enjoyment I get—watching him grow and develop. I can't think of anything that was unexpected during the past year. The most rewarding thing has been watching him grow and develop and seeing him do things that I teach him.

I don't have any advice for a new mother because every baby is different. If a mother asked a specific question, I could give some advice.

My primary concern is that my son grows up and is happy and healthy.

Bonnie

Bonnie, a 28-year-old, black married woman, was not very verbal at the interview. Bonnie is very obese and was casually dressed, with a towel on her head. She moved slowly, had a flat facial expression, maintained poor eye contact, and had very little spontaneous movement, but she gazed out the window thoughtfully when answering questions.

Her active, very mobile daughter played happily around the living room, frequently getting into things. The house was not child-proofed. Bonnie consistently and repeatedly removed her from the china cabinet, said "no," and slapped her hand, without any evidence of anger. Bonnie responded warmly to her daughter, held her on her lap until she wanted to get down. She returned and climbed into Bonnie's lap whenever she wished during the interview. Bonnie's husband arrived home near the end of the interview. He was greeted happily by his daughter, who then stayed in another room with him.

Bonnie discussed her psychiatric history and her therapeutic abortion as being a difficult time for her. She has worked hard to make adjustments to motherhood through counseling. Bonnie would like another child when her daughter is 2½ years old.

Bonnie's future plans for her daughter include music and all areas of creativity. She noted that she would like her to be kind, to treat people well, and to be a happy person.

Bonnie was still working part-time and attending school 1 day a week. Her mother and her husband watch her daughter while she is away.

Bonnie reported that she had not done anything differently as a result of participating in the study but that it had made her feel good to participate. She added that bits of advice from the interviewers (nurses) had helped.

Bonnie said that she had been OK physically, just tired, but that emotionally there were a lot of changes in her life—additional responsibility—and that she was adjusting. She rated her health as very good, and said that prior to the last 6 months she had had a postpartum depression and psychiatric problems in adjusting to motherhood.

She described what it was like for her as a mother:

> Exciting! Busy! Happy, thankful, blessed. Sometimes I want a break. I have a lot of help. I feel the responsibility all the time, even if she's with her grandmother for a day. Since I had a baby I like myself more. I think I'm a responsible adult. I feel more capable, and I'm proud.

> She has changed my life-style a great deal. I have less time for everything. I don't want the same things. I don't have the same interests. She's number one. There is conflict with what I want to do, my value system. I used to dress up, and I had to look glamorous. Now I don't care unless it's something special.

> My husband has been the most helpful to me with mothering. He does the housework. He is so good with her. He watched the birth and was very involved from the beginning.

> She is walking, talking, shows her temper. Plays peek-a-boo and patty-cake. She is aggressive, very individual, independent. She has a sweet disposition. She's grown up. She seems older. She understands a lot and loves to dance and sing and perform. She likes for me to dance, sing, play records, and read to her. I don't have any regular times to play. She tears up the book when I read to her; I try to distract her. I don't always have patience.

> When she wants something she doesn't need I say, "No, no" to her and spank her hand. I rate myself as "seven" in mothering.

> The most difficult thing about mothering now is not being able to go as I would like. Her schedule and mine don't always match. The most difficult thing over the year has been friends—the transition—adjusting to the maturity and the responsibility. The easiest thing about mothering is the fun, the love, the joy. Over the year, loving her and caring for her has been the easiest. The most rewarding thing about motherhood is seeing her grow up.

> The most unexpected thing this first year was getting pregnant again at three months. I had an abortion; I didn't make the decision. My husband did. I was out of my mind. I was sick from three to five months. That was a terrible time; I'm still getting over it.

My advice to a new mother would be to be patient—try to be paient.

My primary concern at this time is her health. I want her to be healthy. [Infant has not been ill.]

Carrie

Carrie, a 33-year-old Anglo-white who was separated from her husband prior to conception, was interviewed at the home where she babysits. She was attractively dressed and had lost weight but looked haggard. She was warm and spirited as she talked about her daughter. Carrie was warm and loving with both infants but did favor her own; the TV was on during the entire interview. Although Carrie encouraged motor skills, she limited her daughter's feeding herself with a spoon because she makes a mess.

Carrie's major role models were her mother and father. She noted that her father played a lot with his children, so she tried to play with Belinda.

Her future plans for Belinda included her working full time and putting Belinda in day care, and good experiences such as dancing lessons, athletics, and having her photographed. She believed that Belinda would complete a minimum of high school and noted that she'd do what she needs to do to get what she wants.

When asked if she planned to have other children, she said, "Yes, but it would require a man who's into sharing the experience."

Carrie's ex-husband had gone to New York without telling her when her daughter was 10 months old and she was finalizing the divorce. Things had been difficult for her the past 4 months because of the legal hassle. She had been to Minnesota to visit her family, had felt fine, and rated her health as good. She wants to go see a dermatologist because of the skin blotches from pregnancy that have not gone away. When asked what it was like for her now as a mother, she was neutral in her response:

I like being a mom. She's older. I'm thinking of day care. I want to get back to work and in the world. [In other interviews Carrie was very positive in her responses to mothering. This change, which had begun at 8 months, appears to be her need to get back to work and be away from the baby.]

Being a mother has made me a stronger person, more compassionate toward my parents. I realize what an enormous task parenting is. I get lots of love from the baby.

She has changed my life-style a great deal. I have to do a lot more arranging. I've paid off bills this year. Now I've grown up. I'm glad I have a baby; it makes you close to others. I'm glad to have a baby need me. It has been a difficult year; intense—but good overall.

My parents have been the most helpful to me the past few months. For awhile I was getting too much attention from bossy friends, so I decreased that and I don't see them now. I was home for Christmas for two weeks. It's knowing that you have someone behind you. Everyone adored her; she was accepted into the family. They were supportive when my husband left me—gave me boxes of clothes, money—very nonjudgmentally. I've had less help than I needed. I wish I had family around so I could go out without paying babysitters.

She can walk with support and stand alone. She tries to feed herself. She says, "Kitty," "Da-da," "Ma-ma," "hi," "baba" [bottle]. She chases the cat, climbs up and down stairs, learns fast, repeats, imitates faces I make, wants what I eat. She likes for me to play with the cat with her, to take her out in the stroller and to socialize with other kids and pets, raise her up over my head and swing her and throw her in the air, likes music, dances, and TV. I spend about one and a half hours a day playing with her. She plays with the other baby and explores a lot [baby that Carrie babysits].

I say "no" when she wants something she doesn't need. I want her to understand; I put flowers on the table, want her to learn she can't take things from others. I move her if she persists or distract her.

I got a letter from the Crippled Children's Society because she was in the ICN at first. I was worried since I was Rh negative and was afraid she was retarded. The doctor said she's normal and healthy, and I called the ICN and they reassured me that all babies who were in the ICN got a letter from the society. So it was good that the doctor could reassure me that she was OK at the last visit.

I first felt like a mother at two weeks. I'd rate myself as a "nine" in mothering.

The most difficult thing about mothering a one-year-old is that they still need your constant attention—one hundred percent responsibility. The most difficult thing over the year was the ending of the relationship with my husband. At four months it looked as though we'd get together but didn't. It was a seven-year relationship; I missed that. My hopes got up and down, and finances are a big concern.

The easiest thing about mothering now is that they are so sweet; don't oppose you—not bratty—all pure learning. Over the year, her affection stands out as the easiest.

The most unexpected event of the year was that her father couldn't appreciate her. It blows my mind. I think there was so much positive aspects of having a baby. The most rewarding thing to me is that she's a gift. The experience of being a mom; the process. It's a whole different type of love. I've learned to take people as they are.

My advice to new mothers would be to be flexible, not to try to do too much—so what if your cleaning doesn't get done, stay involved with friends and people.

My major concern at this time is to get another woman to share a house, pay off my bills. I want to take trips. I want a good-paying job that I like. I want a relationship with a man.

Cathryn

Cathryn, a 36-year-old single woman of Russian heritage, was interviewed in the backyard of her parents' home while her son explored. Cathryn, who has been planning to move out on her own since 4 months, still hasn't made it, although she was continuing with her plans. She doesn't plan ahead and noted that she will check out the babysitting situation after she moves.

Although Cathryn appeared contented, the felt responsibility of motherhood was evident. She continues to be up several times a night with her son. She had age-appropriate toys for her son and was proud of his skills but expected cognitive ability beyond the 1-year level.

Cathryn's future plans for her son included getting him into a play group and continuing with his schooling. She thought that he'd probably complete college one day. Cathryn said that she had not been conscious of any one person as a role model; she specifically noted that she would not say her mother was.

Cathryn stated that the study had caused her to think about things more because of the questions that were asked. When asked if she planned to have other children she said, "It hasn't crossed my mind. It is unrealistic now. I think I might. I'm so close to the labor and delivery experience—like yesterday; it's such a short time. I wouldn't want to repeat it too soon."

Cathryn rated her health as good and noted that she was still quite fatigued. She was still breast-feeding and said that she had a lack of calcium. Her joints have been painful, and the doctor had ruled out arthritis. She was discouraged that her weight remained unchanged despite how little she ate. When asked what it was like for her as a mother, she said:

I feel I have to get prepared for more. I have to set my gears. He's no longer an infant. I have to change my focus, be more prepared. Suddenly you have to be aware of what you are; he can imitate you now. He responds to me, i.e., I can't hang around the kitchen all day smoking; now I must watch it. It's more exciting now. He's practically talking.

I don't have a picture of myself at this stage. I'm not thinking of myself as a mom in a way because I'm not involved in any social life now. I am living a sheltered life, have some friends.

He has changed things a great deal. I'm still aware of the lack of time. I'm too tired in the evening to do anything on my own after he's in bed. No time for my own interests. I used to take classes prior to him moving around. I get too tired now. Am much closer with my family and friends. Am more interested in people with kids.

My mother has been the most helpful to me the past months. She helps with his care—the diapers. She cooks here; she runs the household, which is also a problem. She decides and runs a lot of things. I'm looking forward to living alone with Albert.

He started walking two weeks ago. He climbs upstairs, downstairs, opens doors. Turns on the dishwasher, hands me things. Says, "baba," "Ma-ma," "Da-da," "kaka" [that's me]. He likes for me to play with him —with pots and pans. I like to try to go out and swim. We play peek-a-boo. Likes for me to chase him and roughhouse. He likes to stack rings, boxes. I'm with him all day. I guess I play with him three to four hours a day.

I talk to him mostly when he wants something he doesn't need. I show him and say "no," firmly. [Let him play with teapot during interview, until he broke the lid.]

I felt like a mother at the very beginning. I feel like we're friends. I rate myself as "nine" in mothering—leave a little room for improvement [laughs].

The most difficult thing about mothering is not having enough time for myself. If only he'd sleep more. I'd rather not leave someone else to take care of him. Looking back over the year, time has been the most difficult. The easiest thing now and over the year has been feeding him. Nursing is easy. The most unexpected thing is that it is easy except for the energy and time.

My advice to new mothers would be to have things set up so she can devote a lot of time to the baby and not have to fight a tight schedule. That can be so hard. I met someone who was really frustrated.

The most rewarding thing for me has been to see him change all the time. No, I don't have any concerns at this time about anything.

Cynthia

Cynthia, a 40-year-old, married Anglo-white nurse, was as brief in answering questions at the 1-year interview as she had been earlier. Her mother was visiting from out of state and played with the infant in another room during the interview.

Cynthia continues to work full time and wishes that she had more time to spend with her son. She was casually dressed in slacks and appeared calm, not at all anxious. Her home was very neat; it was child-proofed.

Cynthia's future plans for her son included trying to decide where to send him to nursery school. She thought that he would complete college.

She noted that she would like one more child. Her mother and her sister had been her major role models for mothering. Cynthia rated herself as 8 to 9 in mothering.

Participating in the study had not affected her behavior or mothering.

Cynthia rated her health as very good and noted that she had been fine, in good health since 8 months. When asked what it was like for her as a mother, she said:

> My only problem is that I don't have enough time to do everything. Otherwise it is enjoyable. I have good feelings about myself.

> He has changed our life-style a moderate amount—just in trying to childproof the house and to put everything out of sight.

> My husband has been the most helpful to me with mothering. He helps with a lot of the housework and takes care of Joshua. He's at the licensed day-care center all day; they take care of him most of the time.

> Joshua walks around things; he stood for a few seconds. He likes to play games and to play with his ball and toys in the bath. He opens and closes doors; he gets into cupboards. He likes for me to play with him and to give him his bath. I spend about one to two hours playing with him. He had an ear infection, but it's cleared up.

> When he wants something he doesn't need, I just say "no." Usually we just eliminate the object.

> The most difficult thing about mothering a one-year-old is that I work forty hours a week, and I wish I had more time to spend with him. It was easier when he was three months old and in a crib. Now he's getting into things, but that's normal. The thing that stands out over the year as

the most difficult was leaving him and going back to work at four months.

Feeding him is the easiest thing about mothering now. He eats everything that is in front of him. I can't think of anything that stands out over the year as being the easiest.

Nothing stands out as being unexpected this first year. The most rewarding thing for me is interacting with the child—watching him grow and develop.

My advice to a new mother would be to just relax and enjoy him. I feel more relaxed now. I don't have any concerns.

Carmen

Carmen, a 31-year-old, married woman of Mexican heritage, was casually dressed with her hair in curlers. Her well-furnished home was very neat and clean. Her sister-in-law and 2-year-old niece were visiting.

Carmen was quite vocal and reflective about her relationship with her husband. His high expectations of her and of their son make it difficult for her, and she has continued to feel that she has no time for herself. She frequently commented that she paid no attention to what her husband said, although at other times she said it bothered her, and she indicated that he didn't trust her. Carmen felt that she could do more if she weren't so upset so much of the time about her husband's demands and the degree of protectiveness that he has for his son. She hopes that when they have two children he will be less this way. Carmen is pregnant again and was adamant that two children are all that she wants. She rated herself as 5 in the mothering role.

Carmen had to drop out of school after she became pregnant again. She had planned to return to work at 1 year, but the current pregnancy prevented it. She appeared frustrated that she couldn't even stay in school to keep from being bored.

Carmen's future plans for her son included swimming lessons and teaching him how to play with other children. He now fights. Carmen thought that her child would complete high school. She added that her husband wants him to be a physician, wants to start taking him to the hospital so that he becomes accustomed to the environment, and wants him to start wearing white.

Carmen, who is 5 months pregnant, noted that it came as a surprise to her. She would have preferred to have waited a few more months and finds it really hard now. She rated her health as good.

Participating in the study had stimulated her to read more about child development and to read child-care magazines. The questions asked also stimulated her to think about things more.

When asked what it was like for her as a mother, she said:

Fun. He's now older; has been walking since ten months—very active. I'm not as competent as I should be. Everyone does things differently. I know there are ways of doing things differently than how I do them. I would feel more confident if I had the support of my husband; his demands are unreasonable. He doesn't trust babysitters.

He has changed our life a great deal. He is very spoiled by his father. My number one problem is that my husband doesn't want me to say no; that he's too young. I don't think so. Now my sister-in-law says I need to say no. Carlos wakes up at three a.m. and cries to sleep with us in our bed. I say let him cry; his father won't let me let him cry, but he's going to have to get used to his bed when the new baby gets here.

Relatives from my country [Mexico] have stayed and helped me for a couple of weeks or so and have showed me how to do things. It's good to see how other people do things. But it was a lot less help than I needed.

Carlos crawls up on furniture but can't get down. He turns on the radio and TV. He likes for me to lie down on the carpet and play with him. But it's hard now that I'm pregnant. I play with him a couple of hours a day.

When I say no to the baby for something he doesn't need, he gets upset. My husband thinks his son is perfect. If I try to discipline him, my husband leaves the room saying that he can't watch it.

The most difficult thing about mothering a one-year-old is the discipline, and feeding. I don't know what he should eat many times. The most difficult thing over the year has been that I can't leave him. I can't even go downstairs to do the laundry when he's asleep. My husband says you never know what will happen.

I can't think of anything that's easy now; everything has been hard. The most unexpected thing this year was getting pregnant again. The most rewarding thing for me is to see him walking. Even though I was happy with my career, I'm glad I have a child.

It's hard to give suggestions for anyone else. Everyone reacts differently.

My biggest worry is about his health. [Infant had been well except for a runny nose and fever at 9 months.]

ANALYSIS AND MAJOR THEMES

The joy and fun of interacting with the more social infant expressed by the majority of the women at 1 year were the pay-offs or plusses for being a mother. The 1-year-old can seek out his mother when he needs her, hug and kiss her, and show his attachment to her in many ways. Women were gratified by these responses such that the rewards outweighed the costs of motherhood. Other rewards were evident when women described how the infant had changed their life-styles. One-third saw the infant as bringing them closer to their families and/or friends with infants.

Of importance was the decrease in the level of gratification derived from the motherhood role for teenage mothers. The mobile, individuating infant may threaten the adolescent who is also individuating from parents. The 20- to 29-year-old group of women derived increased gratification in the role at 1 year, with the 30-and-older group continuing to score consistently lower than the other two age groups. The time demands of the infant and isolation from other adults were hardest for the 30-and-older women. These older women had fewer mothers or mothers-in-law in their support network than the younger women had, although they reported having mates and friends more often.

The costs of motherhood in the descriptions of how their life-styles had changed included decreased mobility, increased responsibility, change in routines, and less time for other adults. Half saw the infant's presence as contributing to either strained relationships, less time, and privacy with their mates or decreased interactions with friends. Thus, the infant's greater activity levels and greater demands increased difficulties in parenting and also contributed to the women's felt incompetencies.

The women evaluated their self-change resulting from motherhood as growth-producing or as contributing to their maturation. The essence of this growth and/or maturation, however, was that they were able to assume the *responsibility* for an infant.

The women were no longer satisfied with the all-consuming nature of motherhood and the diffuseness of body boundaries between self and infant. There was a restlessness to regain a sense of self along with a need to resume their usual activities if they had not already done so.

Employment of almost two-thirds of the women increased the possibility for role conflict as well as for stimulation. Many of those who had not returned to work planned to do so soon. Almost one fourth experienced high or very high role strain, yet employment offered desperately needed stimulation and reinforcement of being persons of value for some. Those who saw work as an asset felt that it helped them to be better mothers.

Although the mean score in role strain increased slightly, the percentage of women experiencing high or very high role strain increased from 16% to 21% at 1 year. This needs further examination. Although the increase in high role strain may relate to the increase of women who were employed (from 55% to 62%), other variables need to be examined. For example, one fourth of the women reported negative changes in their relationships with their mates, which could contribute to or cause role strain.

The women's health status may have been another contributing factor to role strain. Over two-thirds of the women had one or more health problem at both 8 and 12 months. Upper respiratory infections and/or flu were the most frequent type of health problem reported. The lingering disappointment about birth experiences was not resolved for several.

The selected vignettes of the 12 women illustrate that generalizations cannot be made about maturation and age. For example, 16-year-old Alma's greatest concern was achieving independence from her parents; 36-year-old Cathryn was struggling with the same goal. However, Alma talked about how she felt more mature and more responsible; Cathryn didn't "have a picture of herself." Deutsch (1967) suggested that pregnancy might be a catalyst in the maturation process for the teenager. Alma's growth and striving for independence would certainly suggest that this was true for her. However, at 36, pregnancy pushed Cathryn back into a dependent position in her parents' home; she was not employed or seeking outside stimulation as one might expect of a person her age.

Carmen continued to have conflict with her husband over disciplining her child. Her husband's high value of a first-born son was overwhelming to her. When she sought outside diversion in school, she became pregnant again and had to quit. Carmen was angry and held a very low opinion of her abilities. She rated herself as 5, just as Amy had done. Both 18-year-old Amy and 31-year-old Carmen saw nothing easy about mothering. Everything about the maternal role was perceived as difficult. Both women seem to feel trapped by motherhood. Both are of a minority culture living within a majority culture. One may question whether the lack of clear-cut cues for

mothering and the ambiguity Amy and Carmen face in seeing assertive Anglo-white women utilize very different feminine and maternal behaviors in the majority culture contributes to their difficulty
with the mothering role.

Single mothers were more concerned about their future roles as
mothers and the problems they faced than they had been at earlier
interviews. Greater overall societal acceptance of single motherhood
has not influenced some of the traditional mothers to accept single
mothers as friends and colleagues. The single woman's need for
someone to back her up was voiced by both Barbara and Carrie.
Regardless of maternal age, a supportive network was critical to the
single mother.

How the woman felt about herself overall was a major predictor
of her feelings about her infant, observed and self-reported maternal
caretaking behaviors. Maternal attitudes, level of functioning (personality disorder), and health status were important predictors of
observed maternal behavior. Having a larger support network was the
only support measure that was predictive of maternal caretaking
behaviors.

INTERVENTIONS

Infant Growth and Development

Knowledge of infant–toddler growth and development as an exciting and rewarding time needs to be strongly laced with how this time
is also challenging and exasperating. As the 1-year-old moves into
toddlerhood, and begins asserting himself with "No," one can imagine even greater concern about how to discipline and foster growth
in this active, delightful youngster.

Parenting groups can provide a feeling of camaraderie that is lacking because many women experienced a decreased amount of time
with friends. In addition, other parents may offer very practical
suggestions. The women stressed flexibility, relaxing, and learning to
trust themselves as helpful suggestions to mothers of 1-year-olds.
However, with increased numbers of women experiencing role strain
and with the overall decrease in self-concept that occurred at 8
months, more than advice to do these things is needed.

Parents need access to good books that describe developmental
changes clearly. They need to know that no one has answers for
each situation, and this is probably one of the greatest difficulties.

There is a lot of trial and error, but if trials are from a sense of love and a sense of fostering growth and development, a few errors will not prove devastating to a child.

Maternal Individuation

Regardless of maternal age, the unity of the mother-infant dyad created frustration that many mothers continued to experience at 1 year. There was overt recognition of the dyadic tie, the tie's impact, and plans to regain one's own personhood. These findings indicate that the process of maternal preoccupation described as occurring during pregnancy and early postpartum (Winnicott, 1958), and the process of polarization described as occurring during pregnancy with an initial break around 1 month, were not fully resolved for all mothers at 1 year. This phenomenon of the attempt to extrapolate the merged self from the mother-infant dyad was called *maternal individuation* since it appears to be analogous to the infant's separation-individuation (Mahler, 1968; Mahler, Pine, & Bergman, 1975).

The infant's individuation does not begin until 4 or 5 months of age, at the peak of his emotional symbiosis, and does not end until sometime during the third year of life, when the child has established a stable sense of self boundaries and has achieved emotional object constancy (Mahler et al., 1975). The mother's individuation seems to parallel this process; however, it would seem that it could be a-chieved sooner than the infant's. The question is raised about whether the woman's sense of separateness from her own mother might also be influential in her individuation process from her infant.

Breast-feeding contributed to both the women's emotional symbiosis with their infants and their state of primary preoccupation with the infant. There was a sense of having their bodies back when infants were weaned; this physical separation may facilitate the psychological individuation of mother and child. The woman's struggle to find herself and to not be excluded from activities important to her was evident at 1 year and included women of all ages.

Women need to be appraised of the dramatic change in life-style that can be expected and the acute sense of oneness that develops between mother and infant with these changes. The preoccupation of the mother with her infant is threatening to relatively new husbands who have not experienced or received in the husband-wife relationship what they observe between mother and infant. The lack of preparation for the intensity of the mother-infant tie and the infant takeover of the mother's time and life may in part account for both the decrease in maternal self-concept at 8 months and the stress from changed mate relationships.

Self-Development

Women don't expect the all-consuming nature of motherhood to extend so extensively over time. Not only does the truth need to be shared about the time and responsibility commitments over time but information needs to be communicated to women that, as a child ages, benefits accrue to the child from interactions with a wide range of people. A few of the women had not used babysitters or had used them very seldom. A feeling of entrapment leads to resentment, and resentment contributes to strain as well as pervading one's over-all feelings toward the child.

The need to mingle with other adults is so great that some women viewed employment roles as therapeutic. However, alternative routes of adult stimulation and self-development must be encouraged. Recreational outlets provided mothers with a sense of renewal, and vacations provided an important change of pace. Time has to be set aside deliberately and consciously for recreational and self-enhancement activities.

If a woman cannot afford a babysitter for one afternoon a week off, perhaps she can exchange babysitting with another mother who also needs the time away. Whether it is a shopping trip, a visit to a museum, or just a walk alone, every mother needs to be en-couraged to plan for an afternoon that is her time each week.

Fostering Positive Relationships with Mate

It takes considerable creativity to make private and special time with the mate as an infant becomes more mobile and more demand-ing of time. However, the positive mate relationship appears to offer the most extensive support available to mothers during the first year, and *this resource cannot afford to be damaged or strained.*

Counseling groups with couples would be an important way of getting some of the practical, "this is the way it is," and "what can be done about it" information across. The isolated nuclear couple feeling stress and strain is usually hesitant to admit or to face up to the disenchantment they are feeling with parenthood amid the social propaganda that is circulated about the joys of parenthood.

Couples need to weigh priorities about what is important to both members of the pair and to establish how to achieve the priorities. An infant benefits tremendously from a harmonious home and suffers little from spending a weekend with a reliable sitter or a relative. Grandparents usually thoroughly enjoy such opportunities to enjoy a grandchild alone. It is time after 8 months or a year for a couple to be enjoying sports and outside activities that a toddler can't keep up with. Again, parents need to know that finding time and a way to have privacy is problematic for all parents (unless they are able to have a housekeeper or other live-in help).

Mothering Doesn't Get Easier

The increased feelings of incompetency in the role indicate that mothering doesn't get easier. Other roles usually become easier with increased time in the role. Again, in an effort to reduce role strain, an honest up-front approach should stress the fact that caretaking tasks and challenges in mothering change with each developmental level of the child and that increased longevity in mothering does not make it easier; this is important information for new parents. Mothers tend to think problems are related to some personal inefficiency rather than to the child's developmental level. Each new developmental behavior introduces something new, even for mothers with several children, because each individual child's temperament and developmental rate are different. What works with one child may not make a dent in the response of another child.

In conveying the fact that motherhood does not get easier, the importance of continued self-development, self-renewal, and increased private moments with the mate are to be stressed as means of being able to cope with the new and exciting challenges.

Maternal Age Differences

The decreased gratification derived by teenagers from mothering emphasizes the importance of long-term follow-up with this group of women. Barnard and Eyres (1979) emphasized that the environmental context did not have an effect on the child's development until approximately 1 year. A teenager who has not been able to mature over the year is extremely unlikely to be able to enjoy a demanding, teasing infant who is trying to manipulate his mother. The teenagers' infants weighing more than older mothers' infants and not being handicapped in motor or social development might not continue over time if their emotional and social milieu does not continue to be supportive. As their mothers derive less gratification in the role, they may suffer.

Fewer teenagers were in school or were employed, compared with older women. Thus, their opportunity for self-development was decreased by comparison. The importance of self-concept and attitudes in mothering behaviors indicate that these young women warrant extensive help in fostering positive growth in both because they scored less favorably than older women in those areas.

The women who were 30 years and older more often seemed bothered by the time demands of the role and the isolation from adult activities that were imposed. This group of women is usually considered mature; thus, they have been largely ignored. The vignettes of Carrie, Cathryn, Cynthia, and Carmen are replete with the time demands and/or feelings of deprivation at 1 year. One cannot assume that older means either more mature or better able to manage.

Group 2 women, who were deriving greater gratification from motherhood, had infants who scored higher on social development. They were also more likely to report greater confidence in themselves as a result of mothering. A reciprocal effect may have been occurring through a transactional process, in which each affected the responses of the other, making it possible for this group of women to provide an optimal overall environment for their children.

CHAPTER 9

Changes in Maternal Role Behaviors over the Year

The pattern of maternal role behaviors has the potential of providing direction as to strategic times for intervention as well as content, based on the kinds of changes that occur over time. At 1, 4, 8, and 12 months, when mothers were interviewed, distinct changes were observed that represented phases in the process of maternal role attainment during the first year of motherhood.

PHASES IDENTIFIED DURING THE FIRST YEAR OF MOTHERHOOD

Gloger-Tippelt (1983) described a process model for the course of pregnancy in which adaptation occurred at biological, psychological, and social levels over four time periods: the *disruption phase,* from conception to 12 weeks; an *adaptation phase,* from weeks 12 to 20; a *centering phase,* from weeks 20 to 32; and the *anticipation and preparation phase,* from weeks 32 to birth. The disruption phase was described as a period of radical change on biological, psychological, and social levels. The adaptation phase was defined as a period of adjustment to the initial disruptions. The centering phase was defined as dominated by the central task of reproduction and production. The final anticipation and preparation phase was defined as the time of active preparation for the birth and life following birth.

Based on the research findings presented thus far, an analogous process model involving three levels of adaptation (biological, psychological, and social) is projected for the first year of motherhood. Adaptation to the maternal role also occurred at biological, psychological, and social levels, which were *interacting* and *interdependent*. The four time periods identified during the first year are as follows: *physical recovery phase,* from birth to 1 month; an *achievement phase,* from 2 to 4 or 5 months; a *disruption phase,* from 6 to 8 months; and a *reorganization phase* that begins after the eighth month and is in process at 12 months.

The *biological level* of adaptation is concerned with infant growth and development and the woman's physical recuperation and general health status. The *psychological level* focuses on the woman's perceptions and evaluations of her emotional reactions to motherhood. The *social level* of adaptation occurs within the social context and alterations of her life-style over the course of the first year of motherhood. The social level includes relationships with the partner, important persons in the family unit and friendship circle, and the broader social environment, such as job settings.

Physical Recovery Phase

During the *physical recovery phase* the biological level dominates the adaptation that occurs; the physiological demand on the mother at childbirth and her recuperation influences the adaptation that can occur on the psychological and social levels. The social support network readily acknowledges the biological demands on the woman during the physical recovery phase, and support is more readily available and forthcoming during the first 2 weeks of this phase than at later times. Mothers or other adult relatives frequently stay with the new mother and infant for 1 to 2 weeks following their return home from the hospital. Health is more closely supervised during this period, and the postpartum checkup along with the infant's first trip to the pediatrician generally occur toward the end of the physical recovery phase.

Physical recovery seems slow because of the constant interruptions in the mother's sleep and her high level of fatigue. Her infant's unpredictable schedule contributes to her fatigue and challenges her resources as she works hard at learning infant cues so that she can respond to the infant's needs.

Achievement Phase

During the *achievement phase,* the psychological and social levels appear dominant but are hindered if there are biological problems for either the mother or the infant. The achievement phase begins following physical recovery, around the second month, and extends through the fourth or fifth months, until the biological development of the infant propels him in action in which he begins to leave his mother for short distances. The achievement phase is characterized by a sense of accomplishment; the woman is skilled in caretaking and feels competent about caring for a young infant. On the biological level, the mother is feeling much better and is no longer as chronically fatigued as she was during the first month. On the social level, many mothers begin joining work forces so that additional roles increase the complexity and role strain in the mothering role. Most infants have settled into a predictable schedule so that coveted time for self can be planned. The socializing skills of the infant at 4 months, in which the spontaneous laughs and vocalizations are easily evoked, greatly increase the mother's pleasure in interacting with the infant.

Disruption Phase

The *disruption phase,* which begins from the fifth to the sixth months and seems to be at a peak at 8 months, is characterized by many changes in the woman's life at the social level. Strains occur in marital relationships as women try to balance mother, wife, and job roles. The infant's developmental changes at the biological level challenge the mother's newly gained competence and organization of the household, so that at the psychological level she once again doubts her capabilities as a "good mother" as she did earlier during the first month. The discontinuity in the level of caretaking skills needed at 8 months, along with other stressors, appears to be totally unexpected. The clash between the infant's evolving self (in the form of greater demands on the mother, clinging to her in unsure situations and willfully exploring, probing, and moving into hazardous situations) and the mother's own need to regain a sense of herself that resembles the prepregnancy period is central to this disruption.

Reorganization Phase

The *reorganization phase* that begins sometime after the eighth month and is evident at the twelfth month following birth is equally dominated by all of the levels; biological changes occur in the woman as she weans her infant and in her infant as he continues to explore and master his environment. At the psychological level the woman has become restless with the all-consuming nature of motherhood in which the responsibility for the infant weighs heavily and totally on her. She is desirous of being recognized as a feminine woman for roles other than the maternal. The diffuseness of boundary between herself and her infant is problematic, and maternal individuation from her infant becomes more evident as the woman feels pressed to regain her usual prepregnancy activities if she has not accomplished this earlier.

The comments of half of the women in the vignettes who were referring to their infants as "he/she" or "the baby," rather than calling a 1-year-old by name, raised questions. This indicates some lack of differentiation of the infant. Reorganization was not complete at 12 months, but this appeared to be the woman's major work.

PATTERNS OF MATERNAL ROLE BEHAVIORS OVER ADAPTATIONAL PHASES

Maternal role behavior was studied for change in pattern over time and whether age group patterns differed (Mercer, 1985a). Only women who completed measures at all test periods were studied for pattern change. A review of the major predictors helps to see which factors were more influential on maternal role behaviors at each specific adaptational phase.

Predictors varied to some extent because some variables were measured at different times and were not entered in predictive models until those times. Role strain, empathy, rigidity, maternal temperament, and infant temperament were not measured until the fourth month. Role strain was measured at each subsequent test period, but measures of the personality variables at 4 months were used for subsequent predictive models because they were considered to be stable characteristics of an individual. Cohler's maternal attitude scale with five major factors was not administered until 1 year. Prior to that time other measures of maternal attitudes were used (see Appendix).

Since maternal age was being tested as a major predictive variable, and the three age groups had differed significantly by race, educational level, and marital status, these three variables were controlled by forcing them into the regression models at the first step. *Maternal age* entered only *one* of the regression models as a predictor of maternal role behavior, with race, educational level, and marital status controlled during the entire year. Age predicted 1.8% of the variance in the growth factor at 4 months and entered the model negatively, i.e., the younger the woman, the greater the infant's growth and development.

Feelings of Love for the Infant

During the achievement phase at 4 months the women's feelings of love for their infants were significantly higher than at the physical recovery phase at 1 month, the disruption phase at 8 months, and the reorganization phase at 1 year. This pattern was the same for all age groups, and there were no significant differences in scores by age group.

Variables predicting feelings about the baby during the recovery phase at 1 month included the following: race, educational level, and marital status, 1%; child-rearing attitudes, 12.6%; infant-related stress, 8.7%; good life events the year prior to birth, 3.6%; and self-concept, 1.6%; a total of 27.5% accounted for.

At the achievement phase at 4 months predictive variables included the following: race, educational level, and marital status, 1.2%; infant-related stress, 13.4%; child-rearing attitudes, 4.8%; infant persistence, 3.6%; empathy, 2.7%; early mother–infant separation, 1.3%; self-concept, 1.2%; and informational support, 1%; a total of 29.2% predicted variance.

At the disruption phase at 8 months, feelings of love for the infant were less predictable than earlier, indicating that factors other than the variables tested were influencing the mothers' feelings about their infants. Predictive variables included the following: race, educational level, and marital status, 0.2%; personality disorder 8.1%; infant-related marital stress, 3.1%; sadistic maternal child-rearing attitudes, 2.4%; and role strain, 1.6%; a total of 15.4% of the variance described.

During the reorganization phase at 1 year, major predictors were as follows: race, educational level, and marital status, 0.0%; self-concept, 11.0%; empathy, 4.0%; infant-related stress, 2.7%; and stress from negative life events, 2.4%; a total of 20% of the variance accounted for.

During the physical recovery phase the woman's feelings about her baby are more influenced by her child-rearing attitudes and the extent of stress that she experiences from infant-related bothersome changes than at the achievement, disruption, and reorganization phases. Self-concept becomes increasingly important over time, and empathy remains consistently important in predicting how a woman feels about her infant. A woman's feelings of love for her infant were influenced little by race, educational level, or marital status during the first 4 months and not at all at 8 and 12 months.

Gratification in the Maternal Role

Gratification in the maternal role was significantly lower at 1 month, during the physical recovery phase, than it was at any of the later phases for the total sample. The pattern of maternal gratification behavior was similar for all age groups at 1 and 4 months but differed significantly after the disruption phase. Groups 1 and 2 experienced a slight decrease in gratification in the role at 8 months, whereas the older women in Group 3 experienced a very minimal increase. At the time of reorganization at 1 year, the teenage group reported a significant decrease in gratification in the role, whereas Group 2 reported an increase, and Group 3 remained the same.

Just over one-fifth of the variance in gratification in the role was predictable at the recovery phase. Major predictors of gratification in the maternal role at one month included the following: race, educational level, and marital status, 9.6%; good life events the year before birth, 7.8%; physical support from mate, 2.7%; and self-concept, 2.1%; a total of 22.2%.

At the achievement phase at 4 months major predictors were as follows: race, educational level, and marital status, 5.0%; empathy, 3.6%; rigidity, 3.0%; child-rearing attitudes, 3.3%; perception of birth experience, 1.6%; appraisal support, 1.4%; and maternal mood quality, 1.6%; a total of 19.5%.

At the disruption phase at 8 months major predictors were as follows: race, educational level, and marital status, 3.2%; role strain, 7.3%; physical support, 5.9%; infant-related marital stress, 3.4%; support network, 2.2%; and empathy 1.7%; a total of 23.7% predicted.

During the reorganization phase at 1 year very little of the variance in maternal gratification in mothering was accounted for (12%). Predictor variables were as follows: race, educational level, and marital status, 0.5%; good life events experienced during the first year of motherhood, 5%; maternal attitude factor of comfort in meeting the infant's needs, 4.1%; and empathy, 2.6%.

An important predictor of gratification at both the physical recovery and reorganization phases was good or positive life events, which contributed to gratification in the mothering role. At the physical recovery phase the positive life events experienced the year prior to birth had positive effects, and at the reorganization phase the positive life events experienced during the first year of motherhood had positive effects. The positive life events seem to serve as a type of support that probably enriches the individual's satisfaction with all roles that she is engaged in. At the disruption phase greater role strain decreased gratification and physical help received increased gratification as major predictors. As the infant moved into toddlerhood and more women were employed and experiencing high role strain, gratification in the maternal role was less predictable.

Higher education has consistently been associated with less gratification in the mothering role. When educational level no longer predicted gratification at 1 year, the maternal attitude factor of comfort in meeting the infant's needs was the second greatest predictor after positive life events. The older women who scored lower on gratification also were achievers who wished to do well in the role. Group 3's dedication in attending prenatal classes (92%) was greater than the younger women's, and their postponement of motherhood could be interpreted as waiting until the ideal time. Their commitment to achieving in the maternal role seemed great, and their gratification in a role may be tied to their comfort or feelings of achievement in a role. Comfort in the mothering role encompasses far more than a broader, more extensive educational background, however. Cohler's maternal attitude scale specifically taps the woman's ability to adapt to meeting the needs of the developing infant and to be comfortable with the infant's increasing assertiveness and sexuality. It is also possible that some women who have postponed motherhood have done so because of unresolved issues around their femininity and sexuality. Group 2 women who increased in gratification at 1 year were not as strongly committed to career roles and held different views about mothering.

Observed Maternal Competency Behavior

The pattern of observed maternal competency behaviors did not vary by age group, but all of the mean scores at 4, 8, and 12 months were significantly higher than scores during the physical recovery phase at 1 month. Means at 4 months were higher than the 12-month means, and 8-month means were higher than 12-month means (Mercer, 1985a). During the first year, observed maternal behavior peaked at the achievement phase and progressively declined at the disruption and reorganization phases. This discontinuity in maternal behavior, in which maternal caretaking skills for a 4-month-old were not appropriate for 8- and 12-month-olds, affected the women's psychological level of adaptation.

The forced variables of race, educational level, and marital status and perception of the birth experience were major predictors of maternal competency behavior at the recovery phase. Predictive variables at 1 month included the following: race, educational level, and marital status, 6.9%; perception of the birth experience, 6.6%; an easy infant, 3.6%; infant health status, 3.3%; child-rearing attitudes, 2.9%; self-concept, 2.1%; and physical mate support, 1.8%; a total of 27.2% accounted for.

At the achievement phase at 4 months many of the same variables were major predictors: race, educational level, and marital status, 13.9%; child-rearing attitudes, 8.0%; self-concept, 4.9%; infant-related stress, 1.5%; infant rhythmicity, 1.1%; maternal health status, 0.8%; and maternal adaptability, 0.9%; a total of 31.1%.

Unlike feelings of love for the infant or gratification in the role, maternal competency behaviors were *more* predictable at the disruption phase. At 8 months the major predictors of maternal competency behaviors were as follows: race, educational level, and marital status, 14.2%; role strain, 19.1%; low boiling point attitude, 4.4%; discipline attitudes, 2.8%; maternal adaptability, 2.1%; emotional support, 1.1%; infant home with mother from hospital, 1.1%; and network support, 0.9%; reaching a total of 45.7% of the variance accounted for.

During the reorganization phase at 1 year the predictive variables were as follows: race, educational level, and marital status, 16.0%; maternal attitude of reciprocity with infant factor, 13.5%; maternal health status, 8.5%; personality disorder, 4.6%; and the size of the support network, 1.3%. A total of 44% of the variance was accounted for.

During the physical recovery and achievement phases an easy infant and infant temperament were predictors of maternal behavior. The perception of the birth experience was a predictor at 1 month only, and this may have been related to recuperation from a cesarean birth; women who had a cesarean also perceived their birth experience less positively (see Chapter 3; Mercer et al., 1983). Some form of social support was predictive at all periods except at 4 months, the achievement phase.

The increased predictability of maternal competency behavior at the disruption and reorganization phases indicates that the woman's performance in the role is more easily predicted than the emotional components of her feelings about her infant or her satisfaction with the role. The forced variables of race and marital status became increasingly important predictors over the year. Being Caucasian and married were predictive of higher maternal competency behaviors. This could mean in part that the measure was biased toward Anglo-whites who made up the Caucasian group. As the child ages, parenting practices may become more culture-specific and varied.

Maternal attitudes from different measures consistently accounted for large portions of the variance in maternal behavior over the year. This supports the conclusion that a woman practices what she believes about child rearing.

The social level of maternal adaptation was more dysfunctional at 8 months. Role strain was the major predictor at the disruption phase. This finding provides additional information about this phase during which adaptation in all maternal role behaviors decreased significantly, and increasingly more women felt incompetent to deal with the infant's changing behavior. This social level of dysfunction, resulting in part from the biological level of infant adaptation, interacted with the mother's psychological adaptation so that she felt incompetent.

The importance of the women's health status to maternal role behavior was not anticipated at 1 year. Health status was the third major predictor at this time. However, this agrees with Rubin's (1984) thesis that early postpartum maternal behavior is influenced by the mother's body image, which includes her own bodily functioning. Realistically, maternal physical stamina is important to keep up with an active toddler.

Ways of Handling Irritating Child Behavior

The pattern of response over the year to self-reported ways of handling irritating child behaviors differed by age group after the disruptive phase at 8 months. All groups showed slightly more positive ways of handling irritating child behaviors from 1 to 8 months. (Ways of handling irritating child behavior was not measured at 4 months.) Group 3 reported handling irritating child behaviors somewhat more positively at the disruption and reorganization phases than at the biological recovery phase. Teenagers handled irritating behaviors less positively at 1 year than they had at either 1 or 8 months. Group 2 tended to handle irritating behaviors slightly less positively at 1 year than they had at 8 months. The more mature Group 3 was able to respond to the child in an increasingly more positive manner despite the stressors experienced at the disruption and reorganization phases.

Although ways of handling irritating child behavior became increasingly more predictable over the year, at 1 month only 10% of the variance could be accounted for. During the biological phase, race, educational level, and marital status accounted for 6% of the variance, and infant-related stress accounted for 3.8%. Being Caucasian and having more education were major predictors of more favorable ways of handling irritating child behavior; marital status was not significant when forced into the model.

At the disruption phase at 8 months, race, educational level, and marital status accounted for 12.1%, disciplinarian attitudes for 9.8%, and infant health status for 1.4%, for a total of 23.3% of the variance explained. Women who reported more strict disciplinarian attitudes handled irritating child behaviors more unfavorably, and infants with a better health status were responded to more positively.

During the reorganization phase at 1 year, one-third of the variance was predictable. Predictive variables were as follows: race, educational level, and marital status, 19.3%; appropriate control of the child's impulses attitude factor, 8%; size of the support network, 2.7%; self-concept, 2%; and closeness to the infant attitude factor, 1.6%.

Over the year, self-reported ways of handling irritating child behavior became increasingly more predictable. The forced variables of race, and educational level became increasingly important as predictors (marital status continued to enter the model at a nonsignificant level). During the physical recovery phase, infant-related stress aroused more unfavorable responses that were less predictable than at later times. The findings were consistent in that mothers' attitudes about discipline and control of the child's normal impulses were put into practice. These attitudes are learned within the woman's cultural or social group, which became an increasingly more important predictor.

Infant Growth

The infant's weight was plotted over the five test periods as an index of growth. The changes over time were significant, as was expected, and the increases at each test period were significant. Infancy is a period of rapid growth. Patterns of weight gain showed small but significant differences between the groups. This interaction is attributed to the teenagers' infants weighing significantly less at birth and having larger weight gains at 1 and 8 months (Mercer, Hackley, & Bostrom, 1984a).

During the physical recovery phase, 16.2% of the variance was predicted in the infant growth and development factor. The forced variables accounted for 6.1%; infant-related stress, 3%; stress from mothering, 4.1%; and informational support, 3%. Race was the only variable that was significant among the forced variables, and being non-Caucasian was associated with greater growth and development.

At 4 months 18.7% of the growth and development factor was predicted. Predictive variables included the following: race, educational level, and marital status, 4.4%; size of support network, 3.4%; physical support, 3.5%; maternal age 1.8%; child-rearing attitudes, 2.0%; informational support, 1.2%; maternal intensity, 1.3%; and emotional support, 1.1%.

During the disruption phase at 8 months, 13.4% of the growth and development factor was predictable. Major predictors included the following: race, educational level, and marital status, 0.5%; low boiling point attitude, 6.9%; maternal mood quality, 3.7%; and role strain 2.4%.

At 1 year 15% of the growth and development factor was predictable. Predictive variables included the following: race, educational level, and marital status, 4.5%; reciprocity with the infant attitude factor, 5.6%; maternal temperament factor, 2.3%; and negative or bad life events experienced the first year of motherhood, 2.3%.

The predictability of the infant's growth and development was consistently from 13% to 19% over time. Stress experienced by the mother was a major predictor of the infant's growth and development at 1 month during the physical recovery phase. Social support (size of the network, physical help, informational and emotional support) was a major predictor of the infant's growth and development during the achievement phase at 4 months.

Maternal attitudes assumed importance at 8 and 12 months as predictors of the infant's growth and development, along with maternal temperament. Importantly, maternal role strain interacted with the infant's growth and development at 8 months. The negative life events experienced during the first year of motherhood interacted with infant growth and development at 1 year but in the opposite direction than would be expected. Greater stress from negative events was associated with greater growth. The question is raised as to whether, when negative events occur, the mother refocuses her energy on her infant as a kind of safe and successful haven; the infant is one area in which she can receive positive feedback.

DISCUSSION AND IMPLICATIONS FOR NURSING INTERVENTION

Social support variables, maternal attitudes, self-concept, empathy, race, and infant-related stress emerged as variables that were consistently predictive of maternal role attainment variables over all four phases of motherhood the first year. Others have emphasized the importance of maternal attitudes toward child care in directly affecting the child's socialization (Cohler & Grunebaum, 1981); a mother's attitudes influence how she views transactions between herself and her child and determine her range of responses. Cohler and associates (1976) also observed that among both well and mentally ill mothers' less adaptive child-care attitudes were related to greater impairment in adaptation to other adult roles.

Although teenagers scored less favorably on maternal caretaking behaviors, their infants scored well on the growth and development factor. Although they were more rigid than older mothers and scored as less adaptive on maternal attitude factors of appropriate control of the child's impulses, encouragement of reciprocity, and acceptance of the emotional complexity of child rearing (see Chapter 2), their infants did not suffer developmentally. This finding agrees with others who observed that teenagers' infants' motor development was positively related to high authoritarian attitudes at 12 months (Camp, Burgess, Morgan, & Malpiede, 1984). Camp and associates postulated high authoritarian attitudes, and the resulting parenting practices may be a strength the first year but become increasingly maladaptive as the child matures. Alternative explanations for Group 1 infants' higher scores may relate to that group's higher proportion of non-Caucasian mothers, and /or different child-rearing practices. Walters (1967) observed that black infants achieved higher motor development than white infants at 12, 24, and 36 weeks as measured on Gesell developmental schedules. A higher proportion of Group 1 was black (41%), compared with Group 2 (12%) or Group 3 (2%).

Critical Periods for Nursing Intervention

Pregnancy One major period for intervention is during the anticipation and preparation phase of pregnancy. Preparing women realistically for expectations during labor and delivery can help avoid disappointment and consequently self-blame during this pivotal period. Childbirth as the formal transition to motherhood is a critical time with long-term effects.

Grossman and associates (1980) concluded that it is a myth that women can expect a problem-free delivery; 55% of the 87 women (43 primigravidas, 44 multigravidas) in their study experienced complications. Entwisle and Doering (1981) reported a 16.7% cesarean birth rate among 120 primigravidas, with only one anticipated, and an additional 12% experienced a variety of serious complications. Fifty percent of the women in this study experienced some complication during labor and delivery. Only 58% had spontaneous vaginal deliveries without any medical intervention; 19% had cesarean births. Thus, it appears that an unexpected event, whether it is a prolonged acceleration phase, second stage of labor, or a perineal laceration, will occur in approximately half of all childbirths.

Labor and Delivery A second period of intervention is during admission to the labor and delivery suite, during labor and delivery, and immediately postpartum. A woman's anxiety is high when she first enters the hospital, and first impressions and how she is treated at this time set the tone for her trust and comfort with staff later.

Staffing of labor and delivery units is very important. Frequently, fewer persons are on night and weekend shifts, so "float" personnel may be sent to those areas when admissions are high. Sensitive staff who enjoy their work will be more involved in keeping women informed during the labor and delivery experience, as well as involved in providing comfort measures and assuring privacy. A routine catheterization is humiliating if the patient is lying naked and is strapped to an operating room table with an audience of physicians and nurses; a woman from Group 2 was still upset by this event at

1 year. In contrast, Bonnie was pleased that "everyone kept saying I was so brave" during what she described as a 6-day labor.

Entwisle and Doering (1981) reported that birth variables (level of awareness or preparation and the quality of the birth experience) appeared more critical to middle-class women's mothering responses. Among lower-class women, breast-feeding and postpartum events played a critical role in predicting mothering, and the birth event had only an indirect effect. They suggested that the closeness of mother to infant during breast-feeding increased their responsiveness to their infants. Comments made by breast-feeding mothers in this study suggest that emotional symbiosis may have been heightened and maternal individuation was more difficult for those who were breast-feeding. Middle-class women may expect more of themselves or of the system than do lower-class mothers. Clarification of expectations, along with presenting realistic events that may occur unexpectedly, are important counseling goals.

Postpartum Hospitalization   Care during the postpartum hospitalization is a third period of important intervention. Unfortunately, women are staying in the hospital for shorter periods, so teaching and counseling time is much shorter. Both the first-time mother and father need all of the counseling about what to expect when they go home that is possible. It is important that they have the phone number of the postpartum unit so that they can call anytime night or day to ask questions of concern. Counseling about the impact of the infant on their life-style and the accompanying infant-related stress is important for both parents. The importance of help from family and friends cannot be overstressed.

Physical Recovery Phase   Ideally, each new mother should have a home visit by a nurse within the first week after discharge from the hospital. Since this service is not possible for all new mothers, part of postpartum follow-up should include telephone calls from a nurse on the postpartum unit who cared for the mother during her hospitalization. This would give the new mother an opportunity to talk with someone who knows her and with whom she feels some comfort in discussing any personal, physical, or emotional problems.

Early discharge programs (mothers and infants leave the hospital within a few hours following birth) often have a nurse visit to examine both mother and infant. This is important because new parents may not detect developing jaundice in their infants early, or may not note the mother's physical problems such as hematomas along episiotomies or developing infections.

The mother's fatigue from lack of sleep and rest during this period can be alleviated only by another person assuming responsibility for the household and helping with infant care. All women should be encouraged to seek out compatible adults who can provide physical help during this period.

Achievement Phase A fifth but almost nonexistent intervention period is around the fourth month following birth. Women need to be counseled about the importance of going for physical examinations if they are continuing to feel fatigued or highly stressed and are having physical problems. Pediatric nurse practitioners and pediatricians are in an excellent position to detect the need for and to direct mothers to appropriate places for health care.

At the achievement phase, mothers also benefit if taught about infant growth and development, how to childproof their homes for the infant's safety, and how to plan to have private time with their mates. Grossman and associates (1980) reported that most couples experienced a strain on their marriage during the first year. Active communication and seeking-out time to spend in couple activities has to be conscious because spontaneity goes out the window with an infant's birth. Increased awareness of this problem can lead to more concerted effort to seek assistance and to work toward alleviating strain as much as is possible.

Lists of excellent, licensed day-care centers, reputable babysitters, telephone hotline numbers, and available parenting classes are important resources for new mothers. Mothers who will be going back to work will benefit from counseling to help them sort out realistic goals for what they can and cannot do in each of the multiple roles as wife, mother, and employee.

Disruption Phase A sixth intervention period is around the eighth month, during the disruption phase. Both the physical and mental health status of the woman should be assessed; if she has not seen a physician since her postpartum checkup, it is a good idea for her to see a physician at this time. Almost two-thirds of the women reported a minor health problem at this time.

Reorganization Phase During the second half of the first year women need to be encouraged to pursue self-enrichment activities that are pleasurable for them. Further counseling regarding her priorities for herself as a person, as well as in relation to her many roles, is important. She will be able to foster her infant's separation-individuation process if she becomes clearer about her own boundaries and regains a sense of self equivalent to or surpassing the pre-pregnancy self.

Parenting groups may offer a special source of support to women or may be "one more thing" to do. Sources for learning about the child's growth and development through toddlerhood are important. Mothers need to be prepared for the toddler's newly learned word, "No," and to learn signs of readiness for toilet and other training.

SUMMARY

Data from this study supported the theory that there are four phases occurring in the process of adaptation to the maternal role over the first year following birth—the physical recovery phase during the first 1 to 2 months, the achievement phase at 4 months, a disruption phase at 6 to 8 months, and a reorganization phase after the eighth month, which is still in process at 1 year.

Three levels of adaptation—biological, psychological, and social—are interacting and interdependent throughout these phases. A problem in one level affects performance or adaptation at the other two levels.

Patterns of maternal responses did not differ by maternal age over the year for feelings of love for the infant and observer-rated maternal competency behaviors. The greatest divergence in maternal age patterns occurred at the disruption and reorganization phases in gratification in mothering and ways of handling irritating child behaviors. In both of these situations, Group 3 remained more consistent in their responses, indicating that they handled the disequilibrium between the social, biological, and psychological levels of adaptation differently.

The emotional components of maternal role attainment—feelings of love for the infant and gratification in the maternal role—become less predictable at the disruption and reorganization phases, whereas the care-taking components—maternal competency behaviors and ways of handling irritating child behaviors—become more predictable at these periods of disequilibrium. The predictability of infant growth and development was consistently low.

CHAPTER 10

Maternal Age Differences Reconsidered

An interaction between biological, psychological, and social levels of adaptation were observed consistently among mothers of all ages over the first year of motherhood. Problems encountered on one level affected adaptation on other levels. Maternal and infant health status and infant growth and development at the biological level both reflected and affected the mother's perceptions and evaluations of her emotional reactions to motherhood. Social support and role strain affected both maternal health status, infant growth and development, and mothers' perceptions and evaluations. Infant-related alterations in women's life-styles affected other areas of social adaptation as well as biological and psychological levels of adaptation.

Different levels of adaptation were more dominant during the four different phases in the first year of motherhood. The biological level of adaptation manifested in part by pervasive fatigue, along with the social support available, dominated the *physical recovery phase.* The psychological and social levels were dominant at the *achievement phase,* which had probably peaked at 4 months. Social and biological levels both dominated at the *disruption phase,* when the majority of the women were employed and the infant's developmental changes challenged the mothers' newly gained competence in mothering a neonate and younger infant, affecting the psychological level by lowered self-evaluations. During the *reorganization phase,* all levels of adaptation seemed about equally dominant.

PREGNANCY AND THE FIRST YEAR
OF MOTHERHOOD

Pregnancy and Birth

Major concerns reported by this sample of women (all ages) during
pregnancy were their body image and feelings of vulnerability.
Women described themselves as ugly or fat, or in general less attractive during pregnancy, and often described their pregnancies in terms
of how many pounds they had gained. The last 2 to 6 weeks of
pregnancy were particularly uncomfortable and restrictive. Feelings
of vulnerability during pregnancy included anxieties about their
infant's size or normality. Previous stillbirths or miscarriages or the
death of family members or friends seemed to increase their feelings
of vulnerability. The concern about body image continued for a
few during the first year of motherhood as they struggled with losing
large weight gains of 50 lb or more.

Fetal movement was first felt around 4 months, with some women
reporting feeling movement as early as 2 months (2%) and others
as late as 6 (3%), 7 (1%), and 8 (1%) months. Most described their
first recognized fetal movements as exciting and making them
realize that a baby was really there. Only 2% of the women said they
had no feelings about this first experience of fetal movement.

Perhaps because of feelings of unattractiveness and vulnerability,
a woman tends to close her world around herself during pregnancy
and to participate in fewer social activities. During labor her world
becomes increasingly narrow as she focuses only on the present and
her imminent needs (Rich, 1973).

The women's labor averaged 13 to 13½ hr, although many had
prodromal labor for some time, and this prodromal labor was not included in the hospital record as actual labor. Short labors less than 3
hr in length tended to scare the women; the frequent, hard contractions began early, and events accelerated so rapidly that they were
unable ever to achieve control.

Following birth, the woman gradually expands her interactions
with the social world. The struggle to get back into the world of
adults and stimulating activities continued throughout the year.
The inability to go out as desired, the increased responsibility of the
infant, and the change in routines all added to their difficulty in regaining admission to their prepregnancy world. This was true for all
women, regardless of maternal age.

Expected and Unexpected Influences on Maternal Role Attainment

Religious Influence Catholics in groups 2 and 3 tended to report greater gratification in the maternal role than non-Catholics ($r =$ .20 and .23), but no significant relationships were observed for maternal behavior, feelings of love for the baby, ways of handling irritating child behaviors, or infant growth and development. Catholics were the largest religious group represented (42%), with 26% reporting no preference, 16% Protestant, 3% Jewish, and 13% other religions. The high value placed on motherhood and the discouragement of contraceptive use by the Catholic church may have been a socializing force that added to women's gratification in the mothering role; motherhood as a highly valued social role increased the women's sense of satisfaction in achieving it.

Slesinger (1981) reported that church attendance was consistently related to good mothering among the low-income women in her study. She postulated two reasons for this finding. Church ties are one type of social bond to social networks outside the family, and church attenders have been identified as financially better off than nonattenders.

Mother's Personality Versus Infant Temperament A woman's mothering was largely influenced by her personality profile (self-concept, empathy, flexibility, low intensity) rather than by her infant's temperament. The infant's growth and development were not predicted by either. During the first year infant temperament may not play as large a role in mothering responses as it does when the child is older. A less stressful infant was associated with higher feelings of maternal love; thus, it may take longer than a year for the decreased emotional investment by the mother to show its fullest impact.

Fatigue Fatigue was high during the first postpartum month, and both physical problems and postpartum blues were experienced well beyond the usual puerperium of 4 to 6 weeks. There was an engulfing feeling that "the baby takes over your whole life," and overall women never had enough time. Talking to other mothers was very reassuring and helpful to the women. Only other women who had children within a couple of years of the ages of their own "could understand how it is" and "offer relevant suggestions."

Infant Care Infant crying was very disturbing to the women, although they realized that this was the infant's way of communicating special needs. However, crying heightened concern and anxiety about whether they could determine the need.

The average feeding time for an infant was 25 to 30 min. Mothers who were breast-feeding reported that they often spent an hour in changing, nursing, and getting the infant back to bed; this recurred every 3 hr the first couple of months and contributed to sleep deprivation.

Although many thought it couldn't happen to them, disagreement with their husbands or mates about how a child should be disciplined was quite common. Most were comfortable with their communication with their mates, however, and worked at reaching agreement.

Uniqueness of Support from Mate As in other research, a good relationship with the mate buoyed the women's feelings about motherhood and the infant. Unmarried women became concerned toward the end of the first year about support systems and lack of a partner to help with the toddler. Although mates provided physical help with the infant and with finances, emotional support appeared to be the key variable they supplied. In the teenagers' support network, made up predominantly of mothers or adult women, informational support was highest. In the older women's network, in which mate support was higher, emotional support was highest. Other women provide valuable information for the role of mothering, but mates provide the reassurance and personal valuing to the woman that seems to be central. Intimate support by mates influences mothers' attitudes, satisfaction with parenting, and positive mother–infant interactions (Crnic, Greenberg, Ragozin, Robinson, & Basham, 1983; Crnic et al., 1984).

Difficult Disruption Phase The disruption phase occurring from 6 to 8 months following the infant's birth is a rough time for all women. The majority are fulfilling employment roles in addition to the maternal role, and the mobile infant requires an entirely new repertoire of mothering skills. In addition, many small and annoying maternal health problems continue, which may be exacerbated by the increased responsibility at this time. Self-concept was lower at 8 months than at early postpartum. This has important implications because self-concept was the major predictor of the maternal role attainment index at 1 year.

Maternal Individuation The struggle for getting back into the mainstream of activities continued throughout the year, and women who had accepted the confinement and intense relationship between mother and infant during the early months became impatient with the impositions posed by this intense relationship at 1 year. This process was labeled maternal individuation because of its parallel to the infant's individuation, and the intense undertone of regaining an identity apart from that of "mother."

However, despite the ups and downs of motherhood, having a second child became more attractive during the first year. Over half of the women said they wanted one or two more children during the early postpartum period; one fourth weren't sure. By the end of the first year of motherhood, two-thirds wanted at least one more child.

MOTHERHOOD'S CONTRIBUTION TO ADULT DEVELOPMENT

Motherhood is commonly referred to as a developmental phase for women. The women viewed motherhood as both transition to adulthood and admission to a new social status. The word that was repeated over and over by the women to describe their personal development that was equated with adulthood was their ability to assume "responsibility." This ability to assume responsibility was equated with adulthood regardless of maternal age. When the women described the reestablishment of priorities in their lives, the priorities always related to the "responsibility" for a helpless infant.

The newly assumed responsibility for another human being was an entirely new experience that weighed heavily on them. This new responsibility was inescapable, and persisted 24 hr a day, even when the infant was spending a weekend with grandparents. However, this new responsibility also commanded a higher, more valued status. In general, first-time mothers perceived that family members viewed them differently and made fewer demands on their time since they became parents. In this sense, an adolescent mother who is elevated to a new status by her family would find the new role highly gratifying.

This facet of personal development that occurred with motherhood came from the women's lived experiences, in which they perceived the transition to adulthood as the assumption of responsibility for another human being. This viewpoint of development is quite different from the intrapsychic perspective of development in which old traumas may be resolved resulting in a more highly integrated personality. The implication is that in the cultural context studied adulthood is reached when an individual proves to be a responsible person. Assuming responsibility for another individual is one very visible and accepted way of demonstrating this developmental change. Motherhood is one role in which this type of responsibility is assumed, and it is one of the most difficult because the duration is longer, never ceases, and it is so central to the individual's self-esteem as well as the child's outcome and survival.

MATERNAL AGE AND MATERNAL ROLE ATTAINMENT

Maternal age was not a predictor of maternal role attainment when race, educational level, and marital status were controlled. Maternal age was a predictor for one of the role-attainment variables, infant growth and development at the 4-month test period, and the prediction was opposite from the expected direction. The younger the woman, the more likely her infant was to score higher on growth and development. However, when the variables predicting maternal role attainment are examined, the majority of teenagers were at a disadvantage. These less advantageous scores on predictor variables are in part a result of both the teenager's level of development and her social context. Slesinger (1981) found that poor socioeconomic conditions were the most important factor related to the woman's mothering ability and the health of her child. Teenagers who had the lowest annual income during the first year of motherhood also had the lowest self-concept, which in turn was the major predictor of the maternal role attainment index at 1 year. Thus, the question posed in Chapter 1 as to whether the problems of teenage motherhood relate to psychosocial deficits rather than maternal age per se can be answered affirmatively.

Dysfunctional parenting has been associated with both separation from parents at an early age and with being a victim of child abuse. Correlations of these two variables with maternal role attainment behaviors were significant in only two instances. Separation from parents before the age of 12 was significantly correlated with less gratification in the maternal role among the teenage group. Women in Group 3 who indicated that they or their sibling had been abused as children tended to score as less adaptive in maternal behavior. A

33-year-old mother illustrated this at 1 year: "I was a battered child —closet child. The hardest thing for me is discipline, and in resolving my own childhood trauma. I don't find motherhood easy; it is a constant struggle." The potential for the kind of intrapsychic development described by Benedek (1959) is high for this mother; when she resolves the issues around her own childhood trauma and discipline of her child, she can achieve a higher level of personality integration.

In order to focus more specifically on maternal age differences, assets and vulnerabilities for assuming the maternal role that were identified by this research are highlighted. Each of the groups enjoyed specific advantages and experienced certain disadvantages. However, Group 2 emerged as having greater advantages and fewer disadvantages.

ASSETS AND VULNERABILITIES THE FIRST YEAR OF MOTHERHOOD

In discussing assets and vulnerabilities by maternal age group, the reader is reminded that the 15- to 19-year-old group of women in this study were *not* incompetent mothers, although some of their maternal role attainment scores were lower and their attitudes were less positive. Rather, the findings should be viewed from the perspective that teenagers were more handicapped in some areas for fulfilling the very complex mothering role; thus, they scored at a lower level of adaptation on the continuum of maternal role behaviors.

Developmentally, the older the age group, the greater their personality integration and their flexibility (see Chapter 2); this finding indicates that these two variables are developmental constructs. Others have found that a personal integration construct was the best discriminator of mothering behaviors both prenatally and at 3 months (Brunnquell, Crichton, & Egeland, 1981). Breen (1975) also reported that women who adjusted more easily to childbearing were more differentiated and were more open in their self-appraisals.

Personality traits that did not change significantly after the teenage years included self-concept, empathy, and the innate temperament traits of high adaptability, low intensity, and positive mood state. Differences were observed in the traits of persistence and distractibility but did not increase or decrease by maternal age. For example, Group 2 was significantly more persistent than the teenagers, whereas Group 3 scored lower than Group 2 but higher

than Group 1. Group 3 was significantly more distractible than
Group 2 but not Group 1. No significant differences were observed
in temperament traits of activity level, rhythmicity, approach-
withdrawal, or threshold to stimulus. The maternal temperament
traits that were predictive of maternal role behaviors were higher
adaptability, lower intensity, and higher or more positive quality
of mood.

Child-rearing attitudes are learned from the cultural context
and vary considerably from one cultural context to another. Further,
the individual's cognitive level of functioning and educational level
also affect attitudes and beliefs. Because adolescence is the period in
which movement from the concrete thinking of childhood evolves
into the ability to conceptualize and view the world more abstractly,
the younger women in Group 1 were less likely to be as facile with
abstract conceptual thought or to have the ability to plan ahead for
the future as the older women. Further, almost half (42%) of the
teenagers had not completed high school; the additional education
the older groups of women had in college and graduate school
had exposed them to a wider range of views and thoughts to expand
their attitudes.

Group 1: 15- to 19-Year-Olds

Assets During pregnancy teenagers reported they thought more
often about having a boy, and in reality they more often had a boy.
Thus, they had fewer adaptations to make in expectations of infant
gender. Teenagers downplayed emotional changes during pregnancy; it is curious whether emotional changes of pregnancy were similar to usual anxieties and emotional changes experienced during
adolescence and not recognized. Their pregnancies tended to be
approximately half a week shorter; going past the due date dampens
perception of the birth experience and contributes to depression
(Entwisle & Doering, 1981). Group 1 labors also began spontaneously (as opposed to induction) more often than those of older women.
The teenager in this population had a normal birth without the
medical intervention of forceps or a cesarean more often than did
older cohorts. This finding supports Merritt et al. (1980) who report
that from a medical viewpoint, 16 to 19 is an optimal time to give
birth.

The lack of time and hectic atmosphere of the first few days home
from the hospital were not as overwhelming to teenagers. Teenagers'

recuperation appeared to progress more smoothly, and they complained of fatigue and depression less often during the first month. Older women were three times more likely to be depressed during their first month postpartum. The teenagers' infants were scored as significantly easier infants at 1 month than the older women's infants. More teenagers had help from their mothers, and this may have contributed to their smoother first month of motherhood. Help from an *experienced mothering person* may be important in reducing fatigue and depression during the first postpartum month. However, the teenager may also use some denial in regard to emotional feelings such as feeling depressed, so this finding merits further study.

Teenagers had more help from their mothers during the entire first year than did older women. Help from mothers tended to be perceived as physical and financial help with the infant and informational help about infant care more than emotional support. At 4 months teenagers reported that they had as much help as or more than they needed more often than did older women.

Motherhood was an important role for these young women. Their gratification in mothering scores was higher than that of other age groups during the first 8 months. During this period their infants surpassed those of older women in areas of physical growth and social or motor development. However, motherhood did not increase Group 1's self-confidence, but it increased their feelings of being more responsible persons as individuals. As was discussed above, all women described a new status as a mother, in which family members respected them more, and that may have been a factor in teenagers' early gratification.

Teenagers were engrossed in and amazed at the rapid growth and development of the infant during the first year. They reported this amazement and pleasure as one of the most unexpected events of motherhood more often than did older women.

Despite Group 1's less adaptable child-rearing attitudes, their infants gained more weight than older women's infants at 1 and 8 months, and their infants weighed more at 1 year. Group 1 infants were more advanced in social and motor development and scored higher on the growth and development factor at 4 months. There are several explanations for this finding. Camp and associates (1984) suggested that high authoritarian attitudes and the parenting practices that result from these attitudes may be a strength the first year of life but become increasingly maladaptive as the child ages. Barnard and Eyres (1979) reported that mothers' psychosocial assets did not begin to have an impact on mother–infant interactions until 8 and 12 months. Another factor may have been the teenagers' feelings of satisfaction and gratification in mothering that conveyed a different emotional climate for the infant.

An alternative hypothesis is that an infant profits from polymatric mothering. Caldwell and associates (1963) studied monomatric (mothering provided by one person) and polymatric (mothering provided by more than one person) families, and their findings do not support this hypothesis. Infants in monomatric families were more dependent on their mothers at 1 year. No significant developmental differences were observed on the Cattell Infant Intelligence or Griffiths Mental Development Scale, although infants from monomatric families scored higher. Thus, type of mothering did not contribute to the infant's level of mental functioning. Monomatric women were more *self-confident* at 6 months; they were more personally involved than intellectually committed to mothering activities and were more dependent on their infants at 1 year. More differences were observed the first half than the last half of the first year, suggesting that differences from type of mothering may diminish as the child ages.

A similar explanation for Group 1 infants' greater weight gain is that their diets were different. Group 1 fed solid foods earlier on their mothers' advice that this practice would help infants to sleep through the night. Although the infants did not sleep through the night earlier, they did gain more weight. In addition, fewer Group 1 infants were breast-fed than other infants; 62% of the teenagers began breast-feeding, 34% continued at 1 month, 21% at 4 months, 16% at 8 months, and 5% at 1 year. Group 2 had 82% begin breast-feeding, with 23% continuing at 1 year; Group 3 had 93% begin, with 28% continuing at 1 year.

The resiliency of the more youthful body in recuperating from an uncomplicated childbirth cannot be denied. The youthful mother's more patent circulatory system appears to be a decided perinatal advantage; analysis of data from 44,386 pregnancies found that perinatal mortality rates increased progressively from 25/1,000 at 17 to 19 years to 69/1,000 after 39 years, due in part to uteroplacental hypoperfusion, placental infarcts, and placental growth retardation (Naeye, 1983). Sclerotic lesions in the myometrial arteries were suggested as a possible cause; these lesions increased from 11% at 17 to 19 years to 83% after 39 years.

This sample of teenagers had access to special programs of prenatal care, and the early adolescent under the age of 15 years, who is at greater psychosocial and physical risks, was not represented. Late prenatal care, smaller maternal stature, and less weight gain during pregnancy have been associated with perinatal complications (Garn & Petzold, 1983; Garn, LaVelle, Pesick, & Ridella, 1984; Lawrence & Merritt, 1981). Also, 61% of the teenagers had delivered at a university hospital that provided a special clinic for teenage mothers in which nurse clinicians, a nutritionist, and social workers provided antepartum care (Neeson, Patterson, Mercer, & May, 1983). Teenagers cared for in this special clinic had significantly more spontaneous deliveries and infants who were average for gestational age than did either teenagers or 20- to 25-year-olds who received care in the general clinic. Their infants were admitted to the intensive care nursery less often than infants in the other two groups.

Vulnerabilities Teenagers were at the lower end of the continuum of personality traits and developmental constructs that were predictive of maternal role behaviors for the entire sample of women over the year—flexibility, personality integration, personality disorder, self-concept, empathy, and temperament traits of adaptability, positive mood quality, and lower intensity. Maternal rigidity was predictive of gratification in the role at 8 months. Personality disorder was predictive of feelings of love for the infant at 8 months and observed maternal behavior at 1 year. Self-concept was predictive of gratification in the role at one month; feelings of love for the infant at 1, 4, and 12 months; observed maternal behavior at 1 and 4 months; and maternal role attainment index and ways of handling irritating child behavior at 12 months. Empathy was predictive of gratification at 4, 8, and 12 months, and of feelings of love for the infant at 4 and 12 months. The temperament trait of a positive mood was predictive of gratification at 4 months. Maternal adaptability was predictive of maternal behavior at 4 and 8 months. Maternal intensity was predictive of infant growth and development at 4 months, and a factor of maternal temperament was predictive of infant growth and development at 12 months.

Fewer teenagers reported having friends visit them in their homes than did older women. Fewer teenagers also reported having someone living in the area that they could call on for any kind of help, which indicated their somewhat greater sense of isolation. Peer groups are important during adolescence in providing social groups to try out new ideas and to practice gender roles. Nonpregnant teenagers participated in sports and other extracurricular activities more often, had more hobbies, and viewed television less than a group of pregnant teenagers (Curtis, 1974). The greater social isolation could have been a predisposing factor to Group 1's pregnancies.

Teenagers were less ready for their pregnancies, as indicated by the greater likelihood of hoping they weren't, being less proud and more worried, and feeling that the pregnancy was not as planned or at a good time. Although their births were more often normal, with fewer medical interventions, Group 1 perceived their childbirth experience less positively. Teenagers reported that they were scared during the childbirth experience more often than did the older women.

Following birth during the hospitalization, teenagers less often described their infants in terms of unique characteristics or identified features as resembling a family member. When comparing her birth experience to her mother's, she viewed her own experience as less satisfying.

Group 1 infants weighed less at birth than infants in groups 2 and 3. Group 1 infants also experienced more illnesses the first month following birth than infants in older groups. However, there were no significant differences in infant health status after that time.

At the disruption phase at 8 months, teenagers reported a significantly less optimal health status than older women. They also expressed more concern about their future security and reported greater financial stress. Their emotional support had decreased from 4 months and was less than that of older women. This was a particularly difficult period for Group 1, and this difficulty may have contributed to their decreasing gratification in mothering.

Teenagers' child-rearing attitudes were also consistently at the lower end of the continuum of scores. Perinatal attitudes—made up of a factor including use of a family-centered program, choosing to breast-feed, attending prenatal class, and knowledge of infant competencies—were lower than those of older women. Although there were no significant age group differences for low-boiling-point attitudes, teenagers were more likely to exhibit role-reversal attitudes and use harsh or unusual punishment (sadistic), and they were less likely to consider the child's needs and feelings in defining acceptable child behavior (strict disciplinarian).

Although there were no differences in maternal attitude factors on two maternal tasks based on specific developmental levels of the infant–toddler, there were differences on three of the attitude factors. No age differences were observed in appropriate versus inappropriate closeness (attains gratification missing in her life through the infant or views the infant as a narcissistic extension of self) and comfort versus discomfort in perceiving and meeting the infant's physical needs (mother understands what the infant wants and provides the needs). Teenagers were *less likely* to have attitudes that children's impulses can be channeled into socially appropriate behaviors, to acknowledge or respond to the infant's ability to communicate and seek social interaction with the mother, and to acknowledge that mothers do not always know best or motherhood is sometimes more work than pleasure.

During hospitalization perinatal attitudes were predictive of perception of the neonate. At 1 month a factor made up of low boiling point, sadistic, and strict disciplinarian attitudes was predictive of feelings of love for the infant, identification of the infant, and observed maternal behavior. At 4 months the same factor was predictive of gratification, feelings about the baby, and observed maternal behavior. At 8 months sadistic attitudes were predictive of feelings about the baby. Low boiling point and strict disciplinarian attitudes were predictive of observer-rated maternal behavior, and disciplinarian attitudes were predictive of self-reported ways of handling irritating child behaviors. Low-boiling-point attitudes were predictive of infant growth and development.

At 12 months the attitude factor of reciprocity was a predictor of maternal behavior, infant growth and development, and the maternal role attainment index factor. The factor, appropriate control of the child's impulses, was a predictor of ways of handling irritating child behaviors and the maternal role attainment index. Thus, maternal attitudes were translated into maternal child-rearing practices.

At 1 year emotional support was significantly related to the teenager's child-rearing attitudes of control of the child's aggressive responses ($r = .44$), encouragement of reciprocity ($r = .56$), and appropriate closeness or not seeing the infant as a narcissistic extension of self ($r = .33$) and to observer-rated maternal behavior ($r = .37$) and self-reported ways of handling irritating child behaviors ($r = -.37$) (Mercer et al., 1984b). These attitudes were strongly correlated with maternal behaviors. A more adaptive response to control of the child's aggressive responses was associated with the teenager handling irritating child behaviors more positively ($r = .62$). More adaptive encouragement of reciprocity was positively related to observed maternal behavior ($r = .46$), feelings of love, ($r = .32$), and ways of handling irritating child behavior ($r = .49$). Thus, emotional support had both direct and indirect effects on the teenager's maternal role behaviors, and teenagers were handicapped by having less emotional support as well as less adaptive attitudes than older mothers.

Differences in conception of what good mothering includes could indicate something of the younger woman's focus or priority. Group 1 stated that a good mother kept her baby clean and dressed the baby appropriately more often than did older women. They less often stated that a good mother teaches the infant, respects the infant's individuality, and takes care of herself. Teenagers more often than older women described a good baby as one who doesn't cry much and is playful. During the achievement phase, when describing the most rewarding thing about motherhood, teenagers reported more often than older women having someone who wouldn't leave them, someone to keep them company, something all their own, or someone to play with (25%, 8%, and 7%).[1] This comment may in part be related to their report of having peers visit them in their homes less often and may indicate their greater social isolation.

Teenagers less often read books or magazines to help them with child care. Fewer reported taking the infant on outings at 1 year. More reported using physical discipline and fewer reported using distraction to divert their infants from something they wanted but couldn't have.

When teenagers compared how they disciplined their children with how their mothers disciplined them, they said that they used more physical punishment than their mother had and less often punished their infant the same as their mothers, more often than older women.

Teenagers scored lower in observed maternal behaviors and in their self-reported ways of handling irritating child behaviors over the entire year. Their interactions with their infants were more rigid and stricter, with more physical punishment than those of older women. In response to how they coped with difficult times with the infant, they more often said they ignored the infant (25%, 5%, and 12%) and stated that they bit or slapped the infant back when the infant bit or slapped (13%, 3%, and 2%). They less often stated that they planned or adjusted their time as a coping strategy. These behaviors can be related in part to less experience with abstract conceptualizations, less experience in general, and less education, all of which influenced their attitudes.

Teenagers also reported higher stress from negative life events experienced during the first year of motherhood, compared with

---

[1] Series of three figures in parentheses indicate percentages for the three groups from the youngest to the oldest, respectively.

older women. This stress in turn was a predictor of the maternal role index, feelings of love for the infant, and infant growth and development at 1 year.

More of Group 1 than older women were separated from their parents before the age of 12 (47%, 26%, and 18%). The father was the parent they were separated from most often (31%), with divorce being the major reason for the separation. Frommer and O'Shea (1973a) observed that women separated from their parents before the age of 11 tended to respond to their infants with either over-anxiety, in attempts to be a perfect mother, or in lack of care. Those who had been separated were also more depressed than those who had not been separated from their parents as a child. Women who denied or had forgotten that they were separated from their parents as children had more marital and management problems than those who had not been separated (Frommer & O'Shea, 1973b).

In summary, these teenage mothers, who had assets at the biological level of adaptation, were disadvantaged at the psychological and social levels of adaptation during the first year of motherhood. Their self-ratings in the mothering role never differed from those of older women; however, their conceptions of the ideal mothering behaviors on which they based their self-ratings were more focused on caretaking. However, despite these disadvantages, Group 1 infants did exceptionally well during the first year. Unlike an earlier study in which adolescents' infants failed to compare favorably with national weight percentiles (Osofsky & Osofsky, 1970), 60% of Group 1 infants in this study were above the 50th percentile for weight at 1 year, compared with 48.3% of Group 2 infants and 39.8% of Group 3 infants (Mercer, 1984). The teenagers' decrease in gratification in the mothering role at 1 year and their additional stress warrants long-term follow-up to assure continuing development for both mother and infant.

Group 2: 20- to 29-Year-Olds

Assets The women in Group 2 were overall more similar to Group 3 and dissimilar to Group 1. Their scores on the developmental constructs, personality integration, and flexibility were significantly higher than the teenagers' yet significantly lower than those of Group 3. Personality trait scores were not significantly different from those of Group 3 but significantly higher than those of Group 1, with two exceptions. Group 2 scored highest in empathy and in the maternal temperament trait of persistence. Both of these traits are very important in the maternal role.

Another asset was that Group 2 had experienced more positive life experiences the year prior to childbirth and during the first year of motherhood. Positive life events seemed to be supportive; among women who reported no emotional, informational, physical, or appraisal support, there was a significant positive relationship between positive life events and the maternal role index. Typical good life events the year prior to birth included marriage, personal achievements, and change of eating habits.

Medical intervention in the labor and delivery experiences of Group 2 women approximated the national norm more so than the other two groups; only 19% experienced cesarean births, compared with 31% of Group 3. Group 2 perceived their childbirth experiences more positively than did other groups. Their higher level of development and more positive scores on personality traits than teenagers, who had even less medical intervention, probably enabled them to feel more positively about their experience.

At 1 month postpartum, Group 2 identified more of their infants' characteristics and traits with either themselves or their mates or other family members. Thus, they seemed to claim their infants as part of a family context more readily. Although they exceeded the teenagers, only half as many in Group 2 as in Group 3 described the baby as taking over their lives (18%, 28%, and 56%). Similarly, in describing the change in their life-styles, fewer in Group 2 than in Group 3 reported changes in their schedules (14%, 25%, and 67%) or household (15%, 16%, and 64%). The woman in her twenties felt less engulfed or consumed by motherhood; her temperament trait of higher persistence may have been helpful in this regard.

At the disruption phase, Group 2 reported fewer changes in their relationships with friends than did the other groups. Women as a whole tend to gravitate toward women with children. Since the modal age for having a first child is during the twenties, Group 2's friendship circle remained more stable. At this time Group 2's conception of an ideal mother more often included the description of loving, giving, and enjoying mothering. Thus, their self-ratings in the mothering role, while not mathematically significantly different from the teenagers, were dramatically different qualitatively; they saw themselves as loving, giving, and enjoying mothering, whereas teenagers saw themselves as keeping their infant clean and dressed appropriately. Also women in their twenties described a good baby as one who has a schedule and is affectionate and loving. This is congruent with Group 2's higher empathy.

Group 2 women scored similarly to Group 3 women on maternal role attainment variables, except for gratification in the mothering role; they were more similar to the younger group of women in this area. Importantly, at 1 year Group 2 scored the highest on gratification in the maternal role. In addition they scored highest on Cohler's well-differentiated satisfaction in the maternal role subscale at 1 year. At this time their infants were ahead of other infants in social development. In describing what had been the most difficult thing in mothering at 1 year, fewer in Group 2 reported role responsibilities. The Group 2 woman's status as a mother and her identity as a loving, giving person who enjoyed mothering seems to be important variables. Is the timing more right in a psychological, cognitive, and social sense for women in their twenties moving into a responsible, adult role? The woman 30 years and older has proved that she is responsible in career roles; does the responsibility of motherhood bring less value, less status, and less pleasure from her perspective because of her earlier accomplishments?

In summary, Group 2 maternal attitudes consistently were more positive or adaptive than Group 1's but less so than Group 3's. Their conception of an ideal mother as one who is loving, giving, and enjoying motherhood, as well as their average score of 8.29 in rating themselves in mothering (ideal = 10), suggests that they viewed themselves in this way. Their higher scores in empathy, i.e., being able to imagine the feelings of others in different situations, and their persistence no doubt contributed to their maternal role attainment.

The cultural environment is such that Group 2 was at decided advantage in some areas of social and psychological levels of adaptation to motherhood. Their network of peers remained more stable when the other two groups were seeking peers who were mothers. Group 2 fit the national norm for type of birth experience, and the birth experience had long-lasting implications. It is noteworthy that only when a group scored higher on the continuum of gratification did their infants surpass other infants in an area of growth or development.

Vulnerabilities Early in motherhood (1 month), more of Group 2 mothers reported feeling the ever-present responsibility in the mothering role as most difficult (11%, 33%, and 22%). However, as noted above, by 1 year Group 2 was less likely to describe the role responsibility as most difficult, which suggests that they had gained much confidence over the year in this area.

Although role strain never differed between age groups, Group 2 employed women experienced more role strain than nonemployed women at the disruption phase. More women in Group 2 were employed at 8 months (40%, 59%, and 55%); this increased to 72% at 1 year. Infants of employed women in Group 2 scored lower on the growth and development factor at 8 months.

Employment roles presented greater difficulty for Group 2 women, who lacked the long-term commitment of the older women to a career, especially when they derived greater satisfaction from mothering. Group 2 women reported greater financial stress than those in Group 3, so they lacked the option of dropping the employment role. Income and subjects' mothers' work histories need to be studied in future research because these characteristics have been associated with mothers' occupational commitment (Riesch, 1984).

Group 3: 30- to 42-Year-Olds

Assets The more flexible, highly integrated women in Group 3 also tended to score more positively or adaptively on personality traits and child-rearing attitudes.

This more highly educated group of women (93% had some college, a baccalaureate or a graduate degree) attended prenatal classes more often than younger women (92%). Their incomes were significantly higher than younger women's; two thirds of Group 1 had annual incomes of $12,000 or less; 60% of Group 2 had incomes of $22,000 or less; and two thirds of Group 3 had incomes higher than $22,000.

Group 3 also chose to breast-feed more often. Many had deliberately postponed motherhood while they pursued education and career roles; thus, when they opted for motherhood, they had planned the pregnancy, were highly motivated, and placed a high value on achieving in this role. Stainton (1985b) observed that self-reliance, achievement, and independence were highly valued among upwardly mobile multiparous mothers over 30, and these values influenced early mothering practices.

During the year, Group 3 consistently scored as more adaptive on observer-rated maternal behaviors (differences were not significant over Group 2) and on self-rated ways of handling irritating child behaviors. These higher competency skills were expected because

of their greater experiences in moving into roles prior to motherhood and their higher level of social and psychological development.

More women in Group 3 reported receiving emotional support
at 1, 4, and 8 months. At 1 month, they more often reported talking
with others as a major coping strategy for handling difficult situations in mothering. A more mature, self-assured individual is more
capable of eliciting and maintaining a support system (Kahn &
Antonucci, 1980).

At the achievement phase, Group 3 less often described problems
with mate relationships than did younger women. They were more
enthusiastic about motherhood and less often described mothering
at this time as harder or busier. This may have been related to
fewer reporting concerns about the infant's growth or development.
They less often described a good baby as one who doesn't cry
but more often described a good baby as one who responds and
vocalizes and is healthy and strong, indicating those qualities as the
ones they valued.

At the disruption phase, Group 3 more often than younger mothers reported that they soothed the infant as a coping strategy during
difficult periods with the infant. Employed mothers in this group
reported more positive feelings of love for their infants than nonemployed mothers. Group 3 was the only group in which *employed*
women's infants scored slightly higher on the growth and development factor, as opposed to Groups 1 and 2, in which employed
mothers' infants scored lower. Recent research indicates that it is
the *home environment rather than mothers' employment* that influences infant growth and development (Squires, 1985); it may be
conjectured that the home environment of employed mothers in
Group 3 was more stimulating and nurturing than that of nonemployed mothers. Group 3's conception of an ideal mother more often
included one who plays with the infant and comforts and nurtures
the infant.

At 1 year Group 3 had less financial stress than younger women.
Their mates and friends were more frequently named in their social
network, and their mothers were named less often. Fewer in this
group reported that *nothing* had been a surprise to them their first
year of motherhood. Importantly, the infant's increased activity level
and beginning individuation from the mother was less bothersome
to Group 3. This finding supports Sander's (1962) thesis that the
mother's maturity is an important variable at this period of infant
development.

Except at the biological level of adaptation, Group 3 had many advantages in the psychological and social levels of adaptation. Their greater maturity fostered greater acceptance of infant activity that required increasing attention. Their higher level of personality integration seemed to make it possible for them to foster their infants' individuality. Infant responsiveness was highly valued by this group. Their greater financial resources meant that they could hire live-in babysitters when they returned to careers and provided them with a choice in doing so.

Vulnerabilities Group 3 experienced significantly more antepartum and intrapartum complications. They had the highest cesarean rate of any age group, and they rated their childbirth experiences less positively than did Group 2 but more positively than Group 1. Their high commitment to preparing for childbirth (92% attending antepartum classes), coupled with their greater than expected cesarean birth rate, may account in part for their resulting disappointment and less positive views about the experience. Fewer in this group met their expectations for achieving a birth experience in which they remained in control and made decisions.

Group 3's higher operative rate at delivery contributed to their poorer health status and greater fatigue at 1 month. They reported more soreness from incisions, episiotomies, and breasts. A lack of time was foremost at 1 month, and changes in their life-styles were greatest regarding scheduling and the household. Group 3 described fewer features of their infants as resembling themselves or a family member.

Group 3 reported significantly less experience in caring for infants prior to the birth of their own infants; 26% reported having had *no* experience at all with young infants. Only 13% reported having had a great deal of experience, compared with 45% of Group 1 and 29% of Group 2.

At the achievement and reorganization phases, more women in Group 3 reported a major concern was balancing career and motherhood roles; the lack of time continued to be difficult for more of Group 3 at these periods and was related to their concern. The motherhood–career role demands that resulted in a lack of time also contributed to isolation from adults reported as the most difficult part of mothering by more of Group 3 women. More women in Group 3, despite their greater readiness for the pregnancy, stated that the infant's birth had changed their life plans such as school or work.

Despite all of Group 3's assets, they consistently reported the least gratification in the maternal role at all test periods. Other researchers reported that more highly educated individuals had less gratification in mothering (Russell, 1974; Steffensmeier, 1982), and that offers one possible explanation here. Group 3 were probably more self-actualized persons prior to motherhood, and the instrument used to measure gratification may have been less salient to them. The instrument was derived from what new parents had described as satisfying in the early 1970s, when fewer women 30 years and older were becoming first-time parents. Group 3 invested more time in preparing for motherhood but experienced more disappointment in their type of birth. This was dissimilar from their experience of preparing educationally for careers in which they had achieved. The significant relationship between Cohler's attitude factor of competence and comfort in meeting the infant's needs and gratification in the role supports the explanation that *competence* in a role is associated with this groups' *satisfaction* in the role. This older group of mothers probably had values similar to those of the older multiparous mothers studied by Stainton (1985b), who reported higher levels of self-reliance, independence, and achievement among these women. Both study samples were from the Bay Area and were largely college-educated, with experience in professions or highly skilled technical positions. With less previous experience in caring for infants, this group with high achievement orientation less often met their own expectations.

LIMITATIONS OF STUDY FINDINGS

The teenage population was largely older adolescents who had received good prenatal care. In addition, over one-third dropped out of the study. Therefore, generalizations cannot be made about *all* teenage mothers from these findings.

The mate relationship offered a unique form of support over the first year of motherhood and therefore must be studied more carefully in order to have better data for counseling families during early parenthood. The mothers' verbal reports of marital-related stress appeared far more pronounced than they were willing to commit to paper on the bother scale items. Future research focusing on mate relationships needs to use an instrument that is developed specifically to measure the dyadic relationship in order to measure more subtle changes in the mate relationship. However, because there may be more freedom in discussing feelings and a hesitancy to rate more negative feelings on paper, a qualitative approach may be more fruitful.

Further study of social support variables is warranted. Different types of support appear more critical from different members of the mother's social network. Other mothers appear to be in a better position to offer informational support, whereas mates are able to provide emotional and appraisal support very well. Several instruments have been developed in recent years since the study was begun, which might prove more discriminating and contribute to the predictive weight of social support.

The pregnancy data that were collected retrospectively at birth were important; this is in agreement with others (Leifer, 1977, 1980; Grossman et al., 1980). Ideally, future longitudinal study would include measures during pregnancy. The tendency of teenagers in this study to have had fewer friends who visited them in their homes suggests a need for prepregnancy assessment in order to know which came first—whether the pregnancy led to fewer social visits with friends or the fewer social visits with friends indirectly led to the pregnancy. In addition, more teenagers than those in the older groups were separated from one or both of their parents before the age of 12; the possible impact of family dynamics on early pregnancy cannot be overlooked.

A strength of the study was in the overall agreement between the qualitative interview data and the quantitative data. An exception related to the stress experienced with the mate was discussed above. There was agreement between observer-rated maternal behavior, maternal self-image in the mothering role, and maternal self-reported ways of handling irritating behaviors that supported the validity of these measures. There was agreement that maternal attitudes were implemented into maternal practices, providing concurrent validity for the different measures. If a woman says that she believes in physical punishment, the health care provider can accept that she will use physical punishment.

IMPLICATIONS

Personal variables that seem to be more discriminating in mothering behavior are not readily accessible to intervention by health care providers. Self-concept, attitudes, negative life events, and other stressors evolve from the societal context, so broader social issues need addressing if a supportive environment is to be experienced by women during early child rearing. Women from Asia and the Pacific Islands were particularly vocal in describing the lack of societal support for new mothers in our contemporary United States society. New families who are isolated from extended families who could help with all types of social support must struggle alone in managing the new parenthood role.

Employment or career roles are no longer options for the average woman having her first child. Financial pressures demand that she juggle work, mate, and mother roles. The lack of well-supported and well-supervised child-care facilities for infants creates a significant problem for mothers. Recent landmark legislation requiring office developers in San Francisco to provide child-care services is one method of meeting the need for working mothers (Sward, 1985). However, a more concerted effort from the state or federal level is needed. Affordable child care centers that are open 24 hours per day, seven days a week, staffed by child development specialists would make it possible for women to seek employment with somewhat less conflict. Such facilities would also provide an opportunity for stressed-out parents to have an evening for special entertainment, or a night for uninterrupted sleep. A short period of time away from an infant provides the change of pace that most parents need to return to their roles with renewed love and vigor.

Emotional, physical, informational, and appraisal support were all important to women in their mothering role. Yet unsolicited attempts at informational support were obnoxious. Women commented that they were amazed that comparative strangers would offer advice. Informational support, however, was particularly important to the older group of mothers. This may have resulted in part from the fact that the majority reported emotional support; however, health care professionals can play large roles in providing relevant, accurate, and current information for all new parents. The importance of all types of support for the teenager make it imperative that much attention is alloted to helping young women identify potential sources of support and helping them to develop social skills in eliciting and maintaining support.

Bother from infant-related stress was associated with both feelings of love for the infant and gratification in mothering. Women just do not know *the extent of the impact of the infant on a family's life-style.* Being forewarned is being forearmed. Part of the distress from infant-related stress was in the lack of being prepared for the extensive change in mate relationships, schedules, and social time for self and others. Tofler's (1970) suggestion of experienced, professional parents taking over child rearing to relieve biological parents of this stress is rather drastic; however, *help* from professional parents is badly needed by young families. Advice that was most highly valued by women in this study was that provided by parents who had a child not more than 2 or 3 years old. Perhaps one way to meet this need is for women who need extra income to free-lance their expertise in child care. Community or church support groups for parents is another way.

Overall, the mothers in this study were highly committed to their children. They worked to foster creativity, independence, integrity, and interpersonal, motor, and intellectual skills in their infants. They worried that they might fall short or do something that would interfere with their infants' optimal development. Even those few who were not major caretakers of their infants saw the extended care from other family members or adults as superior to what they could provide in their current situations. Above all, these mothers wanted their children to have better lives, a better world, and greater opportunities than they had had as children. The challenge is with the health care professional to help them to achieve their goals.

Appendix

MEASURES

Table 1 summarizes the measures administrated at each of the test periods. The battery of instruments administered at each test period was limited as much as possible in an attempt to keep the time required for their completion within 1 to 2 hr.

The personal and social history and the obstetrical and demographic data questionnaires were adapted from Virden's (1981). Some items related to social support and maternal feelings at the time pregnancy was first suspected were from Nuckolls and associates' (1972) The Adaptive Potential for Pregnancy Score. The interview schedules were adapted from Barnard and Eyres' (1979) Family Assessment Interviews in *Child Health Assessment Part 2: The First Year of Life* (pp. 203–210).

A content analysis was done of all open-ended items to derive categories for coding. Initial inter-rater agreement was tested for refinement of the categories. When the categories were established, 12 interview schedules were selected randomly (4 from each of the three age groups) and inter-rater agreement was determined; these ranged from 87% to 89% agreement. After the reliabilities were determined, Mercer coded all of the interviews (Mercer et al., 1982).

Dependent or Predicted Variables

Attachment At early postpartum and 1 month, the Neonatal Perception Inventories (NPI-1 and NPI-2) reported by Broussard and Hartner (1971) were used as a proxy measure of attachment.

TABLE 1 Measures for Variables by Test Period

Variables	Early Post- partum	1 mo	4 mo	8 mo	12 mo
Independent					
Age	x				
Perception of Birth					
Attitudes about labor and delivery questionnaire (Marut & Mercer, 1979)	x				
Early maternal infant separation					
Attitudes about labor and delivery questionnaire	x				
Interview	x	x			
Social stress					
Degree of bother inventory (Broussard & Hartner, 1971)		x			
Life experiences survey (Sarason et al., 1978)	x				x
Checklist of bothersome factors (Hobbs, 1965)		x	x	x	x
Interview, role strain		x	x	x	x
Social support					
Personal and social history	x				
Interview	x	x	x	x	x
Maternal personality traits					
Empathy scale (Hansson, Matthews & Disbrow, 1978)			x		
Perinatal rigidity scale (Larsen, 1968)			x		
Adult temperament questionnaire (Thomas, 1980; Thomas et al., 1982)			x		
Self-concept					
Tennessee self-concept scale (Fitts, 1965)	x			x	
Maternal health status					
Obstetrical and demographic data; hospital record	x				
Interview	x	x	x	x	x

TABLE 1 Continued

| | Test period | | | | |
	Early post-partum	1 mo	4 mo	8 mo	12 mo
Child-rearing attitudes					
Parent attitude scales		x		x	
(Disbrow, Doerr, & Caulfield, 1977;					
Disbrow & Doerr, 1982)					
Maternal attitude scale					x
(Cohler et al., 1970)					
Infant temperament					
Questionnaire			x	x	
(Carey & McDevitt, 1978)					
Infant health status					
Obstetrical and demographic data;					
hospital record	x				
Interview	x	x	x	x	x
Dependent variables, maternal role attainment					
Attachment					
Neonatal perception inventories	x	x			
(Broussard & Hartner, 1971)					
How I feel about my baby		x	x	x	x
(Leifer, 1977)					
Child-trait checklist		x			
(Leifer, 1977, 1980)					
Gratification checklist		x	x	x	x
(Russell, 1974)					
Interview	x	x	x	x	x
Competency					
Ways parents handle irritating behaviors		x		x	x
(Disbrow, Doerr, & Caulfield, 1977)					
Maternal behavior rating scales		x	x	x	x
(Blank, 1964)					
Infant's weight, length, head circum-					
ference, psychosocial and motor skills		x	x	x	x
(Ross Laboratory Scales, 1973)					

The rationale was that a positive perception of the infant would be indicative of attachment. Alpha reliabilities for the average baby early postpartum were reported as .63 for the Average Baby Scale, and .74 for the Your Baby Scale with 100 subjects (Blumberg, 1980). The reliabilities in this study were .56 and .68 for the Average Baby Scale and .61 and .65 for the Your Baby Scale at early postpartum and 1 month.

An attachment factor was derived from interview items that had high validity from reported research for representing attachment at the first test period: emotional response in telling about the infant, how the mother referred to the infant, and the presence of identifying/claiming behaviors. The NPI-1 and the attachment factor had an inverse nonsignificant correlation, indicating that the NPI was not a valid measure of attachment.

Leifer's (1977, 1980) How I Feel About My Baby questionnaire was the measure of attachment at 1, 4, 8, and 12 months. Ten items such as "I feel tenderly towards my baby," and "I feel annoyed at my baby," are rated on a 4-point scale from never, rarely, sometimes, to often. Cronbach alpha reliabilities were .51 ($N = 240$); .65 ($N = 239$); .64 ($N = 228$); and .61 ($N = 222$).

At 1 month Leifer's (1980) Child-Trait Checklist was also used as a measure of attachment because it represents the claiming behaviors described by Gottlieb (1978), Robson and Moss (1970), and Rubin (1961, 1972). The mother identifies characteristics of her infant (hair, complexion, nose, eyes, ears, body build, eating habits, disposition, and other) that resemble herself, mate, her mother and father, mate's mother and father, or other. The number of identifications made by the mother were summed for scoring.

Gratification in the Maternal Role Gratification in the maternal role was measured by an adaptation of Russell's (1974) Gratification Checklist, which was constructed by asking new parents what things they enjoyed most about their new role. Adaptation for this study included changing the items' 3-point scale to a 5-point scale; making two items out of the item "Increased appreciation for family and religious tradition"; and adding the item "Watching baby grow and learn to do new things." Other items were pride in baby's development; fewer periods of boredom; relationship with relatives closer; increased contact with neighbors; more things to talk to mate about; feeling "closer" to mate; feeling of "fulfillment"; new appreciation of my own parents; baby fun to play with; a purpose for living; and enjoy baby's company. The Cronbach alpha reliabilities in this study sample were .80 (N = 240); .78 (N = 240); .78 (N = 231); and .71 (N = 219).

Maternal Behavior Maternal behavior was measured by a self-rated behavioral questionnaire and an observer-rated maternal behavior scale. Mothers rated items on the Disbrow and associates' (1977, 1982) Ways Parents Handle Irritating Behaviors scale, which discriminated abusive from nonabusive parents indicating high content validity for the measure. Eleven child behaviors such as "won't cooperate" or "gets in my way" were checked according to 16 options for handling the behavior. Options included spank with hand, tell him you don't love him, scold or nag, hit with something, shake or shove, yell at him, shame or ridicule, do nothing—my spouse or friend handles it, do nothing—normal behavior, explain why he shouldn't act that way, withhold a privilege or something he wants, put him by himself, pick up and hug, distract him, ignore him, and other categories.

Observer-rated maternal behavior was measured by an adaptation from Blank's (1964) scale. Blank's scales rate mothering behavior from 1 to 5 on items including attentiveness, baby's contact with outsiders, competence, degree of anxiety, intellectual demandingness, training in independence, accuracy of reporting, physical freedom available to child, degree of protectiveness, use of restrictions, willingness to assume motherhood, enjoyment of motherhood, satisfaction with baby's development, and warmth of mother-child relationship. Both the 1 and the 5 represent undesirable behaviors; for this study the scales were modified for a range of 1 to 3 such as was done by Roberts and Rowley (1972). A child development specialist verified the modified adaptation in which the score of 1 was the least competent or adaptive and the score of 3 was the most competent or adaptive.

Inter-rater Spearman Brown reliability means were determined over the year; 35% were $\geqslant$ .90; 44% $\geqslant$ .80 but < .90; 10% $\geqslant$ .70 but < .80; 7% $\geqslant$ .60 but < .70; 2% = .55; and 2% = .48. Cronbach alpha reliabilities for internal consistency at each test period were as follows: .80 (N = 275); .83 (N = 264); .85 (N = 248); and .86 (N = 240).

Infant Growth and Development The infant's weight, length, and head circumference were measured and recorded on Ross Laboratories (1973) forms. Each motor and social development item on the forms was assigned a sequential number (higher numbers indicated a higher level of development in that area), so that mean scores could be determined for motor and social development. A single factor was derived from these measures at each test period. The validity of the infant's growth and development as reflecting mothering has been supported (Pollitt, Eichler, & Chan, 1975; Rutter, 1979).

Maternal Role Attainment Index At 1, 4, 8, and 12 months a principal components analysis of the dependent variables was done to determine whether a single factor could represent maternal role attainment. A factor with adequate weighting by all dependent variables was not found until 12 months.

Independent or Predictor Variables

Maternal Age Maternal age at birth was used throughout the analyses and was entered into the regression models at all test periods.

Perception of the Childbirth Experience Perception of the birth experience was measured by a 29-item questionnaire adapted by Marut and Mercer (1979) from Samko and Schoenfeld's measure (1975), based on pilot data by Marut (1978). The Cronbach alpha coefficient reliability was .87 for 222 cases in this study. Items are rated from 1 to 5, with the higher score indicating a more positive birth experience. Sample items are "How relaxed were you during labor?" "How relaxed were you during delivery?" and "Were you pleased with how your delivery turned out?" This variable was entered into all regression models at all test periods.

Maternal-Infant Separation Four items loaded into one factor to measure early maternal-infant separation: mother's self-report of when she first saw, touched, held, and fed her baby (1 = immediately following birth, 2 = first hour, 3 = from 1 to 2 hr, 4 = from 2 to 8 hr, and 5 = longer than 8 hr). Four modes of contact were included for two reasons. The research studying early mother–infant interactions and the effect of early contact suggests that there are qualitative differences between seeing versus holding the infant. Second, the extent of early mother–infant contact is highly variable, ranging from the woman who breast-feeds immediately following birth to the woman who only sees and touches her infant during the first 8 hr. Mother-infant contact was encouraged and facilitated by nursing staff as soon as maternal and infant conditions permitted. This factor was entered into the regression models at all test periods.

At 1 month, a second measure of mother–infant separation was taken. This was infant hospitalization after the mother's discharge: 1 to 3 days, 4 to 7 days, 8 to 10 days, or 2 to 3 weeks. Although mothers visit their hospitalized infants, extended hospitalization imposes much physical separation and creates anxiety about the infant's welfare. This variable was entered into all regression models at 1, 4, 8, and 12 months.

Social Stress Four measures were used to measure social stress. In the Life Experiences Survey, constructed by Sarason, Johnson, and Siegel (1978), respondents rate life events that have occurred as either good (positive) or bad (negative), and as having either no effect, some effect, moderate effect, or great effect. Test-retest reliabilities with a 5- to 6-week interval among undergraduate students were .19 and .53, p <.001, positive change score; .56 and .88, p < .001, negative change score; and .63 and .64, p <.001, total change score. No further reliability tests were done. However, one known life event that all subjects in this study had experienced was pregnancy, and 95.8% checked this event as occurring during the past year. Total stress scores from positive and negative life events were entered into regression models at test periods 1, 2, and 5.

Hobbs (1965) developed the Checklist of Bothersome Factors to reflect infant-related stress in the transition to parenthood and revised it for a replicated study (Hobbs & Cole, 1976). Items deal with changes such as additional work, meals off-schedule, and physical tiredness. The scoring range of 1 to 3 was changed to a range of 1 to 5, with 1 = not at all, 3 = somewhat, and 5 = very much of a bother. Cronbach alpha reliabilities with this sample were as follows: 1 month, .83 (N = 238); 4 months, .85 (N = 230); 8 months, .87 (N = 218); and 12 months, .86 (N = 208). Infant-related stress was entered into regression models at 1, 4, 8, and 12 months.

A 7-item subscale related to changes in the mate relationship was derived from the Hobbs Checklist. Cronbach alpha reliability for this subscale was .69 at 8 months; it was entered into the regression models at 8 months.

At 1 month, Broussard and Hartner's (1971) Degree of Bother Inventory was used to measure stress related to problematic infant behaviors. Six behaviors are rated—crying, spitting up or vomiting, sleeping, feeding, elimination, and lack of a predictable schedule—on a scale of 1 = none, 2 = very little, 3 = somewhat, and 4 = a great deal of bother. The Cronbach alpha reliability for 240 cases in this

TABLE 2   Maternal Role Strain

None	Absence of discomfort with mothering; able to comply easily with her expectations for the role. Manages extra demands with no difficulty. Feeling of everything under control. Feels good about herself, no concerns about her infant.
Low	Unable to do everything she wishes but expresses little pressure. May say she is a good mom, but too lenient. May describe motherhood as fun but hard. Mentions only one thing as bothering her, overall good. May rate self as 8 on mothering (range, 1-10; 10 = ideal mother).
Moderate	Distressed that she is not keeping up or caught up with everything, frustrated. Occasionally calls husband at work to come home early for help. Conflict or unhappy with career role, concern about meeting increasing demands, may rate self as 7. (A mother may rate self as 10, but if interview reflects one of the above, she is rated as moderate strain.)
High	Feels guilty about something she is or is not doing. Unable to perform adequately or get things done. Disorganized, disheveled appearance—hair uncombed, not dressed late morning or afternoon.
Very high	Distraught, focused on how hard and frustrating mothering is. Responds to infant inconsistently. Decreased self esteem, extremely anxious, worried, guilty, uncomfortable with her situation. Rates self as 5 or lower in mothering role.

study was .63. This variable was entered into all regression models at 1 month.

An adaptation of Burr and associates' (1979) scale of role strain was used as a reflection of stress in the role at 4, 8, and 12 months (see Table 2). Role strain was entered into regression models at those times.

Role strain was scored on the basis of the total interview content. At 12 months there was a significant positive relationship with the Checklist of Bothersome Factors ($r = .30; p = .0001$) and with negative (bad) life events experienced during the first year of motherhood ($r = .15; p = .02$), supporting the conclusion that role strain reflected stress. There was no correlation with positive (good) life events, indicating that positive life events were not stressful.

Social Support   At early postpartum, support during pregnancy and childbirth and anticipated support were used. At 1 month the extent of the help received from both mate and others and whether the help seemed adequate made up support factors used. See Tables 3 and 4 for the support variables that were entered into the regression models at those two periods.

At 4, 8, and 12 months the same interview items were used to derive social support measures for the regression analyses: Who helps you manage the day-by-day situations in mothering? In what way was this person/s helpful? Was this as much help as you needed?

TABLE 3 Factor Loadings for Factors Utilized in Analysis at Early Postpartum

Factor	Factor loading[a]	Final communality estimates	Eigenvalue
Network support			
Number neighbors recognized	-.345	.119	2.07
How often chat neighbors	-.507	.258	
Friends in area	.480	.167	
Outings with friends	-.707	.500	
Frequency friends visit	.714	.510	
Frequency see women friends	.724	.525	
Physical mate support			
Mate attended prenatal class	-.745	.555	2.62
Married to mate	.698	.487	
Mate labor room	.888	.788	
Mate delivery room	.889	.790	
Informational support			
Attend prenatal class	-.745	.555	1.45
Close friends here	.507	.257	
Review birth experiences	.800	.634	
Emotional mate support, factor 1			
How useful mate labor	.915	.843	1.92
How useful mate delivery	.902	.816	
Quality relationship mate	.486	.264	
Quality relationship mother	-.122	.731	
Quality relationship father	-.118	.740	
Emotional parent support, factor 2			
How useful mate labor	.082		1.48
How useful mate delivery	.053		
Quality relationship mate	.166		
Quality relationship mother	.846		
Quality relationship father	.852		

TABLE 3   Continued

Factor	Factor loading[a]	Final communality estimates	Eigenvalue
Mother–Infant separation			
First saw baby	.696	.484	2.27
First touched baby	−.824	.680	
First held baby	.853	.377	
First fed baby	.610	.373	
Perinatal child-rearing attitudes			
Family centered birth program	−.513	.263	1.80
Breastfeeding	−.744	.553	
Prenatal class	.786	.618	
Knowledge infant behavior	.608	.370	
Perinatal health, factor 1			
Problems during pregnancy	.654	.651	1.71
Complications during labor and delivery	.551	.571	
Postpartum complications	.629	.413	
Labor normal	.481	.628	
Number of complications during pregnancy	−.595	.720	
AP, IP health, factor 2			
Problems during pregnancy	−.473		1.27
Complications during labor and delivery	.518		
PP complications	.129		
Labor normal	.630		
Number of complications during pregnancy	.605		
Infant health status			
Apgar 1 min	.870	.757	1.99
Apgar 5 min	.845	.713	
Spontaneous respiration	−.721	.52	
Attachment			
Emotional response	.687	.473	.31
Mother refers to baby	−.643	.413	
Acquaintance behaviors	.659	.421	

[a]Scoring reversed for negative loadings, except when two factors derived.

TABLE 4   Factor Loadings for Factors Utilized in Analysis
at One Month

Variable	Factor loading[a]	Final communality estimates	Eigenvalue
Emotional support			
Number of emotional supports	.669	.447	1.31
Number who bolster morale	.718	.514	
Number of ways person was helpful	.588	.345	
Mate physical support, factor 1			
As much help as needed	–.178	1.000	1.68
How much husband helped	.643	1.000	
Number who help with chores	.222	1.000	
Number of helping actions	.662	1.000	
Physical support, factor 2			
As much help as needed	.670		
How much husband helped	.122		
Number who helped with chores	–.677		
Number of helping actions	.280		
Maternal health status			
Overall feelings previous month	–.841	.707	1.41
Number of problems	–.841	.707	
Infant health status			
Assessment of status	.789	.623	1.25
Sum of illnesses hospitalized	.789	.623	
Infant characteristics easy-difficult			
Length of feeding	.683	.466	1.38
Schedule regularity	–.684	.467	
How feedings go	.666	.444	
Disbrow's parent attitude scale, factor 1			
Low boiling point	.626	1.000	1.62
Sadistic	.850	1.000	
Strict disciplinarian	.711	1.000	
Mothering stress, factor 1			
Child changed environment	.572	.972	1.51
Concerns mate	.473	.931	
Other stressors, sum	.555	.980	
Sum concerns	.470	.712	

TABLE 4   Continued

Variable	Factor loading[a]	Final communality estimates	Eigenvalue
Infant growth and development			
Motor development	.799	1.000	1.99
Social development	.782	1.000	
Weight gain	.653	1.000	
Length grown	.557	1.000	

[a]Scoring reversed for negative loadings.

(1 = a lot more than I needed; 2 = more than I needed; 3 = as much as needed; 4 = less than I needed; and 5 = a lot less than needed.) The kind of help received was categorized into types of support described by House (1981)—physical, informational, emotional, and appraisal. The number of persons who were listed as helpful in day-to-day situations was used as the size of the network.

Empathy A 12-item empathy scale derived from Stotland's 96-item scale by Disbrow's Child Abuse Prediction project (Hansson et al., 1978) was used. The Cronbach alpha reliability for 235 cases in this study was .55. This 4-month score was used for all subsequent analyses and regressions.

Rigidity Rigidity was measured by a 15-item scale constructed by Larsen (1966). Subjects rate a 6-point scale from "agree strongly" to "disagree strongly" for how they feel about dogmatic statements such as "Of all the different ideas of child care which exist there is only one which is correct." The measure was selected for its content validity and brevity. The rigidity score was used for all subsequent regressions and analyses. The Cronbach alpha coefficient for reliability was .81.

Temperament Thomas, Mittelman, and Chess's (1982) 140-item Early Adult Life Temperament Questionnaire was used to measure maternal temperament because of its high content validity and reliability and its isomorphism with the Carey Infant Temperament Questionnaire that was used to measure infant temperament. Alpha coefficients ranged from .72 to .87 in 490 cases. In this sample Cronback alpha coefficients ranged from .64 to .85 for 243 cases.

At 4 months maternal temperament traits of adaptability, intensity of response, mood quality, persistence, and distractibility were entered into all regression analyses. At 8 months adaptibility and mood were entered, and at 12 months a factor of six traits was entered.

Self-Concept The Tennessee Self Concept Scale (TSCS) was selected to measure self-concept, personality integration, and personality disorder. The scale has a reliability coefficient of .88 for the total score. Self-concept was entered into regression models at all test periods. The personality integration scale reflects the level of adjustment and was entered into all regression models at the first three test periods. The personality disorder scale differentiates persons with basic personality defects or weaknesses from those with psychotic states or neurotic reactions (Fitts, 1965) and was entered into the regression models at 8 and 12 months because it had a higher correlation with role attainment variables than integration.

Child-Rearing Attitudes Two measures, the Parent Child-Rearing Attitude Scales developed by Disbrow et al. (1977), and the Maternal Attitude Scale (MAS) developed by Cohler et al. (1970) were used. These scales were selected because they reflect adaptation to the mothering role in different ways, and because of their established validities and reliabilities. The attitude subscales had a split half reliability of .77 with alpha coefficients ranging from .81 to .96 (Caulfield et al., 1977).

In this study the reliability for role reversal was -.16 for 240 cases at 1 month, and this subscale was not used for regression analyses. Other subscale reliabilities ranged from .24 to .58. Items were deleted to improve reliabilities; low boiling point had a final .48, sadistic a .67, and strict disciplinarian had a .61 reliability. A principal components analysis of the three subscales yielded one factor for child-rearing attitudes and was entered into the regression models at 1 and 4 months. At 8 months the role reversal scale was not used again because of low reliability. An item was deleted from each of the other subscales to bring reliabilities to .49 for low boiling point, .51 for sadistic, and .57 for strict disciplinarian. These separate subscales were entered into the regression models at eight months.

The MAS has 233 items that were constructed for mothers with a minimum of a sixth-grade education. The focus of this scale is on tasks confronting the mother the first 3 years of the child's life, with particular attention to the assessment of attitudes regarding reciprocity, encouragement of the child's sense of competence, and the infant's movement away from the mother (Cohler et al., 1970). Alpha coefficients range from .81 to .96 on scales constructed on the basis of items with the highest loadings of the five factors: appropriate control of the child's aggressive impulses; encouragement versus discouragement of reciprocity; appropriate versus inappropriate closeness; acceptance versus denial of the emotional complexity in child rearing; and comfort versus discomfort in perceiving and meeting the baby's physical needs. Validity of these factors has been demonstrated in several studies; they were entered into all regression models at 12 months.

Maternal Health Status At the first test period, data for maternal health status were taken from hospital records and interview (see perinatal health factor that is listed in Table 3 for items that were included). Maternal health status at 1, 4, 8, and 12 months was determined from answers to the following: How have you been feeling since the last interview (since birth/1/4/8 months)? Are you or have you been under a doctor's care (during this time)? Considering what you just described would you consider your overall general health to be (read list): 1 = very good; 2 = good; 3 = fair; and 4 = poor. Maternal health status was entered into all regression models at each test period.

Infant Health Status Items making up the factors for infant health status are shown in Tables 3, 4, 5, and 6 at each test period, except at 4 months when the number of infant illnesses was used. Infant health status was entered into the regression models at all test periods.

Infant Temperament Carey's Infant Temperament Questionnaire (Carey, 1970; Carey & McDevitt, 1978) has 93 statements that the mother rates regarding her infant's activity, rhythmicity, approach, adaptability, intensity, mood, persistence, distractibility, and threshold. A profile of the infant is obtained against standardized scores, and a diagnostic cluster is obtained that describes the infant as either easy, intermediate low, slow to warm up, intermediate high, or difficult. Carey (1981) reported internal consistency of the dimensions of temperament ranging from .49 to .71 with retest reliabilities ranging from .66 to .81. At 4 months the Cronbach reliabilities for 207 cases in this study were disappointing for the categories of intensity (.06), threshold to stimulus (.27), and distractibility (.38). Other categories fell in a more acceptable range: activity, .59; rhythmicity, .73; approach–withdrawal, .62; adapta-

TABLE 5 Factor Loadings for Factors Utilized in Analysis at Four and Eight Months

Variable	Factor loading[a]	Final communality estimates	Eigenvalue
Factors at 4 months			
Maternal health status, factor 1			
Overall general health	.645	.596	1.72
Feelings since one month	.464	.739	
Sum of problems	.717	.711	
Under physician care	.756	.720	
Infant growth, factor 1			
Motor development	.841	.819	1.69
Social development	.841	.819	
Weight gain	.410	.711	
Length grown	.333	.719	
Factors at 8 months			
Maternal health status, factor 1			
Feelings since 4 months	-.610	.393	1.61
Overall health rating	.858	.742	
Sum problems	.704	.497	
Infant health status			
Sum infant illnesses	.877	.786	1.97
Type of medical care	.632	.399	
Number of health problems	.844	.781	
Infant growth and development			
Motor development	.486	.732	1.57
Social development	.566	.727	
Weight	.700	.752	
Length	.736	.752	

[a]Scoring reversed on negative loadings.

TABLE 6 Factor Loadings for Factors Utilized For Analysis at One Year

Variable	Factor loading[a]	Final communality estimates	Eigenvalue
Maternal health status			
Overall health rating	.780	.608	1.69
Feelings since 8 months	.692	.479	
Sum problems	.777	.604	
Infant health status			
Sum illnesses	.813	.661	1.32
Type of medical care	.813	.661	
Infant growth, factor 1			
Motor development	.713	.683	1.48
Social development	.630	.704	
Weight	.541	.654	
Length	.630	.649	
Maternal role attainment index, factor 1			
Maternal behavior	.684	.594	1.53
Feelings about baby	.553	.497	
Gratifications in role	.493	.665	
Ways handling irritating behavior	-.466	.659	
Infant growth	.546	.298	
Maternal temperament adaptability factor			
Approach/withdrawal	.646	.419	2.68
Adaptability	.800	.640	
Intensity	-.627	.393	
Quality mood	.767	.588	
Persistence	.584	.341	
Threshold to stimulus	.552	.305	

[a]Scoring reversed on negative loadings, except for maternal temperament intensity.

bility, .60; mood quality, .58; and persistence, .49. At 8 months the reliabilities were higher, ranging from .43 to .84.

Because of the low reliabilities of several dimensions of temperament at 4 months, the diagnostic clusters were not entered into the regression analyses, but the infant traits of rhythmicity, approach-withdrawal, adaptability, and persistence were used. At 8 and 12 months the diagnostic cluster was used for regression analyses.

STATISTICAL TECHNIQUES

The process of data analysis followed a series of steps. For all nominal data, chi-square tests were done to determine group differences. Kruskal-Wallis chi-square tests were done for testing ranked data, and general linear models procedures that included F tests followed by Duncan's multiple range tests were used for interval data to find where the differences were (SAS Institute, 1979). Reliabilities of measures were established using the Cronbach alpha measure of internal consistency (Nie, Hull, Jenkins, Steinbrenner, & Bent, 1975) where appropriate. Spearman rho correlations were done with ranked variables, point biserial correlations between ranked and interval data, and Pearson Product Moment correlations were utilized for interval data. Several items from the data that were more discriminating in measuring a specific variable, such as support or health, were subjected to principal component analysis to derive a single factor (SAS Institute, 1979). This reduced two or more variables to a more meaningful structure and contributed to more valid measures.

Because of the large numbers of variables under study it was important to rule out the possibility of chance correlations and/or sampling. There was a random selection of two-thirds of the total sample as an index set. The remaining one-third of the sample served as a validation set. Regression functions were derived using the index set and then used to generate predictions for the validation set. Correlations of the observed and predicted values were measures of the success of the regression. Index and validation sets were then combined for a final analysis on the maximum number of subjects to determine the best regression weights. This process was planned for each of the age groups; however, the number of subjects in Group 1 and those with incomplete data on one or more items rendered the tests on groups invalid because of the small number of subjects-to-variables ratio.

At *early postpartum,* correlations between the observed scores (index set) and predicted scores in the validation sets only approached significance: attachment, $r = .20$, $p < .06$; NPI-1, $r = -.20$, $p < .06$. Correlations between the observed scores and predicted scores in the validation sets were all significant at *1 month*: NPI-2, $r = .26$, $p < .03$; gratification, $r = .31$, $p < .006$; maternal behavior, $r = .31$, $p < .006$; feelings of love for infant, $r = .34$, $p < .002$; and ways of handling irritating child behavior, $r = .24$, $p < .03$. At *4 months* predicted scores correlated significantly with observed scores as follows: gratification, $r = .30$, $p = .005$; feelings of love for the infant, $r = .43$, $p = .0001$; and maternal behavior, $r = .43$, $p = .0001$. However, the growth and development factor was not predictable from variables tested in this sample at 4 months, $r = .17$, $p = .11$. At *8 months,* predicted scores correlated significantly with observed scores as follows: observer-rated maternal behavior, $r = .57$, $p = .0001$; ways of handling irritating child behaviors, $r = .42$, $p = .0001$; and gratification in the role, $r = .32$, $p < .003$. The scores for feelings of love for the infant approached significance ($r = .20$, $p < .07$), but the growth and development factor was totally unpredictable ($r = .11$, $p = .34$). At *12 months* correlations between predicted and observed scores were significant for the following: maternal behavior, $r = .56$, $p = .0001$; feelings of love for the infant, $r = .27$, $p < .02$; ways of handling irritating child behavior, $r = .48$, $p = .0001$; and the maternal role index factor, $r = .38$, $p < .002$. Gratification in the role approached significance ($r = .20$, $p < .09$), and the growth and development factor was totally unpredictable as it had been earlier ($r = .11$, $p = .37$).

Stepwise regression analyses rather than hierarchical regression analyses were done because the study was exploratory, seeking to determine the best predictors of the maternal role attainment variables.

In reporting percentages of behaviors observed throughout the book, except for predictive regressions, means, and standard deviations, all numbers were rounded to the nearest whole number.

FACTOR LOADINGS

Tables 3 to 6 include the factor items, factor loading, final communality estimates, and the eigenvalue for each factor for the five test periods. To be acceptable, factors had to have an eigenvalue of 1 or greater.

References

Abernethy, V. D. (1973). Social network and response to the maternal role. *International Journal of Sociology of the Family, 3,* 86–92.

Adams, M. (1963). Early concerns of primigravida mothers regarding infant care activities. *Nursing Research, 12,* 72–77.

Affonso, D. D. (1977). "Missing pieces"—a study of postpartum feelings. *Birth and the Family Journal, 4,* 159–164.

Affonso, D. D., & Domino, G. (1984). Postpartum depression: A review. *Birth, 11,* 231–235.

Ainsfeld, E., & Lipper, E. (1983). Early contact, social support, and mother-infant bonding. *Pediatrics, 72,* 79–83.

Arizmendi, T. G., & Affonso, D. D. (1984). Research on psychosocial factors and postpartum depression: A critique. *Birth, 11,* 237–240.

Arnold, D. (1980). *The adolescent mother: A comparison of her self-concept and her perceived mothering skills.* Unpublished master's thesis, Texas Woman's University, Denton, TX.

Associated Press. (1983, October 11). Women workers increase sharply. *San Francisco Chronicle,* p. 2.

Bakeman, R., & Brown, J. V. (1980). Early interaction: Consequences for social and mental development at three years. *Child Development, 51,* 437–447.

Baldwin, A. L. (1967). *Theories of child development.* New York: John Wiley & Sons.

Ballou, J. W. (1978). *The Psychology of Pregnancy.* Lexington, MA: Lexington Books.

Bampton, B., Jones, J., & Mancini, J. (1981). Initial mothering patterns of low-income black primiparas. *JOGN Nursing, 10,* 174–178.

Barnard, K. (1981). Closing. *Birth Defects: Original Article Series, 17*(6), 285–288.

Barnard, K. E., & Eyres, S. J. (1979, June). *Child health assessment. Part 2: The first year of life.* (DHEW Publication No. HRA 79-25). Washington, D.C.: U.S. Government Printing Office.

357

Barrera, M., Jr. (1981). Social support in the adjustment of pregnant adolescents. In B. H. Gottlieb (Ed.), *Social networks and social support* (pp. 69–96). Beverly Hills, CA: Sage Publications.

Bates, J. E. (1980). The concept of difficult temperament. *Merrill-Palmer Quarterly, 26,* 299–319.

Bates, J. E., Freeland, C. A. B., & Lounsbury, M. L. (1979). Measurement of infant difficultness. *Child Development, 50,* 794–803.

Bell, R. Q. (1974). Contributions of human infants to caregiving and social interaction. In M. Lewis & L. S. Rosenblum (Eds.), *The effect of the infant on its caregiver* (pp. 1–19). New York: John Wiley & Sons.

Bell, S. M., & Ainsworth, M. D. S. (1972). Infant crying and maternal responsiveness. *Child Development, 43,* 1171–1190.

Benedek, T. (1959). Parenthood as a developmental phase. *Journal of the American Psychoanalytic Association, 7,* 389–417.

Berger, A., & Winter, S. T. (1980). Attitudes and knowledge of secondary school girls concerning breast feeding. *Clinical Pediatrics, 19,* 825–826.

Bibring, G. L., Dwyer, T. F., & Valenstein, A. F. (1961). A study of the psychological processes in pregnancy and of the earliest mother-child relationship. *Psychoanalytic Study of the Child, 16,* 9–24.

Birdsong, L. S. (1981). Loss and grieving in cesarean mothers. In C. F. Kehoe (Ed.), *The cesarean experience* (pp. 187–209). New York: Appleton-Century-Crofts.

Bishop, B. (1976). A guide to assessing parenting capabilities. *American Journal of Nursing, 76,* 1784–1787.

Blackburn, S. (1983). Fostering behavioral development of high-risk infants. *JOGN Nursing, May/June Supplement,* 76s–86s.

Blank, M. (1964). Some maternal influences on infants' rates of sensorimotor development. *Journal of American Academy of Child Psychiatry, 3,* 668–687.

Bonica, J. J. (1960). *An atlas on mechanisms and pathways of pain in labor.* North Chicago: Abbott Laboratories.

Boss, P. G. (1980). Normative family stress: Family boundary changes across the life-span. *Family Relations, 29,* 445–450.

Bradley, C. F. (1983). Psychological consequences of intervention in the birth process. *Canadian Journal Behavioral Science/Revue Canadienne Sciences Comportement, 15,* 422–437.

Bradley, C. F., Ross, S. E., & Warnyca, J. (1983). A prospective study of mothers' attitudes and feelings following cesarean and vaginal births. *Birth, 10,* 79–83.

Brazelton, T. B. (1969). *Infants and mothers.* New York: Dell.

Brazelton, T. B. (1979). Behavioral competence of the newborn infant. *Seminars in Perinatology, 3,* 35–43.

Brazelton, T. B., & Als, H. (1979). Four early stages in the development of mother-infant interaction. *Psychoanalytic Study of the Child, 34,* 349–369.

Breen, D. (1975). *The birth of a first child.* London: Tavistock.

Brink, P. J. (1982). An anthropological perspective on parenting. In J. Horowitz, C. B. Hughes, & B. J. Perdue (Eds.), *Parenting Reassessed* (pp. 66–84). Englewood Cliffs, NJ: Prentice-Hall.

Broman, S. H. (1981). Longterm development of children born to teenagers. In K. S. Scott, T. Field, & E. Robertson (Eds.), *Teenage parents and their offspring* (pp. 195-224). New York: Grune & Stratton.

Broussard, E. R. (1976). Neonatal prediction and outcome at 10/11 years. *Child Psychiatry and Human Development, 7,* 85-93.

Broussard, E. R., & Hartner, M. S. S. (1970). Maternal perception of the neonate as related to development. *Child Psychiatry and Human Development, 1,* 16-25.

Broussard, E. R., & Hartner, M. S. S. (1971). Further considerations regarding maternal perception of the newborn. In J. Hellmuth (Ed.), *Exceptional infant* (Vol. 2) (pp. 432-449). New York: Brunner/Mazel.

Brown, C. A. (1978). Teen-age mother's well-child clinic. *Pediatric Nursing, 4*(3), 27-31.

Brown, J. V., Bakeman, R., Synder, P. A., Fredrickson, W. T., Morgan, S. T., & Hepler, R. (1975). Interactions of black inner-city mothers with their newborn infants. *Child Development, 46,* 677-686.

Brown, L. S. (1967). Effectiveness of nursing visits to primigravida mothers. *Canadian Nurse, 63*(1), 45-50.

Bruhn, J. G., & Philips, B. U. (1984). Measuring social support: A synthesis of current approaches. *Journal of Behavioral Medicine, 7,* 151-169.

Brunnquell, D., Crichton, L., & Egeland, B. (1981). Maternal personality and attitude in disturbances of child rearing. *American Journal of Orthopsychiatry, 51,* 680-691.

Bull, M. J. (1981). Change in concerns of first-time mothers after one week at home. *JOGN Nursing, 10,* 391-394.

Bull, M., & Lawrence, D. (1985). Mothers' use of knowledge during the first postpartum weeks. *JOGN Nursing, 14,* 315-320.

Burks, J., & Rubenstein, M. (1979). *Temperament styles in adult interaction: Applications in psychotherapy.* New York: Brunner/Mazel.

Burr, W. R., Leigh, G. K., Day, R. D., & Constantine, J. (1979). Symbolic interaction and the family. In W. R. Burr, R. Hill, F. I. Nye, & I. L. Reiss (Eds.), *Contemporary theories about the family* (Vol. 2; pp. 42-111). New York: Free Press.

Buss, A. H., & Plomin, R. (1975). *A temperament theory of personality development.* New York: John Wiley & Sons.

Caldwell, B. M., Hersher, L., Lipton, E. L., Richmond, J. B., Stern, G. A., Eddy, E., Drachman, R., & Rothman, A. (1963). Mother-infant interaction in monomatric and polymatric families. *American Journal of Orthopsychiatry, 33,* 653-664.

Caldwell, J. C. (1981). Maternal education as a factor in child mortality. *World Health Forum, 2*(1), 75.

Camp, B. W., Burgess, D., Morgan, L., & Malpiede, D. (1984). Infants of adolescent mothers. *American Journal of Diseases of Children, 138,* 243-246.

Campbell, S. B. G. (1979). Mother-infant interaction as a function of maternal ratings of temperament. *Child Psychiatry and Human Development, 10*(2), 67-76.

Campbell, S. B. G., & Taylor, P. M. (1979). Bonding and attachment: Theoretical issues. *Seminars in Perinatology, 3,* 3-13.

Caplan, G. (1959). *Concepts of mental health and consultation.* Washington, D.C.: U.S. Dept. of Health, Education, and Welfare.

Carey, W. B. (1970). A simplified method for measuring infant temperament. *Journal of Pediatrics, 77,* 188-194.

Carey, W. B. (1981). The importance of temperament-environment interaction for child health and development. In M. Lewis & L. A. Rosenblum (Eds.), *The uncommon child* (pp. 31-55). New York: Plenum Press.

Carey, W. B., & McDevitt, S. C. (1978). Revision of the Infant Temperament Questionnaire. *Pediatrics, 61,* 735-738.

Carlson, S. E. (1976). The irreality of postpartum: Observations on the subjective experience. *JOGN Nursing, 5*(5), 28-30.

Carter-Jessop, L. (1981). Promoting maternal attachment through prenatal intervention. *MCN, 6,* 107-112.

Caudill, W., & Weinstein, H. (1969). Maternal care and infant behavior in Japan and America. *Psychiatry, 32,* 12-43.

Caulfield, C., Disbrow, M. A., & Smith, M. (1977). Determining indicators of potential for child abuse and neglect: Analytical problems in methodological research. *Communicating Nursing Research, 10,* 141-162.

Chamberlin, R. W., Szumowski, E. K., & Zastowny, T. R. (1979). An evaluation of efforts to educate mothers about child development in pediatric office practices. *American Journal of Public Health, 69,* 875-886.

Chao, Y. (1983). Conceptual behavior of Chinese mothers in relation to their newborn infants. *Journal of Advanced Nursing, 8,* 303-310.

Charles, A. G., Norr, K. L., Block, C. R., Meyering, S., & Meyers, E. (1978). Obstetric and psychological effects of psychoprophylactic preparation for childbirth. *American Journal of Obstetrics and Gynecology, 131,* 413-428.

Chassan, J. B. (1979). *Research Design in Clinical Psychology and Psychiatry* (2nd ed.). New York: John Wiley.

Chertok, L. (1969). *Motherhood and personality.* London: Tavistock.

Chodorow, N. (1978). *The Reproduction of Mothering.* Berkeley, CA: University of California Press.

Clark, A. L. (1975). Labor and birth: Expectations and outcomes. *Nursing Forum, 14,* 413-428.

Cogan, R., & Edmunds, E. P. (1980). Pronominalization: A linguistic facet of the maternal-paternal sensitive period. *Nursing Research, 29,* 225-227.

Cohen, R. L. (1966). Pregnancy stress and maternal perceptions of infant endowment. *Journal of Mental Subnormality, 12*(22), 18-23.

Cohen, R. L. (1979). Maladaptation to pregnancy. *Seminars in Perinatology, 3,* 15-24.

Cohler, B. J. (1984). Parenthood, psychopathology, and child care. In R. S. Cohen, B. J. Cohler, & S. H. Weissman (Eds.), *Parenthood: A psychodynamic perspective* (pp. 119-147). New York: Guilford Press.

Cohler, B. J., Gallant, D. H., Grunebaum, H. U., Weiss, J. L., Hartman, C. R., & Gamer, E. (1980). Child care attitudes and development of young children of mentally ill and well mothers. *Psychological Reports, 46,* 31-46.

Cohler, B. J., & Grunebaum, H. U. (1981). *Mothers, grandmothers, and daughters.* New York: John Wiley & Sons.

Cohler, B. J., Grunebaum, H. U., Weiss, J. L., Hartman, C. R., & Gallant, D. H. (1976). Child care attitudes and adaptation to the maternal role among mentally ill and well mothers. *American Journal of Orthopsychiatry, 46,* 123-134.

Cohler, B. J., Weiss, J. L., & Grunebaum, H. U. (1970). Child-care attitudes and emotional disturbance among mothers of young children. *Genetic Psychology Monographs, 82,* 3–47.

Colletta, N. D. (1981). Social support and the risk of maternal rejection by adolescent mothers. *Journal of Psychology, 109,* 191–197.

Colletta, N. D., & Gregg, C. H. (1981). Adolescent mothers' vulnerability to stress. *Journal of Nervous and Mental Disease, 169,* 50–54.

Colman, A., & Colman, L. (1973). *Pregnancy: The psychological experience.* New York: Seabury Press.

Colman, L. L., & Colman, A. D. (1973/74). Pregnancy as an altered state of consciousness. *Birth and the Family Journal, 1,* 7–11.

Comer, R., & Laird, J. D. (1975). Choosing to suffer as a consequence of expecting to suffer: Why do people do it? *Journal of Personality and Social Psychology, 32,* 92–101.

Conger, R. D., Burgess, R. L., & Barrett, C. (1979). Child abuse related to life change and perceptions of illness: Some preliminary findings. *Family Coordinator, 28,* 73–78.

Cox, B. E., & Smith, E. C. (1982). The mother's self-esteem after a cesarean delivery. *MCN, 7,* 309–314.

Cranley, M. S. (1981a). Development of a tool for the measurement of maternal attachment during pregnancy. *Nursing Research, 30,* 281–284.

Cranley, M. S. (1981b). Roots of attachment: The relationship of parents with their unborn. *Birth Defects: Original Article Series, 17*(6), 59–83.

Cranley, M. S., Hedahl, K. J., & Pegg, S. H. (1983). Women's perceptions of vaginal and cesarean deliveries. *Nursing Research, 32,* 10–15.

Crawford, G. (1985). A theoretical model of support network conflict experienced by new mothers. *Nursing Research, 34,* 100–102.

Crnic, K. A., Greenberg, M. T., Ragozin, A. S., Robinson, N. M., & Basham, R. B. (1983). Effects of stress and social support on mothers and premature and full-term infants. *Child Development, 54,* 209–217.

Crnic, K. A., Greenberg, M. T., Robinson, N. M., & Ragozin, A. S. (1984). Maternal stress and social support: Effects on the mother-infant relationship from birth to eighteen months. *American Journal of Orthopsychiatry, 54,* 224–235.

Crockenberg, S. B. (1981). Infant irritability, mother responsiveness, and social support influences on the security of infant-mother attachment. *Child Development, 52,* 857–865.

Crockenberg, S. B., & Smith, P. (1982). Antecedents of mother-infant interaction and infant irritability in the first three months of life. *Infant Behavior and Development, 5,* 105–119.

Cronenwett, L. R. (1980). Elements and outcomes of a postpartum support group program. *Research in Nursing and Health, 3,* 33–41.

Cronenwett, L. R., & Kunst-Wilson, W. (1981). Stress, social support and the transition to fatherhood. *Nursing Research, 30,* 196–201.

Curry, M. A. (1983). Variables related to adaptation to motherhood in "normal" primiparous women. *JOGN Nursing, 12,* 115–121.

Curtis, F. L. S. (1974). Observations of unwed pregnant adolescents. *American Journal of Nursing, 74,* 100–102.

Davis, J. H., & Eyer, J. (1984). Sorting out new mothers' learning priorities on home visits. *Home Healthcare Nurse, 2*(2), 38–42.

DeChateau, P. (1976). The influence of early contact on maternal and infant behavior in primiparas. *Birth and the Family Journal, 3,* 149-155.

DeLissovoy, V. (1973). Child care by adolescent parents. *Children Today, 2*(4), 22-25.

Deutsch, H. (1945). *The psychology of women* (Vol. 2). New York: Grune & Stratton.

Deutsch, H. (1967). *Selected problems of adolescence.* New York: International Universities Press.

Deutscher, M. (1970). Brief family therapy in the course of first pregnancy: A clinical note. *Contemporary Psychoanalysis, 7,* 21-35.

Disbrow, M. A., & Doerr, H. O. (1982). *Measures to predict child abuse: A validation study.* Final Report, Project Grant MC-R-530351. Seattle: University of Washington.

Disbrow, M. A., Doerr, H. O., & Caulfield, C. (1977, March). *Measures to predict child abuse.* Final Report, Project Grant MC-R-530351. Seattle: University of Washington.

Disbrow, M. A., Doerr, H., & Caulfield, C. (1977). Measuring the components of potential for child abuse and neglect. *Journal of Child Abuse and Neglect, 1,* 279-296.

Doering, S. G., & Entwisle, D. R. (1975). Preparation during pregnancy and ability to cope with labor and delivery. *American Journal of Orthopsychiatry, 45,* 825-837.

Egeland, B., Breitenbucher, M., & Rosenberg, D. (1980). Prospective study of the significance of life stress in the etiology of child abuse. *Journal of Consulting and Clinical Psychology, 48,* 195-205.

Entwistle, R. R., & Doering, S. G. (1981). *The first birth: A family turning point.* Baltimore: Johns Hopkins University Press.

Erikson, E. H. (1959). Identity and the life cycle. *Psychological Issues* [Monograph]. *1*(1), 1-171.

Fanaroff, A. A., Kennell, J. H., & Klaus, M. H. (1972). Follow-up of low birth weight infants—the predictive value of maternal visiting patterns. *Pediatrics, 49,* 287-290.

Feiring, D. (1976). *The influence of the child and secondary parent on maternal behavior toward a social systems view of early infant-mother attachment.* Unpublished doctoral dissertation, University of Pittsburgh, Pittsburgh. (University Microfilms No. 76-347)

Field, T. (1981). Gaze behavior of normal and high-risk infants during early interactions. *Journal of the American Academy of Child Psychiatry, 20,* 308-317.

Field, T., Widmayer, S., Greenberg, R., & Stoller, S. (1982). Effects of parent training on teenage mothers and their infants. *Pediatrics, 69,* 703-707.

Fillmore, C. J., & Taylor, K. W. (1976). Infant care concerns of primigravida mothers and nursing practice: Two models. *Nursing Papers, 8*(1), 15-25.

Finkelstein, J. W., Finkelstein, J. A., Christie, M., Roden, M., & Shelton, C. (1982). Teenage pregnancy and parenthood: Outcomes for mother and child. *Journal of Adolescent Health Care, 3,* 1-7.

Fitts, W. H. (1965). *Tennessee self concept scale manual.* Nashville, TN: Counselor Recordings and Tests.

Foman, S. J., Filer, L. J., Jr., Anderson, T. A., & Ziegler, E. E. (1979). Recommendations for feeding normal infants. *Pediatrics, 63,* 52-59.

Frommer, E. A., & O'Shea, G. (1973a). Antenatal identification of women liable to have problems in managing their infants. *British Journal of Psychiatry, 123,* 149-156.

Frommer, E. A., & O'Shea, G. (1973b). The importance of childhood experience in relation to problems of marriage and family-building. *British Journal of Psychiatry, 123,* 157-160.

Garn, S. M., LaVelle, M., Pesick, S. D., & Ridella, S. A. (1984). Are pregnant teenagers still in rapid growth? *American Journal Diseases of Children, 138,* 32-34.

Garn, S. M., & Petzold, A. S. (1983). Characteristics of mother and child in teen-age pregnancy. *American Journal Diseases of Children, 137,* 365-368.

Gillman, R. D. (1968). The dreams of pregnant women and maternal adaptation. *American Journal of Orthopsychiatry, 38,* 688-692.

Gloger-Tippelt, G. (1983). A process model of the pregnancy course. *Human Development, 26,* 134-148.

Goode, W. J. (1960). A theory of role strain. *American Sociological Review, 25,* 488-496.

Gordon, R., Kapostins, E. E., & Gordon, K. K. (1965). Factors in postpartum emotional adjustment. *Obstetrics and Gynecology, 25,* 158-166.

Gottlieb, L. (1978). Maternal attachment in primiparas. *JOGN Nursing, 7*(1), 39-44.

Govaerts, K., & Patino, E. (1981). Attachment behavior of the Egyptian mother. *International Journal of Nursing Studies, 18,* 53-60.

Grant, J. A., & Heald, F. P. (1972). Complications of adolescent pregnancy: Survey of the literature on fetal outcome in adolescence. *Clinical Pediatrics, 11,* 567-570.

Gray, J. D., Cutler, C. A., Dean, J. G., & Kempe, C. H. (1980). Prediction and prevention of child abuse. In P. M. Taylor (Ed.), *Parent-infant relationships* (pp. 335-347). New York: Grune & Stratton.

Green, A. H. (1976). A psychodynamic approach to the study and treatment of child-abusing parents. *Journal of the American Academy of Child Psychiatry, 8,* 414-429.

Green, A. H., Gaines, R. W., & Sandgrund, A. (1974). Child abuse: Pathological syndrome of family interaction. *American Journal of Psychiatry, 8,* 882-886.

Green, J. A., Gustafson, G. E., & West, M. J. (1980). Effects of infant development on mother-infant interactions. *Child Development, 51,* 199-207.

Grossman, F. K., Eichler, L. S., Winickoff, S. A., Anzalone, M. K., Gofseyeff, M. H., & Sargent, S. P. (1980). *Pregnancy, birth, and parenthood.* San Francisco: Jossey-Bass.

Grubb, C. A. (1980). Perceptions of time by multiparous women in relation to themselves and others during the first postpartal month. *Maternal-Child Nursing Journal, 9,* 225-331.

Gruis, M. (1977). Beyond maternity: Postpartum concerns of mothers. *MCN, The American Journal of Maternal Child Nursing, 2,* 182-188.

Gunther, L. M. (1963). Psychopathology and stress in the life experience of mothers of premature infants. *American Journal of Obstetrics and Gynecology, 86,* 333-340.

Hall, L. A. (1980). Effect of teaching on primiparas' perceptions of their newborn. *Nursing Research, 29,* 317-322.

Hansson, R. O., Mathews, K. E., Jr., & Disbrow, M. (1978). Empathy as a personality construct. In E. Stotland, K. E. Mathews, Jr., S. E. Sherman, R. O. Hansson, & B. Z. Richardson (Eds.), *Empathy, fantasy and helping* (pp. 87-96). Beverley Hills, CA: Sage Publications.

Hardman, M. (1975). The younger vs. the older adolescent black mother taking on the nurturing-mothering role. *Clinical Conference Papers 1973* (No. G-94 3M 2/75). Kansas City, MO: American Nurses' Association.

Hardy, J. B., Welcher, D. W., Stanley, J., & Dallas, J. R. (1978). Long-range outcome of adolescent pregnancy. *Clinical Obstetrics and Gynecology, 21*, 1215-1232.

Harmon, D., & Kogan, K. L. (1980). Social class and mother-child interaction. *Psychological Reports, 46*, 1075-1084.

Harrell, J. E., & Ridley, C. A. (1975). Substitute child care, maternal employment and quality of mother-child interaction. *Journal of Marriage and the Family, 37*, 556-564.

Harris, B. (1979). Two lives, one 24-hour-day. In A. Roland & B. Harris (Eds.), *Career and motherhood* (pp. 25-45). New York: Human Sciences Press.

Hayter, J. (1980). The rhythm of sleep. *American Journal of Nursing, 80*, 457-461.

Hees-Stauthamer, J. C. (1985). *The first pregnancy: An integrating principle in female psychology.* Ann Arbor, MI: UMI Research Press.

Helfer, R. (1974). Relationship between lack of bonding and child abuse and neglect. In M. H. Klaus, T. Leger, & M. A. Trause (Eds.), *Maternal attachment and mothering disorders: A round table.* Brunswick, NH: Johnson and Johnson.

Henderson, S. (1977). The social network, support and neurosis: The function of attachment in adult life. *British Journal of Psychiatry, 131*, 185-191.

Highley, B. L. (1967). Maternal role identity. In *Defining clinical content in graduate nursing programs in maternal and child health nursing* (pp. 31-34). Boulder, CO: Western Interstate Commission for Higher Education.

Hobbs, D. F., Jr. (1965). Parenthood as crisis: A third study. *Journal of Marriage and the Family, 30*, 367-372.

Hobbs, D. F., Jr., & Cole, S. P. (1976). Transition to parenthood: A decade replication. *Journal of Marriage and the Family, 38*, 723-731.

Hofferth, S. L., & Moore, K. A. (1979). Early childbearing and later economic well-being. *American Sociological Review, 44*, 784-815.

Hogan, D. P. (1980). The transition to adulthood as a career contingency. *American Sociological Review, 45*, 261-276.

Holmes, T. H. (1978). Life situations, emotions, and disease. *Psychosomatics, 19*, 747-754.

Hopkins, J., Marcus, M., & Campbell, S. B. (1984). Postpartum depression: A critical review. *Psychological Bulletin, 95*, 498-515.

Horon, I. L., Strobino, D. M., & MacDonald, H. M. (1983). Birth weights among infants born to adolescent and young adult women. *American Journal of Obstetrics and Gynecology, 146*, 444-449.

House, J. S. (1981). *Work stress and social support.* Reading, MA: Addison-Wesley.

Hubert, N. C., Wachs, T. D., Peters-Martin, P., & Gandour, M. J. (1982). The study of early temperament: Measurement and conceptual issues. *Child Development, 53*, 571-600.

Humenick, S. S., & Bugen, L. A. (1981). Mastery: The key to childbirth satisfaction? A study. *Birth, 8,* 84–90.

Hunter, R. S., Kilstrom, N., Kraybill, E. N., & Loda, F. (1978). Antecedents of child abuse and neglect in premature infants: A prospective study in a newborn intensive care unit. *Pediatrics, 61,* 629–635.

Jarrett, G. E. (1982). Childrearing patterns of young mothers: Expectations, knowledge, and practices. *MCN American Journal of Maternal Child Nursing, 7,* 119–124.

Jimenez, M. G., & Newton, N. (1982). Job orientation and adjustment to pregnancy and early motherhood. *Birth, 9,* 157–163.

Johnson, R. G. (1976). *Tests and measurements in child development handbook II* (Vol. 2, pp. 810–813). San Francisco: Jossey-Bass.

Jones, F. A., Green, V., & Krauss, D. R. (1980). Maternal responsiveness of primiparous mothers during the postpartum period: Age differences. *Pediatrics, 65,* 629–635.

Jordan, A. D. (1973a). Evaluation of a family-centered maternity care hospital program. Part I: Introduction, design, and testing. *JOGN Nursing, 2*(1), 13–35.

Jordan, A. D. (1973b). Evaluation of a family-centered maternity care hospital program. Part II: Ancillary findings and parents' comments. *JOGN Nursing, 2*(2), 15–17.

Jordan, A. D. (1973c). Evaluation of a family-centered maternity care hospital program. Part III. Implications and recommendations. *JOGN Nursing, 2*(3), 15–23.

Josten, L. (1981). Prenatal assessment guide for illuminating possible problems with parenting. *MCN, 6,* 113–117.

Kahn, R. L., & Antocucci, T. C. (1980). Convoys over the life course: Attachment, roles, and social support. In P. B. Baltes & O. Brim (Eds.), *Life-span development and behavior* (Vol. 3, pp. 253–286). New York: Academic Press.

Kellam, S. G., Adams, R. G., Brown, C. H., & Ensminger, M. E. (1982). The long-term evolution of the family structure of teenage and older mothers. *Journal of Marriage and the Family, 44,* 539–554.

Kennedy, J. C. (1973). The high-risk maternal-infant acquaintance process. *Nursing Clinics of North America, 8*(3), 549–556.

Killien, M. G. (1985, May). Sleep patterns and adequacy during the postpartum period. Paper presented at Eighteenth Annual Communicating Nursing Research Conference, Seattle, WA.

Klaus, M. H., Jerauld, R., Kreger, N. C., McAlpine, W., Steffa, M., & Kennell, J. H. (1972). Maternal attachment: Importance of the first postpartum days. *New England Journal of Medicine, 286*(9), 460–463.

Kohn, C. L., Nelson, A., & Weiner, S. (1980). Gravidas' responses to realtime ultrasound fetal image. *JOGN Nursing, 9,* 77–79.

Kontos, D. (1978). A study of the effects of extended mother-infant contact on maternal behavior at one and three months. *Birth and Family Journal, 5,* 133–140.

Kronstadt, D., Oberklaid, F., Ferb, T. E., & Swartz, J. P. (1979). Infant behavior and maternal adaptation in the first six months of life. *American Journal of Orthopsychiatry, 49,* 454–464.

Kutzner, S. K. (1984). Adaptation to motherhood from postpartum to early childhood. Unpublished doctoral dissertation, University of Michigan, Ann Arbor (University Microfilms No. 8422272).

Lamb, M. E. (1982). The bonding phenomenon: Misinterpretations and their implications. *Journal of Pediatrics, 101,* 555-557.

Lamb, M. E. (1983). Early mother-neonate contact and the mother-child relationship. *Journal of Child Psychology and Psychiatry, 24,* 487-494.

Lamb, M. E., Garn, S. M., & Keating, M. T. (1981). Correlations between sociability and cognitive performance among eight-month-olds. *Child Development, 52,* 711-713.

Larsen, V. L. (1966). Stresses of the childbearing year. *American Journal of Public Health, 56,* 32-36.

Larsen, V. L., Evans, T., Brodsack, J., Dungey, L., Elliott, J., Harmon, J., Kaess, D., Kaess, S., Karman, I., Main, D., Martin, L., Ramer, J., & Pearson, J. W. (1966). Attitudes and stresses affecting perinatal adjustment. Final Report. NIMH Grant: MH- 01381-01-02. Washington, DC: NIMH.

Larson, C. P. (1980). Efficacy of prenatal and postpartum home visits on child health and development. *Pediatrics, 66,* 191-197.

Lawrence, R. A., & Merritt, T. A. (1981). Infants of adolescent mothers: Perinatal, neonatal, and infancy outcome. *Seminars in Perinatology, 5,* 19-32.

Lebe, D. (1982). Individuation of women. *Psychoanalytic Review, 69,* 63-73.

Lederman, E., Lederman, R. P., Work, B. A., Jr., & McCann, D. S. (1981). Maternal psychological and physiologic correlates of fetal-newborn health status. *American Journal of Obstetrics and Gynecology, 139,* 956-958.

Lederman, R. P. (1984). *Psychosocial adaptation in pregnancy.* Englewood Cliffs, NJ: Prentice Hall.

Lederman, R. P., Lederman, E., Work, B. A., Jr., & McCann, D. (1979). Relationship of psychological factors in pregnancy to progress in labor. *Nursing Research, 28,* 94-97.

Leifer, M. (1977). Psychological changes accompanying pregnancy and motherhood. *Genetic Psychology Monographs, 95,* 55-96.

Leifer, M. (1980). *Psychological effects of motherhood.* New York: Praeger.

Levenson, P., Hale, J., Tirado, C., & Hollier, M. (1979). A comprehensive interactional model for health education delivery to teenage mothers. *Journal of School Health, 49,* 393-396.

Levine, L., Coll, C. T. G., & Oh, W. (1985). Determinants of mother-infant interaction in adolescent mothers. *Pediatrics, 75,* 23-29.

Levinson, D. J., Darrow, C. N., Klein, E. B., Levinson, M. H., & McKee, B. (1978). *The seasons of a man's life.* New York: Alfred A. Knopf.

Levinson, G., & Shnider, S. M. (1979). Catecholamines: The effects of maternal fear and its treatment on uterine function and circulation. *Birth, 6,* 167-174.

Lewis, M., & Wilson, C. D. (1972). Infant development in lower-class American families. *Human Development, 15,* 112-127.

Lipson, J. G. (1981). Cesarean support groups: Mutual help and education. *Women & Health, 6*(3/4), 27-39.

Lipson, J. G. (1982). Effects of a support group on the emotional impact of cesarean childbirth. *Prevention in Human Services, 1*(3), 17-29.

Lipson, J. G., & Tilden, V. P. (1980). Psychological integration of the cesarean birth experience. *American Journal of Orthopsychiatry, 50,* 598-609.

Lounsbury, M. L., & Bates, J. E. (1982). The cries of infants of differing levels of perceived temperamental difficultness: Acoustic properties and effects on listeners. *Child Development, 53,* 677–686.

Lumley, J. M. (1982). Attitudes to the fetus among primigravidae. *Australian Paediatric Journal, 18,* 106–109.

Lynch, M. A. (1975). Ill-health and child abuse. *Lancet, II*(7929), 317–319.

Lynch, M. A., & Roberts, J. (1977). Predicting child abuse: Signs of bonding failure in the maternity hospital. *British Medical Journal, 1,* 624–626.

Mahler, M. S. (1968). *On human symbiosis and the vicissitudes of individuation.* New York: International Universities Press.

Mahler, M. S., Pine, F., & Bergman, A. (1975). *The psychological birth of the human infant.* New York: Basic Books.

Majewski, J. L. (1983). *The impact of perceived role conflict on the transition to the maternal role.* Unpublished doctoral dissertation, University of California, San Francisco.

Manly, P. C., McMahon, R. J., Bradley, C. F., & Davidson, P. O. (1982). Depressive attributional style and depression following childbirth. *Journal of Abnormal Psychology, 91,* 245–254.

Marut, J. S. (1978). Special needs of the cesarean mother. *MCN American Journal of Maternal Child Nursing, 4,* 202–206.

Marut, J. S., & Mercer, R. T. (1979). Comparison of primiparas' perceptions of vaginal and cesarean births. *Nursing Research, 28,* 260–266.

May, K. A. (1980). A typology of detachment/involvement styles adopted during pregnancy by first-time expectant fathers. *Western Journal of Nursing Research, 2*(2), 445–453.

McClellan, M. S., & Cabianca, W. A. (1980). Effects of early mother-infant contact following cesarean birth. *Obstetrics & Gynecology, 56,* 52–55.

McLanahan, S. S., Wedemeyer, N. V., & Adelberg, T. (1981). Network structure, social support, and psychological well-being in the single-parent family. *Journal of Marriage and the Family, 43,* 601–612.

Mead, G. H. (1934). *Mind, self, and society.* Chicago: University of Chicago Press.

Medinnus, G. R., & Curtis, F. J. (1963). The relations between maternal self acceptance and child acceptance. *Journal of Consulting Psychology, 56,* 52–55.

Melges, F. T. (1968). Postpartum psychiatric syndromes. *Psychosomatic Medicine, 30,* 95–108.

Meltzoff, A. N., & Moore, M. K. (1983). Newborn infants imitate adult facial gestures. *Child Development, 54,* 702–709.

Melzack, R., Kinch, R., Dobkin, P., Lebrun, M., & Taenzer, P. (1984). Severity of labour pain: Influence of physical as well as psychologic variables. *Canadian Medical Association Journal, 130,* 579–584.

Mercer, R. T. (1977). *Nursing care for parents at risk.* Thorofare, NJ: C. B. Slack.

Mercer, R. T. (1980). Teenage motherhood: The first year. *JOGN Nursing, 9,* 16–27.

Mercer, R. T. (1981a). A theoretical framework for studying factors that impact on the maternal role. *Nursing Research, 30,* 73–77.

Mercer, R. T. (1981b). The nurse and maternal tasks of early postpartum. *MCN The American Journal of Maternal Child Nursing, 6,* 341–345.

Mercer, R. T. (1984). Health of the children of adolescents. In E. R. McAnarney (Ed.), *The Adolescent Family* (pp. 60–66). Columbus, OH: Ross Laboratories.

Mercer, R. T. (1985a). The process of maternal role attainment over the first year. *Nursing Research, 34,* 198–203.

Mercer, R. T. (1985b). Relationship of the birth experience to later mothering behaviors. *Journal of Nurse-Midwifery, 30,* 204–211.

Mercer, R. T. (1986a). The relationship of developmental behaviors to maternal behavior. *Research in Nursing and Health, 9,* 25–33.

Mercer, R. T. (1986b). Predictors of maternal role attainment at one year post birth. *Western Journal of Nursing Research, 8*(1), 9–32.

Mercer, R. T., Hackley, K. C., & Bostrom, A. (1982). *Factors having an impact on maternal role attainment the first year of motherhood.* (Final Report of Grant MC-R-060435). San Francisco: University of California, Department of Family Health Care Nursing.

Mercer, R. T., Hackley, K. C., & Bostrom, A. G. (1983). Relationship of psychosocial and perinatal variables to perception of childbirth. *Nursing Research, 32,* 202–207.

Mercer, R. T., Hackley, K. C., & Bostrom, A. (1984a). Adolescent motherhood: Comparison of outcome with older mothers. *Journal of Adolescent Health Care, 5,* 7–13.

Mercer, R. T., Hackley, K. C., & Bostrom, A. (1984b). Social support of teenage mothers. *Birth Defects: Original Article Series, 20*(5), 245–290.

Mercer, R. T., & Marut, J. S. (1981). Comparative viewpoints: Cesarean versus vaginal childbirth. In D. D. Affonso (Ed.), *Impact of cesarean childbirth* (pp. 63–84). Philadelphia: F. A. Davis.

Mercer, R. T., & Stainton, M. C. (1984). Perceptions of the birth experience: A cross-cultural comparison. *Health Care for Women International, 5,* 29–47.

Merritt, T. A., Lawrence, R. A., & Naeye, R. L. (1980). The infants of adolescent mothers. *Pediatric Annals, 9,* 100–110.

Miller, B. C., & Sollie, D. L. (1980). Normal stresses during the transition to parenthood. *Family Relations, 29,* 459–465.

Millor, G. K. (1981). A theoretical framework for nursing research in child abuse and neglect. *Nursing Research, 30,* 78–83.

Milne, L. S., & Rich, O. J. (1981). Cognitive and affective aspects of the responses of pregnant women to sonography. *Maternal-Child Nursing Journal, 10,* 15–39.

Minde, K., Trehub, S., Corter, C., Boukydis, C., Celhoffer, L., & Marton, P. (1978). Mother-child relationships in the premature nursery: An observational study. *Pediatrics, 61,* 373–379.

Moore, K. A., & Waite, L. J. (1977). Early childbearing and educational attainment. *Family Planning Perspectives, 9,* 220–225.

Naeye, R. L. (1983). Maternal age, obstetric complications, and the outcome of pregnancy. *Obstetrics & Gynecology, 61,* 210–216.

Nakashima, I. I., & Camp, B. W. (1984). Fathers of infants born to adolescent mothers. *American Journal of Diseases of Children, 138,* 452–454.

Neeson, J. D., Patterson, K. A., Mercer, R. T., & May, K. A. (1983). Pregnancy outcome for adolescents receiving prenatal care by nurse practitioners in extended roles. *Journal of Adolescent Health Care, 4,* 94–99.

Neugarten, B. L., Moore, J. W., & Lowe, J. C. (1965). Age norms, age constraints, and adult socialization. *American Journal of Sociology, 70,* 710–717.

Neumann, C. G., & Alpaugh, M. (1976). Birthweight doubling time: A fresh look. *Pediatrics, 57,* 469–473.

Newton, L. D. (1983). Helping parents cope with infant crying. *JOGN Nursing, 12,* 199–204.

Newton, R. W., Webster, P. A. C., Binu, P. S., Maskrey, N., & Phillips, A. B. (1979). Psychosocial stress in pregnancy and its relation to the onset of premature labour. *British Medical Journal, 2*(6187), 411–413.

Nie, N. H., Hull, C. H., Jenkins, J. G., Steinbrenner, K., & Bent, D. H. (1975). *SSPS Statistical Package for the Social Sciences* (2nd ed.). New York: McGraw-Hill.

Ninio, A. (1979). The naive theory of the infant and other maternal attitudes in two subgroups in Israel. *Child Development, 50,* 976–980.

Norbeck, J. S., & Tilden, V. P. (1983). Life stress, social support, and emotional disequilibrium in complications of pregnancy: A prospective, multivariate study. *Journal of Health and Social Behavior, 24,* 30–46.

Norr, K. L., Block, C. R., Charles, A., Meyering, S., & Meyers, E. (1977). Explaining pain and enjoyment in childbirth. *Journal of Health and Social Behavior, 18,* 260–275.

Nuckolls, K. B., Cassell, J., & Kaplan, B. H. (1972). Psychosocial assets, life crisis, and the prognosis of pregnancy. *American Journal of Epidemiology, 95,* 431–441.

Nye, F. I., & Gecas, V. (1976). The role concept: Review and delineation. In F. I. Nye (Ed.), *Role structure and analysis of the family* (pp. 3–14). Beverley Hills, CA: Sage Publications.

Oakley, A. (1980). *Women confined.* New York: Schocken Books.

O'Connor, S., Vietze, P. M., Sherrod, K. B., Sandler, H. M., & Altemeier, W. A. III. (1980). Reduced incidence of parenting inadequacy following rooming-in. *Pediatrics, 66,* 176–182.

O'Hara, M. W., Neunaber, D. J., & Zekoski, E. M. (1984). Prospective study of postpartum depression: Prevalence, course, and predictive factors. *Journal of Abnormal Psychology, 93,* 158–171.

O'Hara, M. W., Rehm, L. P., & Campbell, S. B. (1983). Postpartum depression: A role for social network and life stress variables. *Journal of Nervous and Mental Disease, 171,* 336–341.

Oppel, W. C., & Royston, A. A. (1971). Teen-age births: Some social, psychological and physical sequelae. *American Journal of Public Health, 61,* 751–756.

Osofsky, H. J., & Osofsky, J. D. (1970). Adolescents as mothers: Results of a program for low-income pregnant teenagers with some emphasis upon infants' development. *American Journal of Orthopsychiatry, 40,* 825–834.

Paykel, E. S., Emms, E. M., Fletcher, J., & Rassaby, E. S. (1980). Life events and depression: A controlled study. *Archives of General Psychiatry, 136,* 753–760.

Persson-Blennow, I., & McNeil, T. F. (1981). Temperament characteristics of children in relation to gender, birth order, and social class. *American Journal of Orthopsychiatry, 51,* 710–714.

Peterson, G. H., & Mehl, L. E. (1978). Some determinants of maternal attachment. *American Journal of Psychiatry, 135,* 1168–1173.

Pickens, D. S. (1982). The cognitive processes of career-oriented primiparas in identity reformulation. *Maternal-Child Nursing Journal, 11*, 135-164.

Pollitt, E., Eichler, A. W., & Chan, C. K. (1975). Psychosocial development and behavior of mothers of failure-to-thrive children. *American Journal of Orthopsychiatry, 45*, 525-537.

Porter, L. S. (1984). Parenting enhancement among high-risk adolescents. *Nursing Clinics of North America, 19*(1), 89-102.

Porter, R. H., Cernoch, J. M., & Perry, S. (1983). The importance of odors in mother-infant interactions. *Maternal-Child Nursing Journal, 12*, 147-154.

Pridham, K. F. (1981). Infant feeding and anticipatory care: Supporting the adaptation of parents to their new babies. *Maternal-Child Nursing Journal, 10*, 111-126.

Ragozin, A. S., Basham, R. B., Crnic, K. A., Greenberg, M. T., & Robinson, N. M. (1982). Effects of maternal age on parenting role. *Developmental Psychology, 18*, 627-634.

Ralph, K. C. S. (1977). *Maternal ability to adapt to infant cues of temperament.* Unpublished doctoral dissertation, Arizona State University. University Microfilms No. 7732420.

Rees, B. L. (1980). Measuring identification with the mothering role. *Research in Nursing and Health, 3,* 49-56.

Rich, O. J. (1973). Temporal and spatial experience as reflected in the verbalizations of multiparous women during labor. *Maternal-Child Nursing Journal, 2*, 239-325.

Riesch, S. K. (1984). Occupational commitment and the quality of maternal infant interaction. *Research in Nursing and Health, 7,* 295-303.

Roberts, F. B. (1983). Infant behavior and the transition to parenthood. *Nursing Research, 32*, 213-217.

Roberts, C. J., & Rowley, J. R. (1972). A study of the association between quality of maternal care and infant development. *Psychological Medicine, 2*, 42-49.

Robertson, J. (1962). Mothering as an influence on early development. *Psychoanalytic Study of the Child, 17*, 245-264.

Robson, K. S., & Moss, H. S. (1970). Patterns and determinants of maternal attachment. *Journal of Pediatrics, 77*, 976-985.

Rock, D. L., Green, K. E., Wise, B. K., & Rock, R. D. (1984). Social support and social network scales: A psychometric review. *Research in Nursing and Health, 7,* 325-332.

Roosa, M. W., Fitzgerald, H. E., & Carlson, N. A. (1982a). Teenage and older mothers and their infants: A descriptive comparison. *Adolescence, 17*(65), 1-17.

Roosa, M. W., Fitzgerald, H. E., & Carlson, N. A. (1982b). A comparison of teenage and older mothers: A systems analysis. *Journal of Marriage and the Family, 44*, 367-377.

Ross Laboratories. (1973, February). Girls/Physical Development: Birth to 56 Weeks: Girls/Adaptive Social Development: Birth to 56 Weeks; Boys/Physical Development: Birth to 56 Weeks; Boys/Adaptive Social Development: Birth to 56 Weeks, Forms. Columbus, OH: Ross Laboratories.

Rothenberg, P. B., & Varga, P. E. (1981). The relationship between age of mother and child health and development. *American Journal of Public Health, 71*, 810-817.

Rubin, R. (1961). Basic maternal behavior. *Nursing Outlook, 9,* 683–686.

Rubin, R. (1967a). Attainment of the maternal role: Part 1. Processes. *Nursing Research, 16,* 237–245.

Rubin, R. (1967b). Attainment of the maternal role: Part 2. Models and referrants. *Nursing Research, 16,* 342–346.

Rubin, R. (1970). Cognitive style in pregnancy. *American Journal of Nursing, 70,* 502–508.

Rubin, R. (1972). Fantasy and object constancy in maternal relationships. *Maternal-Child Nursing Journal, 1,* 101–11.

Rubin, R. (1975). Maternal tasks in pregnancy. *Maternal-Child Nursing Journal, 4,* 143–153.

Rubin, R. (1977). Binding-in in the postpartum period. *Maternal-Child Nursing Journal, 6,* 67–75.

Rubin, R. (1984). *Maternal identity and the maternal experience.* New York: Springer.

Russell, C. S. (1974). Transition to parenthood: Problems and gratifications. *Journal of Marriage and the Family, 36,* 294–301.

Rutter, M. (1979). Maternal deprivation, 1972–1978: New findings, new concepts, new approaches. *Child Development, 50,* 283–305.

Saltzer, E. B., & Golden, M. P. (1985). Obesity in lower and middle socioeconomic status mothers and their children. *Research in Nursing and Health, 8,* 147–153.

Sameroff, A. J., Seifer, R., & Elias, P. K. (1982). Sociocultural variability in infant temperament ratings. *Child Development, 53,* 164–173.

Samko, M. R., & Schoenfeld, L. S. (1975). Hypnotic susceptibility and the Lamaze childbirth experience. *American Journal of Obstetrics and Gynecology, 121,* 631–636.

Sander, L. W. (1962). Issues in early mother-child interaction. *Journal of the American Academy of Child Psychiatry, 1,* 141–166.

Sandler, I. N. (1980). Social support resources, stress and maladjustment of poor children. *American Journal of Community Psychology, 8,* 41–52.

Sarason, I. G., Johnson, H. H., & Siegel, J. M. (1978). Development of the life experience survey. *Journal of Consulting and Clinical Psychology, 46,* 932–946.

SAS Institute. (1979). *SAS user's guide: 1979 edition.* Cary, NC: SAS Institute.

Schectman, K. W. (1980). Motherhood as an adult developmental stage. *American Journal of Psychoanalysis, 40,* 273–282.

Scholl, T. O., Decker, E., Karp, R. J., Greene, G., & DeSales, M. (1984). Early adolescent pregnancy: A comparative study of pregnancy outcome in young adolescents and mature women. *Journal of Adolescent Health Care, 5,* 167–171.

Shainess, N. (1980). The working wife and mother—a "new" woman? *American Journal of Psychotherapy, 34,* 374–386.

Sheehan, F. (1981). Assessing postpartum adjustment: A pilot study. *JOGN Nursing, 10,* 19–23.

Shereshefsky, P. M., & Yarrow, L. J. (1973). *Psychological aspects of a first pregnancy and early postnatal adaptation.* New York: Raven Press.

Sherwen, L. N. (1981). Fantasies during the third trimester of pregnancy. *MCN, 6,* 398–401.

Siegle, E., Bauman, K. E., Schaefer, E. S., Saunders, M. M., & Ingram, D. D. (1980). Hospital and home support during infancy: Impact on maternal attachment, child abuse and neglect, and health care utilization. *Pediatrics, 66*, 183-190.

Silverman, P. R. (1982). Transitions and models of intervention. *Annals of the American Academy of Political and Social Science, 464*, 174-187.

Simonds, M. P., & Simonds, J. F. (1981). Relationship of maternal parenting behaviors to preschool children's temperament. *Child Psychiatry and Human Development, 12*(1), 19-31.

Slavazza, K. L., Mercer, R. T., Marut, J. S., & Shnider, S. (1985). Anesthesia, analgesia for vaginal childbirth: Differences in maternal perception. *JOGN Nursing, 14*, 321-329.

Slesinger, D. P. (1981). *Mothercraft and infant health.* Lexington, MA: Lexington Books, D. C. Heath.

Smith, L. (1983). A conceptual model of families incorporating an adolescent mother and child into the household. *Advances in Nursing Science, 6*(1), 45-60.

Snyder, C., Eyres, S. J., & Barnard, K. (1979). New findings about mothers' antenatal expectations and their relationship to infant development. *MCN, The American Journal of Maternal Child Nursing, 4*, 354-357.

Sosa, R., Kennell, J., Klaus, M., Robertson, S., & Urrutia, J. (1980). The effect of a supportive companion on perinatal problems, length of labor, and mother-infant interaction. *New England Journal of Medicine, 303*, 597-600.

Squires, S. (1985, August 28). Child development unhampered if Mom works. *The Washington Post, Health—A weekly journal of medicine,* 7.

Stainton, M. C. (1985a). The fetus: A growing member of the family. *Family Relations, 34*, 321-326.

Stainton, M. C. (1985b). *Origins of attachment: Culture and cue sensitivity.* Unpublished doctoral dissertation, University of California, San Francisco.

Stechler, G., & Kaplan, S. (1980). The development of the self. *Psychoanalytic Study of the Child, 35*, 85-105.

Steffensmeier, R. H. (1982). A role model of the transition to parenthood. *Journal of Marriage and the Family, 44*, 319-334.

Stern, L. (1973). Prematurity as a factor in child abuse. *Hospital Practice, 8*(5), 117-123.

Stewart, W. A. (1977). *A psychosocial study of the formation of the early adult life structure in women.* Unpublished doctoral dissertation, Columbia University, New York.

Strang, V. R., & Sullivan, P. L. (1985). Body image attitudes during pregnancy and the postpartum period. *JOGN Nursing, 14*, 332-337.

Sumner, G., & Fritsch, J. (1977). Postnatal parental concerns: The first six weeks of life. *JOGN Nursing, 6*(3), 27-32.

Svejda, M. J., Campos, J. J., & Emde, R. N. (1980). Mother-infant "bonding": Failure to generalize. *Child Development, 51*, 775-779.

Sward, S. (1985, September 7). Feinstein signs new S.F. law on child care. *San Francisco Chronicle,* 1.

Taub, J. M., & Berger, R. J. (1974). Acute shifts in the sleep-wakefulness cycle: Effects on performance and mood. *Psychosomatic Medicine, 36*, 164-173.

Taylor, B., Wadsworth, J., & Butler, N. R. (1983). Teenage mothering, admission to hospital, and accidents during the first 5 years. *Archives of Diseases in Childhood, 58*, 6-11.

Taylor, S. E. (1983). Adjustment to threatening events: A theory of cognitive adaptation. *American Psychologist, 38,* 1161-1173.

ten Bensel, R. W., & Paxson, C. L. (1977). Child abuse following early post-partum separation. *Journal of Pediatrics, 29*(3), 490-491.

Thomas, A., & Chess, S. (1977). *Temperament and development.* New York: Brunner/Mazel.

Thomas, A., & Chess, S. (1980). *The dynamics of psychological development.* New York: Brunner/Mazel.

Thomas, A., Mittelman, M., & Chess, S. (1982). A temperament questionnaire for early adult life. *Educational and Psychological Measurement, 42,* 593-600.

Tilden, V. P., & Lipson, J. G. (1981). Cesarean childbirth: Variables affecting psychological impact. *Western Journal of Nursing Research, 3,* 127-149.

Toffler, A. (1970). *Future shock.* New York: Random House.

Tocco, T. S., & Bridges, C. N. (1973). The relationship between the self-concepts of mothers and their children. *Child Study Journal, 3*(4), 161-179.

Turner, J. H. (1978). *The structure of sociological theory* (rev. ed.). Homewood, IL: Dorsey Press.

Uddenberg, N. (1974). Reproductive adaptation in mother and daughter. *Acta Psychiatrica Scandinavica,* (Suppl. 254), 5-115.

Uddenberg, N., & Nilsson, L. (1975). The longitudinal course of para-natal emotional disturbance. *Acta Psychiatrica Scandinavica, 52,* 160-169.

Van Meter, M. J. S., & Agronow, S. J. (1982). The stress of multiple roles: The case for role strain among married college women. *Family Relations, 31,* 131-138.

Vaughn, B. E., Taraldson, B. J., Crichton, L., & Egeland, B. (1981). The assessment of infant temperament: A critique of the Carey Infant Temperament Questionnaire. *Infant Behavior and Development, 4,* 1-17.

Ventura, J. N. (1982). Parent coping behaviors, parent functioning, and infant temperament characteristics. *Nursing Research, 31,* 269-273.

Virden, S. B. (1981). *The effect of information about infant behavior on primiparas' maternal role adequacy.* Unpublished doctoral dissertation, University of California, San Francisco.

Walters, C. E. (1967). Comparative development of Negro and white infants. *Journal of Genetic Psychology, 110,* 243-251.

Wandersman, L. P. (1978). Parenting groups to support the adjustment to parenthood. *Family Perspective, 12*(3), 117-127.

Wandersman, L., Wandersman, A., & Kahn, S. (1980). Social support in the transition to parenthood. *Journal of Community Psychology, 8,* 332-342.

Watson, J. (1977). Who attends childbirth classes? A demographic study of CEA classes in Rhode Island. *JOGN Nursing, 6*(2), 36-39.

Werner, H. (1948). *Comparative psychology of mental development.* New York: International Universities Press.

Werner, H. (1957). The concept of development from a comparative and organismic point of view. In D. H. Harris (Ed.), *The concept of development* (pp. 125-148). Minneapolis: University of Minnesota Press.

Westbrook, M. T. (1978). The reactions to child-bearing and early maternal experience of women with differing marital relationships. *British Medical Journal Psychology, 51,* 191-199.

Winget, C., & Kapp, F. T. (1972). The relationship of the manifest content of dreams to duration of childbirth in primiparae. *Psychosomatic Medicine, 34*, 313-320.

Winnicott, D. W. (1958). *Primary maternal preoccupation. Collected papers: Through Paediatrics to psychoanalysis* (pp. 300-305). London: Tavistock.

Wise, S., & Grossman, F. K. (1980). Adolescent mothers and their infants: Psychological factors in early attachment and interaction. *American Journal of Orthopsychiatry, 50*, 454-468.

Woodrow, K. M., Friedman, G. D., Siegelaub, A. B., & Collen, M. F. (1972). Pain tolerance: Differences according to age, sex, and race. *Psychosomatic Medicine, 34*, 548-556.

Wylie, R. C. (1974). *The self-concept* (Vol. 1). Lincoln, NE: University of Nebraska Press.

Yogev, S. (1981). Do professional women have egalitarian marital relationships? *Journal of Marriage and the Family, 43*, 865-871.

Zambrana, R. E., Hurst, M., & Hite, R. L. (1979). The working mother in contemporary perspective: A review of the literature. *Pediatrics, 64*, 862-870.

Zongker, C. E. (1980). Self-concept differences between single and married school-age mothers. *Journal of Youth and Adolescence, 9*, 175-184.

Zuckerman, B., Winsmore, G., & Alpert, J. J. (1979). A study of attitudes and support systems of inner city adolescent mothers. *Journal of Pediatrics, 95*, 122-125.

Zuckerman, B., Alpert, J. J., Dooling, E., Hingson, R., Kayne, H., Morelock, S., & Oppenheimer, E. (1983). Neonatal outcome: Is adolescent pregnancy a risk factor? *Pediatrics, 71*, 489-493.

Index